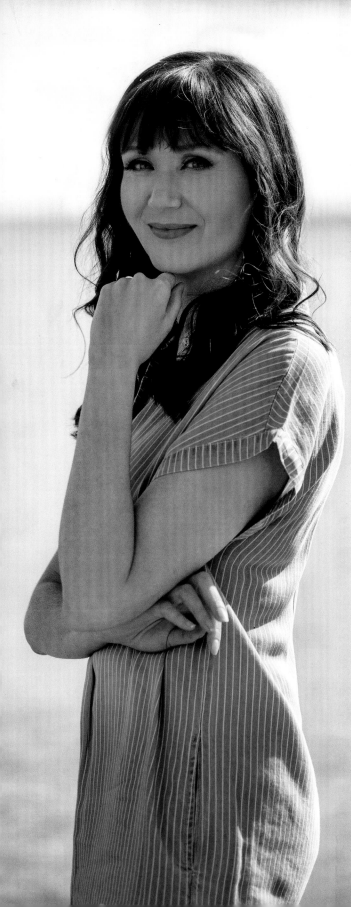

Becoming
Sugar-Free

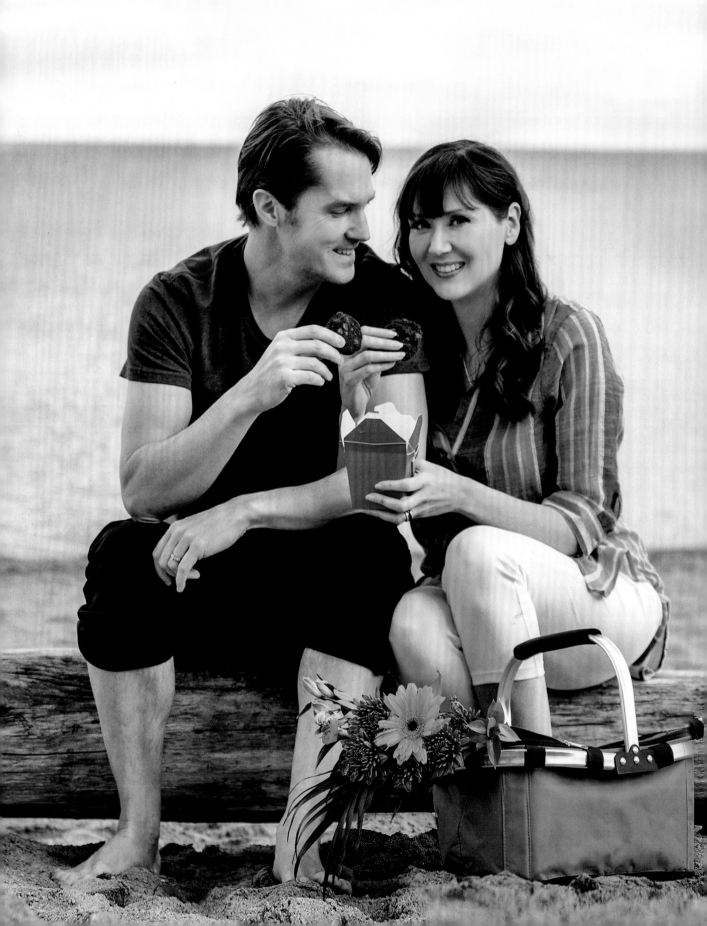

Becoming Sugar-Free

How to Break Up with Inflammatory Sugars and Embrace a Naturally Sweet Life

Julie Daniluk, R.H.N.

PENGUIN
an imprint of Penguin Canada, a division of Penguin Random House Canada Limited

Canada • USA • UK • Ireland • Australia • New Zealand • India • South Africa • China

First published 2021

www.penguinrandomhouse.ca

Library and Archives Canada Cataloguing in Publication

Title: Becoming sugar-free : how to break up with inflammatory sugars and embrace a naturally sweet life / Julie Daniluk.
Names: Daniluk, Julie, author.
Identifiers: Canadiana (print) 20200404288 | Canadiana (ebook) 20200404296 | ISBN 9780735240537 (softcover) | ISBN 9780735240544 (EPUB)
Subjects: LCSH: Sugar-free diet. | LCSH: Sugar-free diet—Recipes. | LCGFT: Cookbooks.
Classification: LCC RM237.85 .D36 2021 | DDC 641.5/63837—dc23

Cover and interior design by Emma Dolan
Cover photography by Nat Caron
Interior photography by Alan Smith, with Julie Daniluk, Bethany Bierema and Nat Caron.
Photography assistance by Joanna Wojewoda and Mike Rees.
Prop and food styling by Tanya Scata, Laura Ricci, Stuart Vaughan and Carol Dudar

Printed and bound in China

10 9 8 7 6 5 4 3 2 1

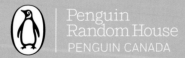

Penguin
Random House
PENGUIN CANADA

Dedication and Gratitude

I wrote this book for you because I want you to believe that finding your health through nutrition is delightful and a worthwhile pursuit. Trust that healing your relationship with food is not only possible but also delicious. Even if we have not met, I think fondly of you because I know the beautiful journey you have in store and the contribution you will make once you share this knowledge with your circle!

I also dedicate this book to my family because they made it possible to bring you this volume in half the time and with twice the enjoyment than if I'd had to create it on my own.

My hubby, Alan Smith, makes every recipe test, every photograph and every edit better than I ever thought it could be. You hold the whole project in your capable arms so I can play and create inside the secure container you willingly carry. Words can't describe how grateful I am that you walk with me through life. I love you to the moon and back!

My sister, Lynn Daniluk, not only showed me how to create a recipe in the early days, but also handles every email while I am working to meet book deadlines. Thank you so much for all your wisdom and intuition. I look forward to getting stronger and more adventurous together as the years flow by.

My mom, Elaine Daniluk, and father, Neil Daniluk, decided to change the course of my life by eliminating sugar and artificial foods from our diet when I was only seven years old. Thank you. I owe you my life, my joy and my ability to write clearly.

My brother and yoga instructor, Yogi Shambu (Steven Daniluk), calls me every single morning to set my day off on the right foot. He can calm anxiety and clarify the mind in a way that feels like the world is a kind and optimistic place, and I am forever grateful for his guidance.

My nephews and nieces give me great joy and purpose. I love to cook for them and treat them to many exotic foods. I am grateful that they are brutally honest when something "tastes funny" because it pushes me to create kid-approved recipes and hide some brain-building nutrition so I can pay forward the gifts my parents gave me all those years ago. Big love goes out to Christian, Kaydn, Taevan, Eli, Aiden, Finn, Colton, Jade, Audrey, Avery, Ashlyn and Amelie.

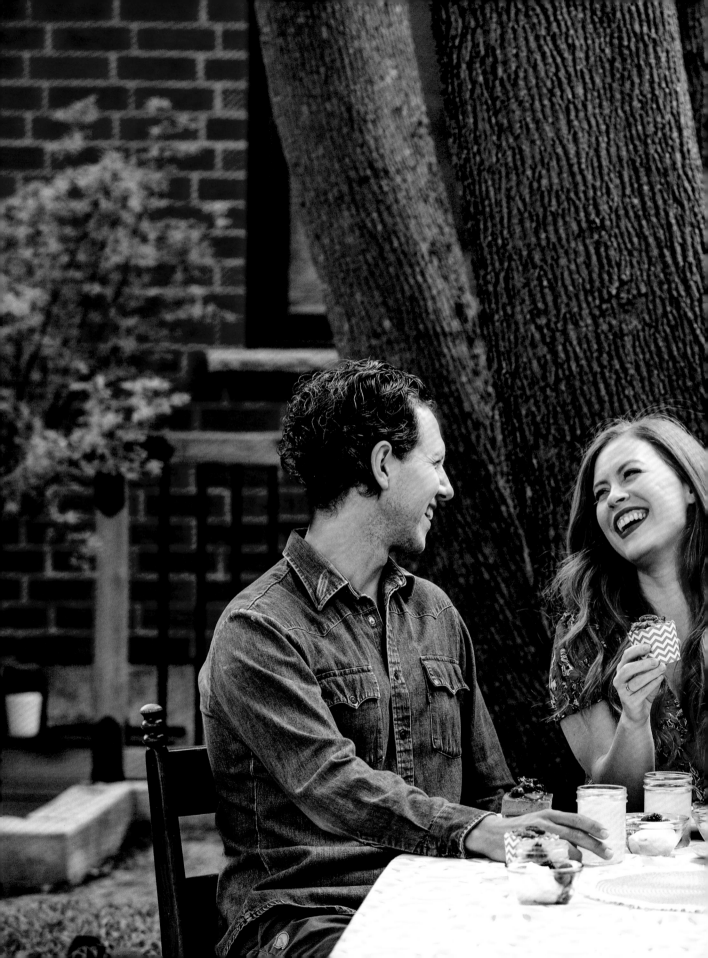

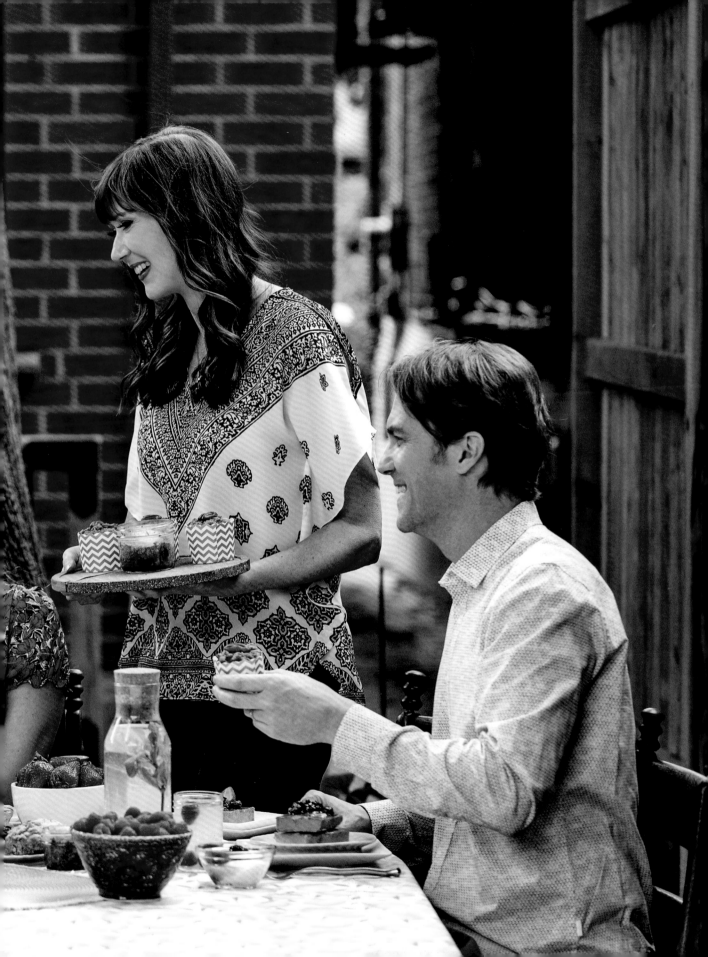

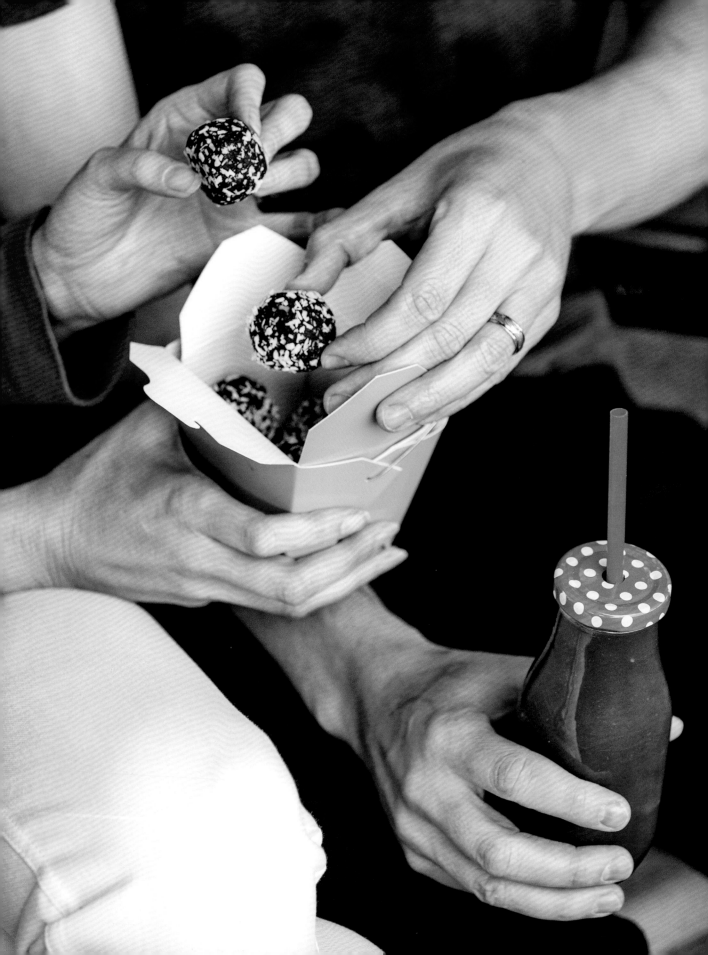

Contents

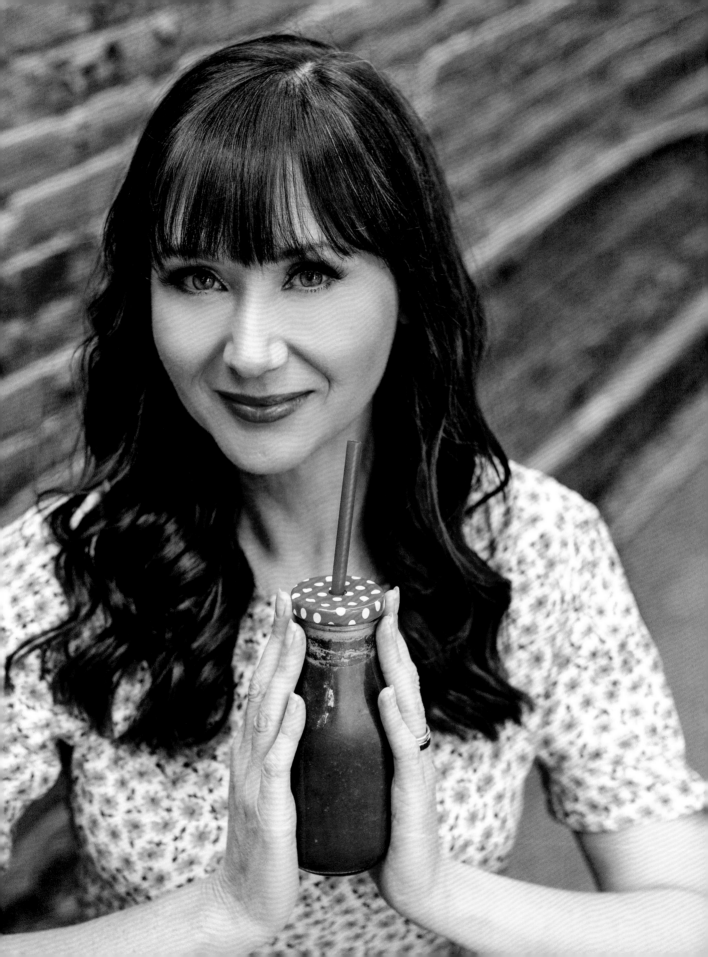

Introduction

I want to begin by thanking you for picking up this book. If you are reading this, my guess is that you already know that sugar is running the show. What may surprise you is that sugar is now in more than 74 percent of packaged products on the grocery shelf! I hope that the information provided in this book will be the inspiration you need to give up the white stuff. You may have wanted to for a while but didn't know how to make that leap. This book is designed to close the gap between your knowledge about sugar's impact on your health and your daily actions of actually going sugar-free.

I wrote this book to encourage you to take back your taste buds and feel the liberation of positive moods and mental clarity that will put you back in the driver's seat of your life. This is your opportunity to stop allowing sugar to rule you and instead choose that the next bite you eat will be authentic, honest and, most importantly, delicious. This book is for everyone. Even if you don't think you have a problem with sugar, listen to your body. Your symptoms or conditions might tell you otherwise. Whether you have a predisposition to anxiety or depression, dementia or attention-deficit/hyperactivity disorder (ADHD), mood imbalances or low energy, these all can result from brain inflammation that is linked to high blood sugar levels. By decreasing and ultimately removing sugar from your diet, you will reduce inflammation in your entire body and create an improvement in overall health. It can be one of the first steps in relieving the struggle and pain of arthritis, bursitis, colitis, heart disease, weight gain, memory loss, chronic fatigue, fibromyalgia and a myriad of other inflammatory conditions.

Why did I decide to write this book about breaking up with sugar? I have had a very long journey to living sugar-free that started when I was a little girl. I was seven years old when my mother realized that I was intolerant to cane sugar. My body could not efficiently break down sucrose, the type of sugar found in good old white table sugar. It was exacerbating my insomnia and ADHD and increasing the symptoms of my auditory learning disability. It was causing neuroinflammation. I have memories of feeling trapped in my little anxious body. I would get so hyperactive that I drove my older sister, Lynn, crazy. I would cry at my birthday parties after eating the sugary cake. I would have a collosal meltdown after Halloween, Christmas and Easter because my brain couldn't think clearly after the sugar binges. In love and desperation, my parents decided to conduct an experiment in which they would eliminate refined sugar, artificial dyes and preservatives from my diet and choose to sweeten my food with honey or dates. My sleep improved in a few days, and my grades skyrocketed from Ds to As within the month. My moods and confidence improved, and I could smile again.

I owe all my success to their brave decision. I can only imagine what my life would have become if they had never taken that big dietary leap. This was the first step, but not the last, in my dangerous dance with sugar.

As I became a teenager, the forbidden foods of my childhood found their way back into my life when times got tough. I rebelled hard, eating whatever I wanted. Having control over my diet made me feel powerful, plus I loved the feeling of flying high on a sugar-dopamine rush. My go-to comfort food was sugary baked goods. I knew these items were bad for me and caused mind and body issues similar to those I had experienced as a child, but I felt powerless to stop.

My insomnia and problems with focus returned, along with a whole host of other issues. Lack of confidence, rampant negative self-talk, energy depletion, acne, premenstrual syndrome (PMS) and emotional outbursts all came as a result of my binge eating. And it was a vicious cycle: the more sugar I ate, the worse I felt, and the worse I felt, the more sugar I wanted to eat. The self-hatred that came with this cycle was overwhelming.

Then something magical happened. One day, I met a therapist who helped me stop binge eating by addressing my true feelings. After giving up the sugar-crazed eating sessions, my self-loathing and negative self-talk disappeared. Then my energy returned, my skin cleared up and my weight balanced out. My confidence improved, and the PMS and emotional outbursts dramatically reduced. All of my symptoms started to go away, and I knew it was because I was no longer eating mass amounts of the white powdered drug we call sugar.

I don't believe in diets, as they can make you want to break out of food prison. I do believe in establishing healthy boundaries with food. A firm boundary can reduce anxiety because you don't become exhausted by the decisions about which foods you can or cannot eat. When I was on my honeymoon in Mexico fourteen years ago, I read a study on how sugar drives the production of advanced glycation end products (AGEs) inside your body. AGEs are produced because sugar causes inflammation on a cellular level. I realized at that moment that sugar causes pain. I immediately put down the pina colada I was sipping and set a firm boundary for myself that the one thing I cannot eat is sugar. I declared to myself (and my new husband): "I am sugar-free." And that was it: I have never intentionally eaten refined white sugar again.

Fast-forward to my life now and the difference is profound. It feels like the world is filled with opportunity and hope. I feel positive (almost) all the time, and I am connected to my loved ones without any raging outbursts or mood swings. My confidence, energy and motivation are sky-high, and the negative self-talk is a thing of the past. How do I know this is all thanks to my low-carb, sugar-free, nutrient-rich menu? If I happen to eat something with cane sugar, I immediately feel my mood start to decline. My energy is zapped, and my brain becomes foggy. I feel like my health is affected, and it's not worth it. I'd much rather live free of refined sugars and enjoy the natural sweetness that life has to offer. Does this seem too good to be true? I feel confident that if you try it for yourself, you will understand how exciting it is to live life with a youthful spring in your step.

It might seem hard, or even impossible, but you can do it. The weight struggles, the hormonal fluctuations, the skin issues, the blood sugar swings, the energy crisis, the horrible moods: it's all connected to the poison that is sugar. I know what's on the other side of this sugar compulsion, and I'm holding out my hand to help you climb aboard the sugar-free train.

There is sweetness on the other side, and there is joy. You'll find self-acceptance and freedom from the addiction that's ruining your efforts to be happy and healthy. The only thing you have to do is give up one of the things that's destroying your health, and that is sugar. The great news is you don't have to give up sweetness, just refined sugar and carbohydrates. As this book will show you, you can have delicious treats without the aftertaste of guilt.

Now it is your turn. I have spilled the goods on my sordid affair with sugar. It is time to see how much sugar relates to your life by first completing the Sugar Sensitivity Quiz on page 11.

What else will be covered in this book? I am going to walk you through everything from why sugar is the most harmful food ingredient to how to make easy swaps for healthy sweeteners. I'm going to share what happens in your brain when you eat sweets and how to conquer emotional eating and kick sugar to the curb. You will enjoy more than fifty ways to help you on your journey, including different tools you can incorporate to maximize your sugar-free lifestyle. I am going to provide both a slow and a fast plan to break up with sugar, and most important, I am going to provide such delicious recipes that you won't miss sugar at all.

Right now, living sugar-free might seem impossible, like a theoretical concept and a promise that feels unattainable. All I ask is that you try it on. Shambu, my brother who is an amazing yoga instructor, has a great saying that I use frequently when faced with doubt. He says, "Don't believe me, just suspend your disbelief long enough to try it on." And this is my request to you: give sugar-free living a month of your life and you will be pleasantly surprised with how much more energy and joy you feel. It's as simple as that. What have you got to lose?

Organically yours,
Julie

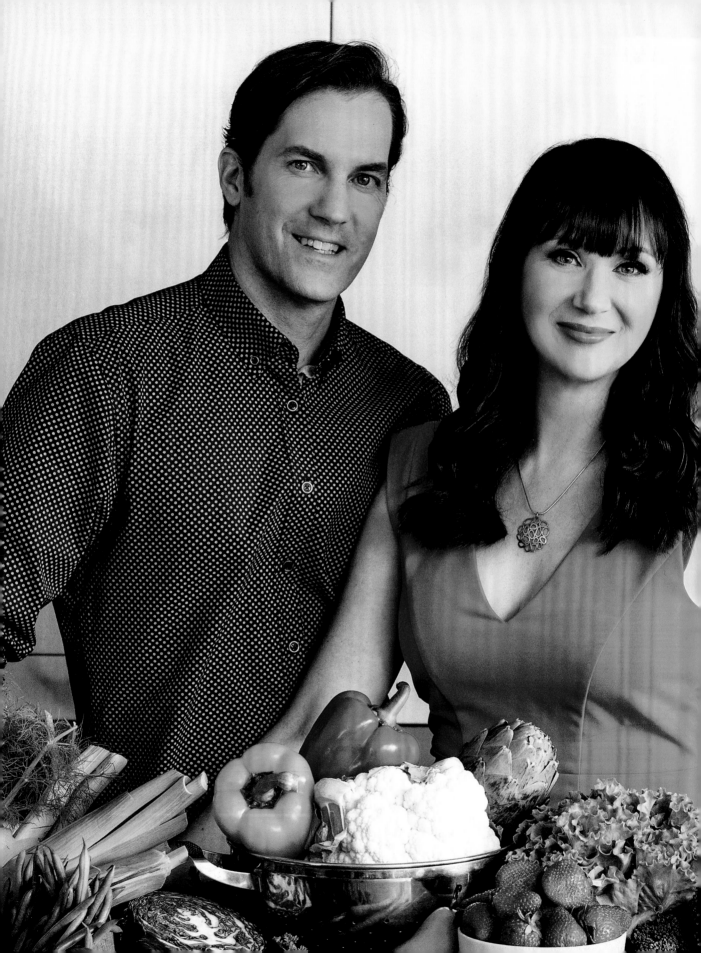

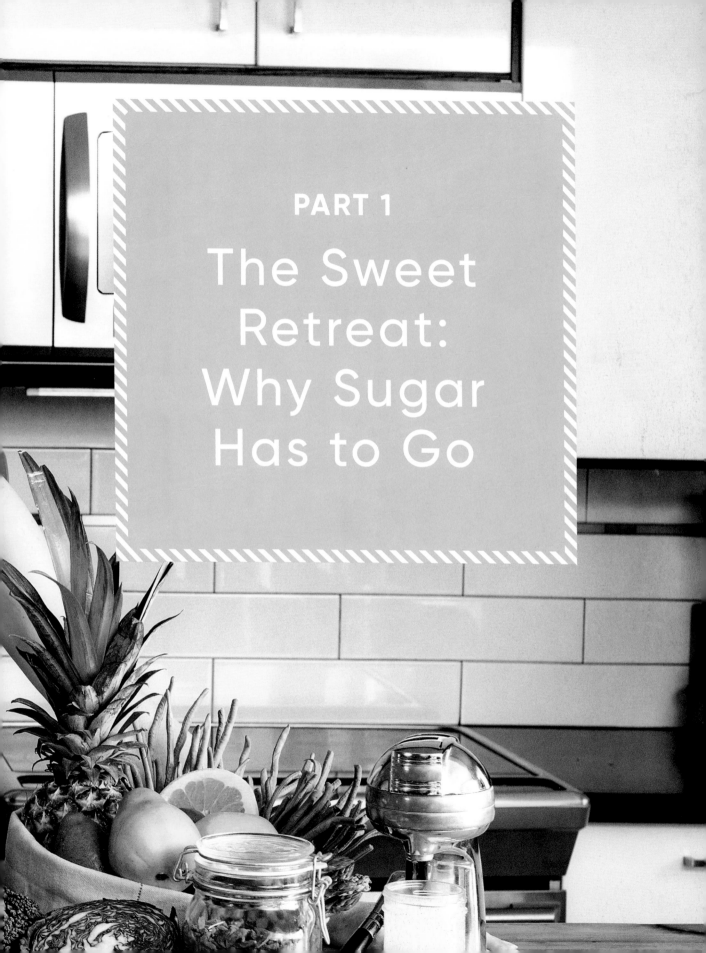

PART 1

The Sweet Retreat: Why Sugar Has to Go

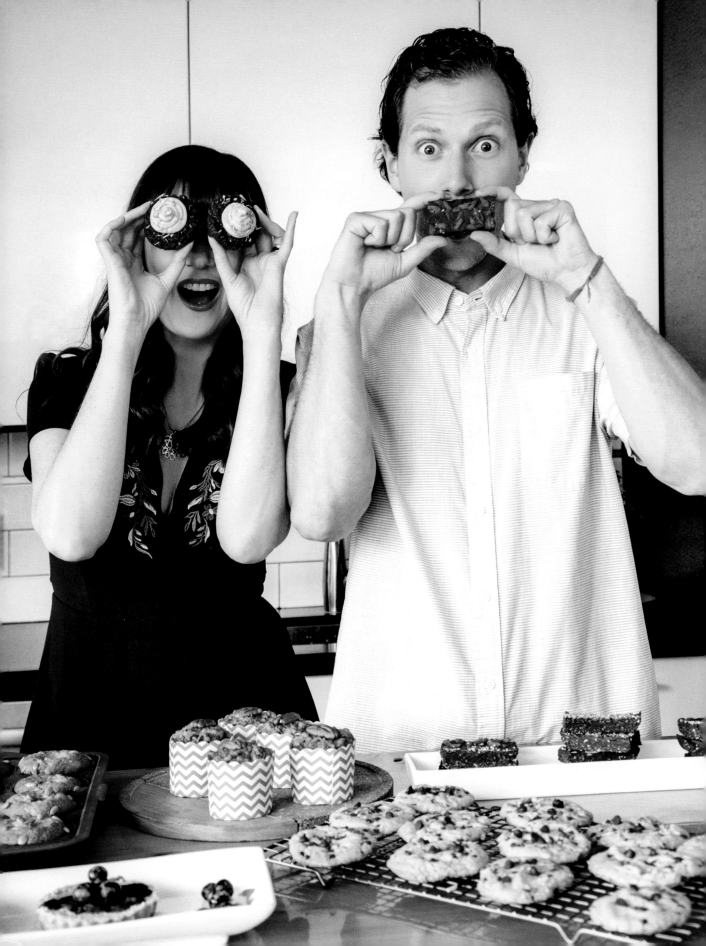

1
The Impact of Sugar on the Body

This book isn't just about giving up sugar—it's about gaining freedom. The freedom to take control of your life and what you eat; the freedom to let go of cravings, mood swings and energy slumps; the freedom to eat real, delicious, naturally sweet foods without feeling deprived.

You may be asking how all of this can come from letting go of sugar. The simple answer is that sugar has a grip on society. It is estimated that Canadians eat, on average, 26 teaspoons of sugar per day, which translates to a shocking 88 pounds of sugar per year. The World Health Organization recommends that women eat less than 6 teaspoons of sugar per day and men eat less than 9 teaspoons because of its negative impact on health. How can we go from consuming that much sugar to cutting it out altogether? I am going to give you two options for how to break up with sugar, and I think you will be amazed at how tasty sugar-free treats can be. More importantly, I am going to provide savoury foods that can help you banish your sweet tooth. Sugar is a highly refined substance that triggers the reward hormone dopamine, giving you a temporary but blissful high every time you consume it. It can be so easy to become addicted to this feeling, this false happiness that sugar brings. But soon after the initial blush fades and your blood sugar falls, the mood swings come on, the exhaustion and sadness hit, and all you want is to feel on top of the world again—so you eat more sugar. The cycle continues—and will continue—until you break it.

Once the cycle is broken, you will find that your moods level out, and you won't need to rely on sugar to give you the happiness high anymore. Your energy will remain stable all day long, and your focus, memory and attention will sharpen. You'll feel empowered to take control of your mental and emotional faculties. When you naturally feel good all the time, you won't need sugar to give you a boost.

People don't understand how good they can feel when they remove the influence of sugar from their lives. Sugar is like a wet blanket that dampens your experience. When you throw it off and stand with a clear head and feel joy in your heart that isn't attached to a substance, you can begin to be the unshackled person you are meant to be.

I want to give you a snapshot of the benefits of a sugar-free lifestyle that are backed up by science. Keep this page handy for when your willpower needs a boost.

BENEFITS OF A SUGAR-FREE LIFESTYLE

1. **Look younger.** When you eat sugar, your collagen cross-links and glycation occurs, rendering your collagen fibres incapable of easy repair, thus creating wrinkles on your skin that make you look older. Skip the sugar and look (and feel) much younger.

2. **Reach your ideal weight.** Excess amounts of sugar can create insulin resistance within the cells in our body. Giving up sugar and flour helps reset your metabolism, allowing you to burn energy more efficiently and creating the conditions for natural weight balance.

3. **Improve your gut health.** Sugar is guilty of feeding the wrong types of bacteria and yeast that cause gut dysbiosis and can lead to a host of gastrointestinal (GI) and digestion issues. For instance, high doses of a fructose solution were shown to elevate *Enterobacteriaceae*, which are associated with gut and brain inflammation, as well as poor cognition. When we get off sugar and eat more sweet vegetables, such as cabbage, onions, sweet peas and peppers, that are rich in prebiotics, we feed the good bacteria in our gut. This benefits all areas of our health, including mental health. Because more than 90 percent of our serotonin is made in our gut lining, eating too much sugar can cause an overpopulation of harmful bacteria and yeast that increases mood disorders such as anxiety and depression. Supporting the right kind of bacteria with healthy whole foods will create a healthier GI environment that will positively affect cognitive health and your mood.

4. **Enjoy happy, balanced moods.** When you consume sugar, you experience a massive spike in dopamine, which triggers your brain's reward centre. As with any reward, you immediately go back for more and more, chasing the "high" that allowed you to feel great or to avoid the pain you were feeling. Like a drug, it can lead to addiction. You may feel great at the moment, but when you lose that dopamine high, your moods become unbalanced. Your blood sugar levels are like a roller coaster, continually flying and crashing with your sugar binges. When we go off sugar, the emotion centres in the brain stay balanced, which can positively affect all other areas

of your life. A happy mood leads to better concentration, higher productivity, positive relationships, less stress, improved self-confidence and so much more.

5. **Protect your memory.** An insulin resistance can happen in your body and in your brain when your blood sugar levels spike over and over again after eating refined sugar. Your brain requires large amounts of glucose, and if it becomes resistant to insulin, neurons can become inadequately nourished and injured. *Type 3 diabetes* is a term that has been proposed by scientists to explain the hypothesis that Alzheimer's disease, a leading cause of dementia, can be triggered by insulin resistance and dysfunction of insulin-like growth factor in the brain. If you want to have a healthy mind filled with your beautiful memories, you should be mindful of your sugar intake.

6. **Enjoy pain-free movement.** When you eliminate refined sugar and flour, inflammation levels in your body will start to go down, and the pain you may feel in your joints, knees, knuckles and so on will go down with it. People who work with me report feeling a reduction in pain in as little as two weeks when following a sugar-free (and flour-free) menu.

7. **Recalibrate your taste buds.** Natural sweetness (the sweetness that occurs naturally in foods) becomes pleasurable. When you give up sugar, your taste buds for sweet tastes intensify. As your taste buds go through this adjustment phase, you will find that a berry tastes much sweeter than it did before. It's much more complex than just being at the level of your taste buds because your gut is involved as well. The sweet receptors in the gut can also influence blood sugar, hunger and appetite through the release of hormones.

8. **Get your nutrients back.** Refined sugars are empty calories that require nutrients to be processed, nutrients that your body needs to function optimally. Therefore, the more added sugars you consume, the more nutritionally depleted you may become. By opting for natural sweeteners such as unrefined coconut sweetener or dates that contain vitamins and minerals instead of empty refined sugar, you gain nutrients instead of losing them.

9. **Achieve hormonal balance.** Cane sugar and corn syrup can overwhelm your liver. Corn syrup is mostly fructose, and cane sugar is equal amounts glucose and fructose. Glucose is a burden on its own, but your liver needs to convert fructose into glucose for use in the body, creating an even heavier burden. The liver

becomes overwhelmed and may begin to store the sugar as liver fat. If left unchecked, it can lead to fatty liver syndrome and elevated liver enzymes, even if you're not over-weight or a heavy drinker. A burdened liver cannot function as well as it should and can cause hormonal imbalances, such as estrogen dominance, poor skin and much more. If you want clear skin and balanced hormones, skip the sugar.

10. **Protect your heart.** When sugar overwhelms the liver, it produces some-thing called very-low-density lipoprotein (VLDL) cholesterol particles. The kidneys also raise blood pressure when sugar is high. By reducing sugar and flour, you can quickly reduce the risks associated with high blood pressure and bad cholesterol.

11. **Reduce your risk of cancer.** German scientist Otto Warburg noticed that tumour cells in a Petri dish consume more glucose than non-dividing normal tissue. His research was developed into technology for cancer diagnosis (a positron emission tomography [PET] scan with radioactive glucose) using his "Warburg effect." In essence, the effect shows how cancer cells use sugar to produce a substance called lactate, which provides an abundant source of usable energy for cancer cells that allows them to rapidly replicate and tumours to grow.

If the benefits listed here haven't convinced you that getting rid of sugar might help resolve many of your health struggles, consider taking the following quiz to see how sugar may be affecting you.

SUGAR SENSITIVITY QUIZ

Are you vulnerable to refined carbohydrate intolerance or sugar addiction? This quiz is a great gauge of how serious your battle with sugar and starch is. I developed it as a motivational tool, not a diagnostic one. If you end up with a high score, I suggest contacting your health care provider to have further testing done to check your blood sugar levels and metabolism. If you are struggling emotionally, I recommend getting a referral for a mental health professional trained in food addiction to assess your issues and suggest more in-depth solutions. It is important to note that some people don't have a sweet tooth, but rather a starch tooth, and that starch (found in bread, pasta, pastry, corn, potatoes and so on) breaks down to sugar within seconds thanks to the enzymes within the saliva in your mouth. Take the time to think about your answers because they will be very insightful on your path to healing.

1. As a child, were you rewarded or bribed with sugar or starchy treats?

- Never
- Rarely
- Occasionally
- Frequently
- Constantly

2. As a child, did your parents withhold sweets or starchy treats as punishment?

- Never
- Rarely
- Occasionally
- Frequently
- Constantly

3. As a teenager, did you suffer from disordered eating—for example, bingeing, heavy dieting, purging, or overeating?

- Never
- Rarely
- Occasionally
- Frequently
- Constantly

4. Do you suffer from headaches, migraines or eye pain?

- ○ Never
- ○ Rarely (or in the past)
- ○ Occasionally
- ○ Frequently
- ○ Constantly

5. Do you suffer from brain fog, attention deficit, memory loss or moodiness?

- ○ Never
- ○ Rarely (or in the past)
- ○ Occasionally
- ○ Frequently
- ○ Constantly

6. Do you often crave starchy carbohydrates like bread, pasta, rice or potato?

- ○ Never
- ○ Rarely
- ○ Occasionally
- ○ Frequently
- ○ Constantly

7. Do you eat when you're not hungry because you're craving a certain food?

- ○ Never
- ○ Rarely
- ○ Occasionally
- ○ Frequently
- ○ Constantly

8. Do you feel guilty after eating?

- ○ Never
- ○ Rarely
- ○ Occasionally
- ○ Frequently
- ○ Constantly

9. Do you still feel hungry after eating an appropriate amount of food?

- Never
- Rarely
- Occasionally
- Frequently
- Constantly

10. Do you feel sleepy or brain fogged one to three hours after eating a meal or snack that contains sugars or starches?

- Never
- Rarely
- Occasionally
- Frequently
- Constantly

11. Do you tend to gain weight around your waist?

- Never
- Rarely
- Occasionally
- Frequently
- Constantly

12. Do you have symptoms of low blood sugar, such as feeling shaky, panicky, irritable, anxious or light-headed, when you're hungry or if you don't eat every two to three hours?

- Never
- Rarely
- Occasionally
- Frequently
- Constantly

13. Do you crave ice cream, milk, yogurt, cheese or other dairy products?

- Never
- Rarely
- Occasionally
- Frequently
- Constantly

14. Do you wake up at night with difficulty getting back to sleep unless you eat something sweet or starchy?

- Never
- Rarely
- Occasionally
- Frequently
- Constantly

15. Do you get irritable, restless, anxious or pensive before dinner?

- Never
- Rarely
- Occasionally
- Frequently
- Constantly

16. Do you have a hard time limiting how much alcohol, sugar or starch you consume?

- Never
- Rarely
- Occasionally
- Frequently
- Constantly

17. Do you struggle to lose weight, or does your weight fluctuate?

- Never
- Rarely
- Occasionally
- Frequently
- Constantly

18. Would you consider yourself an emotional eater? In other words, do you eat down your feelings or eat as a way to cope with feeling stressed or sad?

- Never
- Rarely
- Occasionally
- Frequently
- Constantly

19. Do you or anyone in your immediate family deal with obesity, high blood pressure, high cholesterol or diabetes?

- ○ Nobody (score 0 points)
- ○ 1 person (score 1 point)
- ○ 2 people (score 2 points)
- ○ 3 people (score 3 points)
- ○ Almost everyone (score 4 points)

20. Do you binge on sweets, such as candy, sugary drinks, ice cream, cookies and cupcakes, or prefer starchy choices, such as bread or pasta, over all other types of food?

- ○ Never
- ○ Rarely (or in the past)
- ○ Occasionally
- ○ Frequently
- ○ Constantly

21. Would you consider yourself obsessed with food?

- ○ Never
- ○ Rarely
- ○ Occasionally
- ○ Frequently
- ○ Constantly

22. Are you a cyclical dieter—that is, are you always trying to restrict calories and then fall off the diet wagon?

- ○ Never
- ○ Rarely
- ○ Occasionally
- ○ Frequently
- ○ Constantly

23. Have you been diagnosed with an eating disorder, such as anorexia, bingeing and purging, bulimia or consistent overeating?

- Never (score 0 points)
- Some symptoms but never diagnosed (score 1 point)
- I need help but have not reached out (score 2 points)
- Diagnosed and working on treatment (score 3 points)
- Diagnosed but it is still heavily impacting my life (score 4 points)

24. Do you feel panic or hunger or faint while exercising?

- Never
- Rarely
- Occasionally
- Frequently
- Constantly

25. Do sweet and starchy foods make you feel temporarily less anxious or depressed?

- Never
- Rarely
- Occasionally
- Frequently
- Constantly

Calculating your score:

Never = 0 points
Rarely = 1 point
Occasionally = 2 points
Frequently = 3 points
Constantly = 4 points

How did you score? The higher the score, the greater the likelihood that sugar has a firm grip on you.

YELLOW ALERT Score of 1 to 19

You may be sensitive to carbohydrates or developing an intolerance. It is best to avoid refined carbohydrates to prevent health issues.

If you scored low (less than 5), you are one of the lucky and metabolically blessed individuals who handle carbohydrates efficiently. You do not show signs of chronic disease at the moment, but you may still want to consider that refined sugar and flour can have a negative impact on your future health. Our insulin receptors become less receptive over time, making us increasingly intolerant of refined carbohydrates as we age. If we go through a stressful life event or hormonal shift, our ability to tolerate processed foods plummets. It is easy to dismiss our long-term health needs, but it is important to remember that our health gives us greater access to everything we want to create in our life. If you want more ease, joy, brainpower and confidence, letting go of refined sugar and starch is a sure-fire way to stack the deck in your favour. If you scored higher in the yellow range, then read on.

ORANGE ALERT Score of 20 to 55

You likely have a carbohydrate intolerance and/or addiction. You could be insulin resistant and should seriously consider cutting back on all refined carbohydrates in your diet.

If your score is in the orange range, do you have to stop eating all sweet and starchy foods to feel better? The good news is that you don't have to jump to a low-carb menu right away. Most people feel better by just avoiding refined sugar, flour and dairy containing foods. By preventing a spike in insulin, the body can use its stored fuel by converting fat back into energy. This book is going to give you many options so that you can scale up or down the amount of unrefined slow-burning carbohydrates you consume. The questions in this quiz look for clues in the symptoms you are experiencing. Meet with your primary health care provider and discuss the blood work or testing needed for a proper diagnosis. You'll want to ask for both a fasting blood sugar test and a hemoglobin A1C blood test to measure how your blood sugar is managed over time. You might also want to have your thyroid hormones tested to rule out other hormone-related symptoms that may affect your blood sugar and metabolism.

If you scored higher in the orange range (35 to 55), you may want to avoid as many added sugars and starches as possible and embrace the wonderful sugar-free substitutions that will keep you satisfied. The good news is that your metabolism (and endocrine system, including thyroid, adrenals and sex hormones) can be balanced. I have hundreds of testimonials from people who have turned their health around when they found themselves in a similar situation. They now have found the energy and joy they long thought they had lost.

RED ALERT Score of 56 or higher

You most likely have a strong carbohydrate intolerance or a full-blown sugar addiction, and it is time to seek help to resolve this issue.

Breaking up with sugar and other refined carbohydrates is imperative to your short- and long-term health. If you scored in the red range, you may already agree or acknowledge that you are a sugar and starch addict, and it is essential that you get help to ensure a long and happy life free of inflammatory conditions. If you don't prioritize changing your eating habits, you may find that diabetes, heart disease, cancer and/or fatty liver disease are probable. If you already have a metabolic-related health problem, it is critical to trust your body's power to heal. It turns out that our body can heal very quickly when given the right nourishment. Reducing carbs may be your most powerful ally in turning things around.

I am here to help you look closely at your relationship with food. As a recovered sugar addict, I know this can feel like a battle of will. It is possible to find a new way to cope that is forever gratifying in a way that sugar never can be. Sugar creates the void, so it cannot be the solution to fill that void. The answer lies inside you, and it is time to take the first step. Don't worry, you will have many tools on this path to healing, and you will look back at this moment with great fondness as the time you decided to treat yourself so well that you willed your wellness into being.

Whatever score you got on this quiz, the most important thing to keep in mind is that it is always a great idea to remove harmful sugars and starches from your diet. Thankfully, the solutions are sweet.

THE DARKER SIDE OF SUGAR

Refined sugar has a whole host of adverse effects on the body that directly create inflammation. Inflammation has five fundamental symptoms of pain, heat, redness, swelling and loss of function. The problem is that we often experience only loss of function (for example, memory loss), so this silent inflammation is easy to ignore. I hope the information outlined below will encourage you to pay closer attention to the signals your body is trying to give you that sugar has got to go.

Digestive Tract Impact

Refined sugar (sucrose) is made of one molecule of fructose and one molecule of glucose. This makes it a very difficult thing for many people to digest because their bowel lining lacks the digestive enzyme needed to break down larger sugars into smaller ones. If your body cannot split the sugar into its two molecules, it will irritate your bowel. From there, a condition called leaky gut or intestinal hyperpermeability can develop. This is where food particles can enter the bloodstream directly through the bowel. This is not supposed to happen and can negatively affect your health. If you are unable to break down sugars, you likely will have symptoms of irritable bowel syndrome (IBS) such as diarrhea or constipation.

There's also such a thing as sucrose intolerance. The digestive enzyme sucrase assists in a person's ability to digest certain sugars. The absence or low levels of this enzyme disrupts the digestive process and can cause symptoms upon eating foods containing sugars. If you suffer from malnutrition, diarrhea, gassiness, abdominal distention and pain, you may also have a sucrase deficiency known as SI deficiency, disaccharide intolerance, and congenital sucrase-isomaltase deficiency (CSID). It's rare, but if you can't find answers to your digestive woes, it's a good idea to try removing sucrose from your diet and see if your symptoms improve.

Mental Minefield

Sugar does more than cause digestion issues. In fact, even though I had IBS and sugar exacerbated it, that wasn't the main reason I cut sugar from my diet. Sugar negatively affects my mind. It triggers feelings of self-loathing, insecurity, sadness and anger. It makes me feel bad about myself. I didn't realize this until I cut it out and experienced how much better I felt. And now, people know me as a person of compassion, confidence and joy. I know that I am this way partly because I broke up with sugar for good.

Aside from digestive and mood issues, sugar affects a whole range of other things. It suppresses the activity of a hormone called brain-derived neurotrophic factor (BDNF) that is low in individuals with depression and schizophrenia. Furthermore, it appears to worsen anxiety symptoms, increases your risk of depression and impairs the body's ability to cope with stress. A 2017 study found that men who consumed a high amount of sugar each day were 23 percent more likely to receive a diagnosis of depression. A study in animals found a definite link between sugar intake and anxiety symptoms. While dietary changes alone cannot cure anxiety, they can minimize symptoms, boost energy and improve the body's ability to cope with stress.

Cognitive function also takes a hit from the sugar train, as sugar may compromise learning and memory. And all those colds and cases of flu you're getting? Sugar plays a role there by suppressing the immune system. A study published in the *American Journal of Clinical Nutrition* showed that when people consumed the amount of sugar in two sweetened beverages, their immune responses were lowered by 50 percent for up to five hours afterwards.

You may have heard this terrible saying: "Nothing tastes as good as skinny feels." That doesn't promote a healthy body image, so what if we say instead, "There isn't a dessert that tastes as sweet as my happy mood" or "There isn't a dessert that is tasty enough to warrant me feeling badly"? Let's turn the conversation on its head and look at it that way. It's not just about being skinny or losing weight—it's about how we feel about ourselves. The sugar is not worth the hours of self-doubt or indigestion that follow. I believe that "Nothing tastes as good as healthy feels!"

DON'T AGE YOURSELF

Right about now, some people might be thinking: *Okay, we get it, sugar should go, but isn't it a fuel source, a carbohydrate? How can it cause all of these problems?* Sugar is indeed our fastest and most common fuel source, but that does not make it the best or the only option we have. In nature, sugar (as in fruit) has always been bound with so much fibre that it's dispensed slowly in your system, much like how a time-release capsule works. But in today's world of highly processed food, we have stripped sugar of its fibre and refined it to the point that it's no longer absorbed slowly. It enters the body and spikes our blood sugar so quickly that insulin needs to pump out at a high rate to get the sugar into our cells to be used as "fuel." This rapid fuel source is not ideal because it indirectly robs your body of valuable resources, such as vitamins and minerals, in order to be metabolized. But the rate at which we consume sugar and the amounts we consume have caused an issue. There's too much sugar in the body, and eventually the glucose transporters are overloaded and cannot allow for sugar transport into the cells.

Think of it this way: Imagine that your cells are a popular club, and sugar is the people trying to get into that club. When the club first opens for the night, people can get in with no problem. Similarly, our cells allow sugar access when they need fuel. But as the night wears on and the club gets busier, it cannot let people in at the same rate because the lineups get longer and only a couple of doors can be used to get inside. Eventually, the club has to close its doors because it's at capacity, even though there are crowds waiting outside. That's what happens when we have too much sugar. Our cell membrane says, "No, we're too full, we can't handle any more!" and we end up overproducing and under-responding to insulin, leading to a condition called insulin resistance. And when sugar stays outside the cell, that's where it gets dangerous. It starts attacking areas outside the cell, and we end up with dysfunction and glycation (the bonding of a sugar molecule to a protein or lipid molecule). Sugar attacks our joints, and we get inflammation and arthritis; it attacks our skin, and we get wrinkles; it attacks our arteries, and we get plaque and heart disease. It literally ages us from the inside out.

When glycation occurs, advanced glycation end products are formed, appropriately abbreviated as AGEs because glycated molecules cause cells to age. AGEs age cells because they ignite and stoke the flames of inflammation. The health consequences can be profound. Glycated proteins can't function properly, and therefore they're unable to maintain essential bodily processes efficiently.

The following conditions demonstrate how inflammatory AGEs can lead to accelerated cell aging and eventually cause tissue damage or degenerative diseases.

Weathered Skin

Ever wonder why some people have very wrinkled skin by age fifty while others retain their radiant, youthful skin? This has nothing to do with the skin creams they use. Beauty is more than skin deep. A daily sugar spike in the bloodstream will cause glycation of the skin's collagen (collagen is the most abundant protein in the skin). Collagen contains a lot of water, and this is why it keeps skin elastic, supple, hydrated and youthful.

When sugar attaches to collagen, it is called glycated; it's like a hardened rubber band—it once could stretch and shrink back but over time has lost its flexibility. Collagen can break down because of AGEs, overexposure to ultraviolet (UV) rays and other free radicals, chronic dehydration, local or blood-borne infections or toxins, local inflammation, poor nutrition, lack of sleep and changes in hormones (especially estrogen). A diet that promotes AGE formation will lead to early wrinkles and loss of skin elasticity. If you want to keep your skin supple and firm, steer clear of refined carbohydrates and avoid spiking your blood sugar.

Arthritis

Collagen is also the viscous, gel-like protein in all of your joints that pads the space between your bones. When glucose attaches itself to collagen in the joints, they become stiff. To remain flexible, joints require a lot of healthy, well-hydrated collagen. AGEs gum up your joints, impair joint movement and can lead to arthritis. AGEs can also make joints more prone to injury because they hinder collagen's ability to bind water and function as a lubricant. Think twice about that doughnut in today's staff meeting—it might cause tomorrow's aches and pains.

Heart Disease

High concentrations of glucose in the blood can glycate the collagen found in arterial walls and transform it into malfunctioning AGEs. This creates small leaks in the arterial walls, which in turn alerts the body to repair the damage. When artery walls are weakened or damaged, cholesterol is used to help patch up the small lesions. Over time, this results in the arterial plaque we know as atherosclerosis (hardening of the arteries). Blood doesn't flow freely through atherosclerotic blood vessels, and this strains your heart. It also means that tissues receive less oxygen and nutrients and get stuck with toxins that cannot be properly flushed. This can lead to the development of various deep-seated, chronic disorders, including chronic systemic inflammation.

Cataracts

AGE accumulation can also affect the eye and cause structural damage to the lens. When glucose attaches to proteins in the eye lens, it can change the lens cells from transparent and clear to slightly opaque or cloudy, leading to cataract formation. In fact, studies report diabetes or poor sugar regulation as a major risk factor for the development of cataracts.

What does all of this mean? Simply put: sugar causes us pain. It causes our body to lose its function and shortens our life. But it doesn't have to be this way. You can avoid and reduce AGEs by cutting sugar out of your diet—for good.

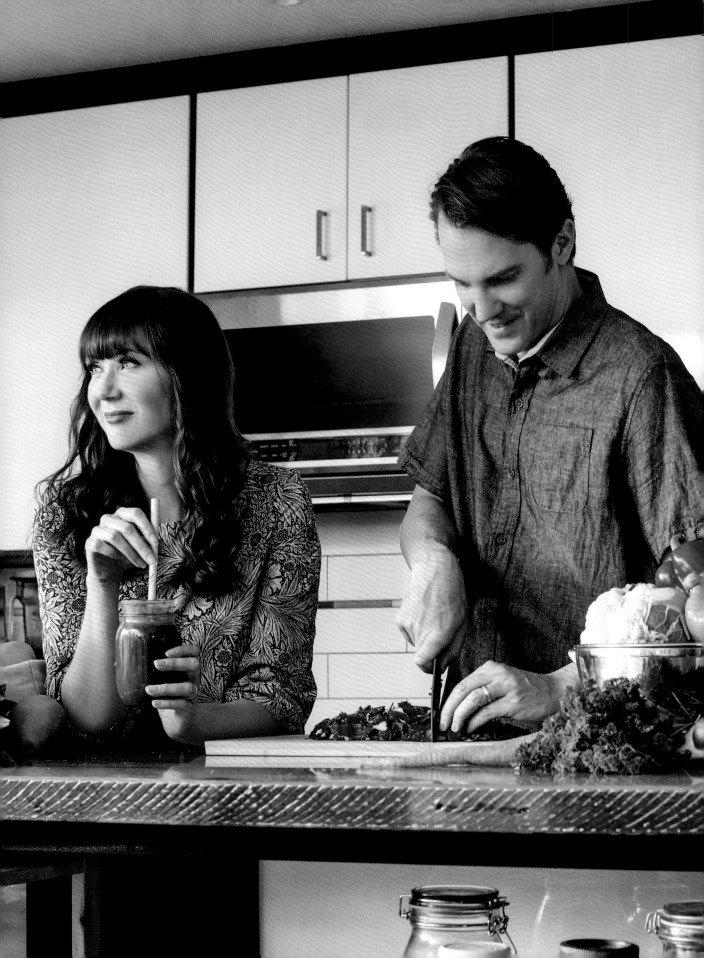

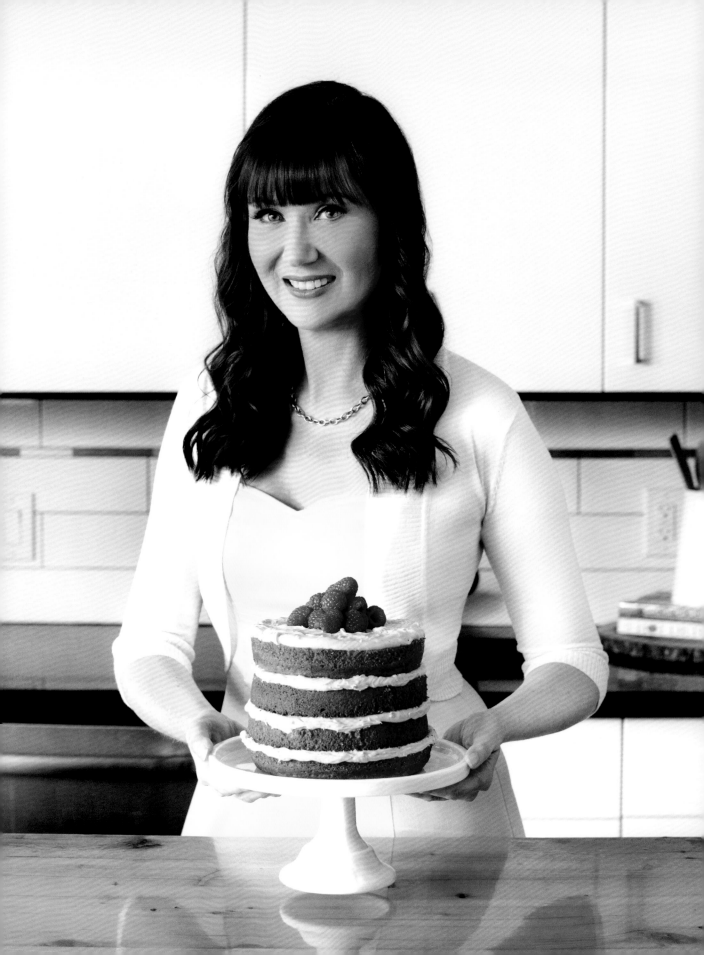

2
Understanding Sugar

The easiest way to describe sugar is that it is a unit of simple carbohydrate, a compound that contains both hydrogen and oxygen in equal measure. Sounds innocent when I describe it that way, doesn't it? Unfortunately, that could not be further from the truth. For example, a teaspoon of white sugar (also known as sucrose) seems harmless, tastes good and contains only fifteen calories. However, when you take a closer look at how the body metabolizes sugar, you'll see that a tremendous effort is needed for the body to use those fifteen calories as fuel.

You may have heard the saying "A calorie is a calorie." Let's dispel that myth right now. Refined sugar is not the same as the naturally occurring sugars found in fruits or vegetables. For one thing, refined sugar has its fibre package stripped away, so it doesn't carry any nutrients, minerals, fibre or other beneficial constituents with it. It's just glucose and fructose, and that's it. Without any fibre, it releases quickly into your bloodstream, giving you that immediate sugar rush. Even more important is that, over time, the gut lining can become inflamed and more permeable, and eventually it gets harder to digest sugars (disaccharides) and starches (polysaccharides). We can be missing the enzymes needed to break down the longer starches and disaccharides, and so after the initial high, your body starts to reject them and feel the effects of undigested sugar, such as gas, bloating, pain and diarrhea. This will also move the disaccharides undigested into the large intestine, where they can feed unfriendly microbes in the gut and continue the cycle of damage.

ARE ALL SUGARS CREATED EQUAL?

The short answer is no. There are many types of sugars, but let's first focus on letting go of refined white sugar that is filled with a type of sugar called sucrose. Conventional, refined sugar comes from the sugar cane plant or sugar beet root. Even though both plants are rich in vitamins and minerals in their whole form, they're reduced to simple sucrose—stripped of all valuable nutrients—once they're refined. This means that after the body uses its bank of stored nutrients to metabolize the sugar, it receives no payback.

Refined carbohydrates are like credit cards because after they've been digested, they provide little or no micronutrients. They are "borrowing" micronutrients and creating debt that eventually will need to be paid off by whole foods. When sugar is eaten in very small amounts, such as in accordance with the World Health Organization's recommendation of 6 to 9 teaspoons per day, our body may be able to handle it before inflammation begins, as long as we have a good metabolism. However, the average Canadian eats up to 26 teaspoons of sugar a day. The trouble begins when the body's insulin sensitivity drops because of overexposure to sugar. Just because our body can handle the sugar doesn't make it a good thing. Our body shouldn't have to handle things—it should be able to thrive. In these high amounts, sugar isn't just a simple carbohydrate, but a very dangerous simple carbohydrate. This is why the main sources of sugar that we eliminate first are refined white sugar (sucrose made from sugar cane and sugar beet) and refined fructose (made from corn).

DANGERS OF SUCROSE FROM REFINED SUGAR CANE AND SUGAR BEET

Sucrose is a simple sugar disaccharide made of glucose and fructose molecules. We have all been fed the myth that sucrose is natural; however, although it is derived from plants, sugar cane and sugar beet require processing to turn them into refined sugar. Upon digestion, each sucrose molecule is separated into one glucose molecule, which is rapidly absorbed into the bloodstream, and one fructose molecule, which is transported to the liver. The liver converts fructose to glucose so that it can then be used as fuel for cells. Micronutrients such as chromium, magnesium and vitamin B1 are needed for all of these steps in the metabolism of sucrose since refined sucrose doesn't come with these micronutrients.

Unfortunately, there is more to say about beet sugar. It is estimated that close to 95 percent of all sugar beets are genetically modified to resist insects and to grow quickly. Although promoted as a solution for economic and production stability, understandable concern is being raised about the potential of genetically modified organisms (GMOs) potentiating antibiotic resistance, food allergies and digestive issues. Moreover, even when organic sugar beets are processed into sugar, it nurtures the wrong type of microbes in the gastrointestinal (GI) tract and can increase the symptoms of irritable bowel syndrome (IBS) and inflammatory bowel disease (IBD).

DANGERS OF CORN

High-fructose corn syrup has been used as a sweetener for decades, but because of its high fructose content, it has been shown to harm our health. To understand this better, we should discuss how it is produced. As you'd expect, it is derived from corn, which is usually genetically modified. The corn is first milled to produce corn starch and then processed into a syrup. Then, enzymes are used to convert glucose into fructose to achieve different concentrations, some as high as 90 percent fructose.

The problem with fructose is that only the liver can metabolize it. If your liver is overloaded because it is busy processing other things such as toxins, hormones or drugs, it converts fructose into fat, which can contribute to health concerns and chronic conditions such as insulin resistance and non-alcoholic fatty liver disease (NAFLD). High-fructose corn syrup has also been linked to increased triglycerides, metabolic syndrome, obesity and type 2 diabetes.

The *National Health and Nutrition Examination Survey* (NHANES) study in 2014 showed that drinking one can of fructose-sweetened soda per day is equivalent to aging 4.6 years faster, which is similar to the effect of cigarette smoking. Fructose affects the release of leptin, a hormone that lets us know when we are full and not hungry. It appears that fructose doesn't stimulate as much insulin release as glucose does, and insulin is needed to release leptin. This means that compared to sugar sources that are predominantly glucose, fructose is more likely to lead to higher food intake.

I also encourage you to avoid using corn flour or corn starch in recipes because the protein in corn, called zein, is so similar to wheat gluten. It can bind easily to the human leukocyte antigen (HLA DQ2 or DQ8) and be presented to immune cells, triggering a full-blown immune response, similar to the one seen when exposed to wheat gluten (autoimmune response against the intestinal lining). Therefore, zein is able to induce an inflammatory and immune response in the intestinal lining of patients with celiac disease. When corn isn't eliminated, total symptom remission may not be achieved in all individuals and the intestinal mucosa continues to be damaged.

If you find that you still suffer from digestive symptoms despite adhering to a strict gluten-free diet, it might be time to consider that corn might be the culprit. If you choose the elimination route, get familiar with reading ingredient lists and avoiding things like corn syrup, corn starch, corn alcohol, corn oil, maize, zein and corn gluten; even flavouring, aspartame and citric acid can contain hidden corn.

DO YOU HAVE A STARCH TOOTH INSTEAD OF A SWEET TOOTH?

Some people don't have a sweet tooth but rather a starch tooth! The starch found in corn, bread, pasta, pastry, potatoes and more breaks down to sugar within seconds when mixed with the digestive enzyme amylase found in your saliva.

When people are looking to let go of sugar, it is easy to switch to flour and starchy favourites, but unfortunately this action will undo all of your hard work.

THE ROLE OF CARBOHYDRATES

Now that you know about the dangers of sugar, which are derived from carbohydrates, the question that often follows is, "Do I really need carbs to thrive?" Unrefined carbohydrates can provide a clean-burning energy source and an important source of fibre (also known as roughage), which promotes elimination of solid wastes and cleanses the intestinal tract. Our body requires four essential macronutrients: carbohydrates, proteins, fats and water.

Sadly, at the height of the low-fat diet craze, carbohydrates replaced the vilified fats as a way to spike the flavour in food. Before you go low carb, it is a good idea to explore whether it is enough to remove refined carbohydrates. That is normally sufficient to ensure that we maintain blood sugar balance and healthy digestion.

I believe that the complete elimination of any macronutrient can be an unhealthy approach in the long term. However, it might be necessary for some people to tailor their ratios of macronutrients to treat certain medical conditions. For example, seizure disorders and certain cancers respond well to a ketogenic diet, which focuses on a low-carb, high-fat menu. If you are intolerant to exercise, it is important to scale down your carbohydrate consumption to match your energy output. The wholesome carbohydrates found in fruits and vegetables can be part of a balanced diet—as long as you can digest it. On the other hand, refined carbohydrates like white flours and sugars can leave you vulnerable to the painful symptoms of inflammation.

When we take a closer look at carbohydrates, we discover that all carbs are made of sugar molecules linked together. Carbohydrates are classified based on their structure, size, type of constituent sugars and arrangement of the sugar molecules. They range from simple (such as monosaccharides and disaccharides) to complex (such as polysaccharides).

You may have been told that the more complex the carbohydrate, the better it is for your health. The only problem is that if you cannot break down the bonds between the sugars easily, this type of carbohydrate may cause you major havoc. Some people lack the enzymes needed to break down longer carbohydrate chains into simple sugars, causing digestive

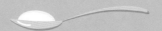

We Eat Sugary Foods That Contain Disaccarides (Sucrose, Lactose and Maltose)

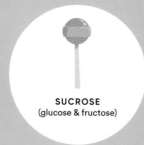

SUCROSE
(glucose & fructose)

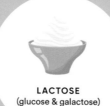

LACTOSE
(glucose & galactose)

MALTOSE
(glucose & glucose)

Enzymes Break Disaccharides into Various Types of Monosaccharides

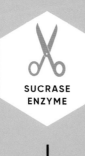

SUCRASE ENZYME

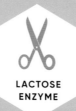

LACTOSE ENZYME

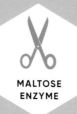

MALTOSE ENZYME

↓

↓

↓

GLUCOSE MOLECULE

GLUCOSE MOLECULE

GLUCOSE MOLECULE

FRUCTOSE MOLECULE

GALACTOSE MOLECULE

GLUCOSE MOLECULE

distress and inflammation. For example, lactose is composed of a molecule of glucose and a molecule of galactose. To split this double sugar (disaccharide) into single sugars (monosaccharides), you need an enzyme called lactase. If lactase is deficient, you will experience symptoms of indigestion such as bloating, gas, diarrhea, constipation and so on.

Lactose intolerance is experienced by close to 65 percent of the population and between 70 and 95 percent of people of Asian and African descent. And what if you are unable to digest other types of disaccharides, such as those found in sugars and grains? In the 1920s, Dr. Sidney Valentine Haas created the Specific Carbohydrate Diet to address these concerns and found great success with people suffering from IBD, including Crohn's disease and colitis. Dr. Campbell-McBride furthered this work, which led to the Gut and Psychology Syndrome (GAPS) Diet for brain disorders. Both doctors provided solid case studies of people who followed a low-disaccharide menu—for example, removal of grains, refined sugars and carbs and lactose-containing foods—and experienced not only relief of their digestive symptoms but also a significant improvement in their mental health.

The good news is that you don't need to cut out these difficult-to-digest carbohydrates for a lifetime but just until the lining of your digestive system heals. What I like about these dietary interventions is that they allow for honey, as it has been predigested by bees into simpler sugars. They also encourage fermented foods because the good bacteria work to break down carbohydrates for you, allowing for easier assimilation. Plus, by increasing foods that contain good bacteria, you accelerate the repair of your digestive tract, which can improve both mental and physical health.

THE HORMONES THAT MAKES SUGAR IRRESISTIBLE

I want to take you on a journey so that you can understand what happens inside your body when you eat sugar. To begin, imagine that you are being served your absolute favourite sweet thing for your birthday. Maybe it's an extraordinary chocolate lava cake, a maple pecan fudge cheesecake or another sweet treat. This treat likely has been created with a very specific combination of flavours referred to as the bliss point: a perfect ratio of sugar, salt and fat that has you hooked.

Simply looking at the sweet treat starts your mouth watering. This is because your brain signals your mouth to make extra saliva that will help dissolve sugar molecules as the first step of digestion. Next, with the first bite the "sweet" taste buds (pods with tiny hair-like fronds that are concentrated near the tip of the tongue) trigger a dizzying amount of lightning-fast chemical and electrical messages (via neurotransmitters along neural pathways) to the forebrain of the cerebral cortex.

When the forebrain perceives sweetness, it sends signals to your brain's reward centre, the substantia nigra (sub-STAN-sha NY-grah), a little strip of tissue on either side of the base of your midbrain, which tells you to keep eating that sweet treat you've found. In ancient times, when humans were hunter-gatherers, a sweet food signalled the presence of carbohydrates, an important source of quick and sustaining energy. The reward centres of our brain would release "feel-good" hormones, such as serotonin and dopamine, which made us feel happy and safe. We would eat more of the sweet stuff and feel more reward when doing so.

This feedback loop played an essential role in our survival, and our species thrived because of it. Plus, when our ancestors ate a sweet food, it often carried with it important vitamins and minerals. Sweet and starchy foods became fast favourites during our evolution, as they indicated that food is safe to eat and provided much-needed nutrition.

In the modern world, refined sugars and starches are playing tricks on the brain. Sugar- and flour-filled treats are abundant and readily available to eat, creating a crisis of overstimulation of our brain's reward system that we just cannot seem to control. Our brain has simply not caught up to our technological prowess, as we have only been refining flour and sugar for the masses since 1815.

Why Do We Love Sugar?

Did you know that children do not develop a taste for salt until four months of age, but our taste for sweet happens the minute we are born? It turns out that sugar is a type of temporary analgesic. A 2005 study showed that children can keep their hands in cold water for longer if they have a sweet in their mouth.

Sugar is so seductive that scientists have recently revealed through brain scans that our brain lights up when we eat sugar in a similar way as it does when we ingest strong drugs such as cocaine. Many mind-altering substances, including OxyContin, ecstasy, heroin, alcohol and marijuana, overactivate the dopamine reward system. Dopamine, our major reward hormone, tells us things like "Great job, do it again, you're successful, you're awesome." It's released when we do things we enjoy, such as getting together with friends, winning an award, being successful at work and so on. It's also released when we consume sugar.

To make matters worse, dopamine receptors may become insensitive to the presence of dopamine because of being triggered continuously. If you constantly spike your dopamine, you'll need to do more and more of an extreme action to get to the same "reward" that a less extreme action elicited before. In other words, your brain becomes resistant to the dopamine hit, creating more and more extreme behaviour. Because dopamine is the major hormone involved in addiction, you can see how it can be running in the background of your sugar addiction whether you're aware of it or not.

You will get some of the dopamine response every time you eat a sweet treat, but you will need to increase the amount of sugar you eat in order to feel the same rush over time. Sugar elicits the greatest dopamine response of any food on the planet, which is fascinating when compared to other notably pleasurable foods that do not stand a chance at holding our attention. I wish that broccoli would generate the same reward response, but compared to refined sugar, your reward centre simply gets bored with healthy food. Sugar is addictive because we never get tired of being rewarded, and as the reward lessens with each hit, we chase it more and more.

Let's revisit that bite of the chocolate lava cake. It's so joyful that your reward centre is screaming, "Yes, that's a great idea! Do that again!" We often enjoy treats like this when we're doing other joyful things. For example, if it's our birthday, we are usually socializing with friends and having other pleasurable substances like alcohol or caffeine that give us a huge dopamine rush. There's an old saying in neuroscience: "Neurons that fire together, wire together." This means that the more you run a neural circuit in your brain, the stronger that circuit relationship becomes. If you continue to chase dopamine with sugar and combine that behaviour with other pleasures, this stacking of multiple rewards that feels good in the moment may create some long-term health effects. This chapter looks at the ways in which you can create new behaviours that will stack the health cards in your favour. When you learn healthy ways to stimulate dopamine, you won't need refined sugar or flour anymore.

Why Does Sugar Make Me Feel Better in the Moment?

I understand that you feel you may want to dive headfirst into a box of sugary cookies when you are sad. It is common to crave refined carbs when you are depressed and/or angry. It is interesting that we might feel as if we would do anything for a cinnamon bun when "hangry," so why can't we find the same passion for a bunch of kale?

It turns out that insulin, the hormone responsible for shuttling sugar into our cells, plays a critical role in promoting the absorption of L-tryptophan, an amino acid we require to make our happiness hormone, serotonin. Refined carbohydrates cause large amounts of insulin to be released, which increases tryptophan absorption, especially when you eat carbs with high-tryptophan foods. The increased amount of tryptophan in the blood causes more serotonin to be produced, which is why eating a dessert after a high-protein meal may give you a temporary mood lift.

It may also allow you to sleep better because tryptophan boosts melatonin, our sleep hormone. However, to not risk snoozing during the day, it is best to have a protein-rich breakfast and lunch, saving your carbohydrates for your last snack or meal, when they will best help to improve serotonin and melatonin synthesis. The good news is you don't need refined carbs to promote happy hormones. Eating berries, sweet potato or squash will help with your mood balance without the crash you experience with sugar.

If you are following a lower-carb menu, here are things you can do to boost serotonin:

- Exercise is a fast track to making more serotonin. If you are exercise intolerant, start in the pool!

- Go outside or stand at a window for 10 to 15 minutes first thing in the morning to shut off meletonin and have a serotonin boost. If you can't get outside, consider buying a light therapy box to reduce Seasonal Affective Disorder (SAD) that is caused by lack of direct sunlight in the winter months.

- Expose the skin on your arms to bright sunshine (without sunscreen) for 20 minutes a day to make extra vitamin D, the vitamin responsible for serotonin synthesis. In northern climates from November to May, the sun is often not strong enough to make enough vitamin D, so ask your health care provider if a vitamin D supplement would be beneficial for you.

- Increase probiotics and fibre-rich foods, as new research shows that both play a role in boosting serotonin production via the gut-brain axis. (See Part 3, Recipes Using Sugar Alternatives on page 139.)

How Does Sugar Affect Your Brain over Time?

The brain uses more glucose as fuel than any other organ. It is the most metabolically active organ, consuming about 120 grams of glucose daily (about 420 calories), accounting for 60 percent of the glucose needed by the whole body in a resting state. This doesn't mean you should eat refined sugar. Your body creates the glucose it needs at the right pace from the healthy foods you consume. High glycemic foods (foods that break down into glucose quickly) such as sugar and white flour can overactivate the amygdala, an almond-shaped brain structure involved with the experiencing of emotions.

Regular sugar consumption can change gene expression and the availability of dopamine receptors in the midbrain and frontal cortex. Specifically, sugar increases the brain's excitatory receptor (D1) and decreases the inhibitory receptor (D2). In other words, the brain's reward pathway can develop tolerance, which means that you need to eat more sugar to activate dopamine receptors. It's a vicious cycle and a classic feature of addiction. Other ways in which the brain is affected include sleep disturbances, memory and attention decline, and mood swings as discussed in more detail on page 34.

In addition, there is recent evidence that overconsumption of sugar and refined flour may be implicated in bipolar disorder. You've probably heard of uric acid and its link to causing painful gout. Uric acid does so much more than that. It plays a role in appetite, cognition, memory, impulsivity. It also seems to be associated with bipolar disorder.

Data published in 2019 suggests that high serum uric acid levels may predict conversion to bipolar disorder in those diagnosed with major depressive disorder. High levels of insulin, caused by too much sugar, is associated with a decreased excretion in urinary uric acid from the kidneys.

The study showed that people hospitalized with a major depressive disorder who also had high levels of uric acid in their blood were more than 34 times more likely to go on to develop bipolar disorder in the next 8 to 11 years. Men with uric acid levels higher than 5.35 mg/dL (or 318 micromoles/litre) and women with uric acid levels higher than 4 mg/dL (or 241 micromoles/litre) were associated with increased risk for bipolar disorder. For people with a family history of bipolar disorder, this knowledge should inspire and empower you to reduce your sugar, flour and alcohol intake.

You Sleep Poorly

Frequent consumption of sugar is associated with poor sleep quality. A 2016 study found that a group that consumed significantly more sugar and fat spent less time in deep, slow-wave sleep, the sleep stage essential for the body's physical restoration and healing. This group also took longer to fall asleep and experienced a more restless sleep with frequent awakenings throughout the night.

Your Memory and Attention Decline

When it comes to memory and cognition, even a single instance of elevated glucose can be harmful and cause cognitive deficits in memory and attention. If you have consistently high blood sugar, the glucose can become a slow-acting corrosive agent, which destroys the insides of the blood vessels of the eyes, heart and brain.

One study followed more than four thousand individuals and found that those who consumed more sweetened drinks had poorer memory and reduced overall brain volume, especially in the hippocampus, the area known for processing short-term memory. Sugar can age the brain more rapidly as well, with a study showing that consuming two sugary drinks per day led to brains that appeared eleven years older than normal.

Your Moods Drop

Let's get back to that chocolate lava cake. I bet it felt good for a little while, but after a few hours, you probably felt tired, moody and maybe even brain fogged. That's because sugar can increase your risk of developing anxiety and depression—and if you already have these conditions, they can feel a lot worse.

It's interesting that we self-medicate with sweets when they can actually negatively affect our mental health. It seems that consuming foods that are high in carbohydrates tend to temporarily raise serotonin levels (our happiness hormone), but this response diminishes over time. In fact, sugar has been linked to chronic inflammation, and we know that inflammation is linked to depression. Recall the study that found that people who consume a high amount of sugar were 23 percent more likely to receive a diagnosis of depression.

We also know that sugar and anxiety are related. Sugar causes spikes and drops in dopamine, which directly affects mood and can exacerbate feelings and symptoms of anxiety.

If you need to do extreme things to feel pleasure, are unmotivated or procrastinate, have energy and memory issues, feel apathetic or have lost your zest for life, then you may suffer from low dopamine levels.

How to Naturally Raise Your Dopamine

As we can see, dopamine plays an important role in our health, so how can we increase it naturally and in a balanced way? As discussed, we first want to avoid harsh stimulants, refined sugar and starch, drugs and risky or repetitive behaviours that trigger the overproduction of dopamine. Second, we want to increase the nutrients and activities that create a steady, balanced stream of dopamine in our bodies, such as the ones outlined in the following chart.

THINGS WE CAN EAT	
Tyrosine	The amino acid tyrosine is the major building block of dopamine, and we need a lot of it. Tyrosine is used as a building block for thyroid hormones, so if you have weak thyroid function, it's even more important to have increased levels of tyrosine. We can find tyrosine in all animal-based proteins, such as chicken, eggs, beef and fish, and find smaller amounts in legumes, nuts and seeds. One of the highest plant-based sources of tyrosine is pumpkin seeds.
Caffeine	We know that caffeine stimulates dopamine, but it's important to use caffeine every few days for maximum performance. A recent study of sprinters showed that caffeine improved repeated sprint performance only if the athlete had low habitual caffeine consumption. I only use it for meeting deadlines, media performances and special occasions where I want that extra sparkle. If breaking up with daily caffeine feels too hard, try kinder sources of caffeine such as an organic green or yerba mate tea. These drinks will give you the lift and focus you're craving without overstimulation.
Resveratrol	Resveratrol not only helps prevent heart disease but also helps make dopamine. Most people associate resveratrol with wine, but where do we find it if we don't want to drink alcohol? The good news is that Concord grapes contain resveratrol, which has many beneficial properties for cardiovascular health. You can also get decent amounts of resveratrol in blueberries, cranberries, and even a red-skinned peanut or the red tinge on a pistachio; the deep red colour indicates the presence of resveratrol.

THINGS WE CAN EAT

Omega-3	Omega-3 is important for the production of dopamine. In fact, virtually all disorders of the brain (including dopamine-related disorders) are associated with reduced levels of a type of omega-3 called DHA (docosahexaenoic acid) in brain tissue. Omega-3s help increase both dopamine and serotonin neurotransmission in the brain. It also helps prevent type 2 and type 3 diabetes that can contribute to brain inflammation and mental illness. The best source of omega-3 is tank-grown algae because of its low environmental toxicity, but small oily fish like mackerel, sardines, herring, lake trout and arctic char are also excellent sources.
Vitamin D	Vitamin D facilitates the production of both dopamine and serotonin and also helps increase the number of dopamine receptors. Vitamin D and omega-3 come together when you eat fish, but you may need to supplement to ensure that you get enough. We make vitamin D in our skin when the sun is very bright. In northern countries like Canada, we get bright enough sun to make vitamin D only from May to November. If you are unsure about your levels, ask your primary health care provider for a vitamin D test during your next visit.
B Vitamins	If you are dealing with memory loss, anxiety, depression, mood issues, premenstrual syndrome (PMS), emotional ups and downs or sleep disturbances, B vitamins are absolutely critical to help turn things around. Many people rely on folic acid, but not everyone is able to metabolize it into the bioavailable form that your brain and liver need. Folate, the naturally occurring and more absorbable form of vitamin B9, is found in the food we eat like most green leafy plants. Vitamins B12, B1 (thiamine) and B3 (niacin) also play important roles in maintaining optimal mental health and energy production.

THINGS WE CAN DO

Consider a Dopamine Detox	You may help increase your dopamine receptors (D2) by refraining from activities that give you a sharp spike of dopamine. We want healthy levels of dopamine but without the extreme highs and lows as this can lead to negative behaviours such as seeking sugar and overeating. If you are a person who seeks unhealthy levels of dopamine consistently then consider a break from strong dopamine stimulators (i.e. TV, social media and gaming). This is often called a dopamine detox. Consider intermittent fasting at night, as outlined on page 125 and cognitive behavioral therapy techniques, as outlined on page 106.
Touch	You may know that hugging increases the love hormone oxytocin, but it also triggers our dopamine. That's why caressing, hugging and shaking hands are ways in which we can have our dopamine needs met. Look for ways to touch and be touched, and always make sure to max out your health benefits. How many people let their massage benefits expire without using them up? Dopamine is expressed through massage and also reduces stress. This applies for pets, too—hugging your pet or stroking its belly or head will raise your dopamine level and theirs.
Sleep	We need sleep to keep the dopamine receptors in our brain responsive and plentiful. Consider switching to a sunrise alarm that uses a gentle light shift instead of a harsh alarm sound that jolts you out of bed. Harsh alarms should be used only for catching planes. Avoiding the blaring buzzer helps keep your stress hormone cortisol down in the morning so that you can wake up calmer and happier.
New Habits	Similar to finding new foods, our brain is rewarded when we discover new avenues of satisfaction. Try these new experiences to help increase dopamine if they're not already part of your regular habits. • Meditation teachers found a 64 percent increase in dopamine production after meditating for one hour, compared to when resting quietly. • Listen to music, especially new songs or stations that you've not heard before. The brain loves new things.

THINGS WE CAN DO

New Habits (continued)	• Try to make your own music. As someone who never played an instrument, I was awestruck when my husband and nephews gave me a ukulele for my birthday. I learned to play it using an app and was amazed by how much I enjoy it. • Learn a language. I decided to learn French using an app so that I could better connect with my Québécois nieces. I couldn't believe how fun and gamified it was. When you learn through gamification, you are rewarded with bells and whistles and "good job" rewards. Regardless of your age, your brain is going to love that sort of reward.
Complete Tasks	Overachievers unite! Completing tasks and closing circles create a wonderful dopamine response. Completion is a big thing for dopamine and why creating lists is so powerful. List-making helps break large tasks into smaller ones, freeing up attention and creating a sense of calm (this is why doing a mind dump the night before a big day can help you sleep). Making a list allows many opportunities for dopamine hits as you complete tasks. I even have subdivisions within my to-do list. I've got lists for work, home, friends and family, creative projects and more. All of these lists have checkmarks and clickable boxes so that when I complete a task, I check it off and collect my hit of dopamine.
Gamification	Do you love it when you establish a streak? The reward and feedback can help build your commitment to something. For example, when I started using an intermittent fasting app on my phone, day 1 through 30 was no big deal. But now that I'm on day 927 (at the time of printing this book), I am committed to not breaking that streak because it's just too rewarding and fun to see how long the streak can last! Each day adds to the total, and the game keeps me interested and motivated. That's what's really cool about gamification. People may think that negative habits are more ingrained and harder to change, but it's just a matter of choosing to be consistent and finding a fun way to train it into a habit. When positive actions become automatic habits, you move from conscious competence to unconscious competence, and that's when healthy lifestyle actions go on autopilot.

THINGS WE CAN DO

Cold Exposure	Surprisingly, cold exposure spikes your dopamine by 250 percent. I dislike cold showers, so instead I practise cold immersion by putting my limbs in cold water. Hydrotherapy is a process whereby you pulse cold and warm water exposure to improve your circulation. Want to try it? Put your feet in a warm-water bucket for a few minutes, then plunge them into a cold-water bucket for 1 minute and then move them back to the warm water. When I do this, my endorphins spike so high that I can't help but be happy. I'm so full of dopamine and happiness that I typically want to run around.
Exercise	For hundreds of thousands of years, we walked ten to thirty kilometres a day to ensure that our food needs were met. Our need to walk is in our DNA, and we have lost our way in the modern day. Sitting is not only the new smoking but also an absolutely sure-fire way to dip your dopamine production. Can you consider a standing desk or walking desk? My walking desk has totally changed my life. I purchased a second-hand treadmill, and my husband designed a piece of wood that goes atop the handlebars, so that I could write this book while I walked. Exercise helps the body in so many ways, but it is important for us to keep it fun or the brain will not produce as much dopamine. If you despise running, don't run. Don't force yourself! It's very important to find out what kind of exercise lights you up. For me, I can dance anytime if you put the right music on. And when you interact with a person or pet while exercising, it compounds the dopamine effect. Exercise classes are great because you're surrounded by people doing the same thing as you and have an instructor encouraging you.
Take Breaks	I get mini hits of dopamine throughout my day because I take work breaks, such as taking 20 minutes to run around the block or taking 10 minutes to practise French on my online app. By taking short breaks, you shake up your routine and keep things fresh. This helps build healthy habits while allowing you to have fun and accomplish big things over time.

OXFORD COUNTY LIBRARY

The Importance of Insulin Balance

Insulin is the hormone made in the beta cells of your pancreas that helps you regulate blood sugar levels. Insulin shuttles the sugars from your bloodstream across the cell membrane so that they can be used as a source of energy. To recap, constant exposure to sugar can leave you with a condition called insulin resistance, in which insulin binds to the cell receptors but the signal isn't sent into the cell and therefore the cell does not take up glucose. This results in high blood glucose levels and advanced glycation end products (AGEs) that can cause damage to cells and organs over time.

Glucagon is a hormone that is produced by alpha cells of the pancreas. It works opposite to insulin to raise the concentration of glucose in the bloodstream. It is the main catabolic (breakdown) hormone of the body, responsible for encouraging the use of stored fat for energy instead of glucose, which may be in short supply in the blood.

It is good to keep in mind that when your insulin is high, your fat-burning hormone glucagon cannot be expressed, making it very hard to burn fat. That is why some people can restrict calories on a diet without any results. If they continue to spike insulin, glucagon is unable to do its job. You may want to avoid insulin-spiking carbohydrates by following the fast breakup on page 121.

When you are digesting your food, and the nutrients enter the intestines, a similar hormone called glucagon-like peptide-1 (GLP-1) keeps blood sugar levels stable and makes you feel full. You make more GLP-1 when eating anti-inflammatory protein choices such as oily fish and omega-3-rich seeds (flax and chia).

For you to understand where your hormone levels are at, you need to have some blood work done. By running some important tests, you will know whether your cells are being overburdened by too much sugar. For more information on blood sugar testing, consult your doctor and check out our sugar-free online program at www.JulieDaniluk.com.

HOW TO IMPROVE INSULIN SENSITIVITY

Avoid Foods That Harm	The number one thing you can do is avoid all refined food (for example, white sugar, wheat flour, corn flour, corn syrup, etc.). Make sure to avoid foods you are sensitive, allergic or intolerant to.
Include the Anti-Inflammatory Rainbow	After you take out the bad things, enjoy an anti-inflammatory rainbow of foods to get the vitamins and phytonutrients that you need. For example, foods that are orange in colour often contain high levels of vitamin A. Vitamin B foods are often green in colour and vitamin C is most often found in red and purple coloured foods. When you ensure you have a colourful plate of vegetables and fruit, you ingest the nutrients you need to keep your blood sugar and inflammation balanced, which is most important to prevent and manage diabetes.
Nutrients	Which nutrients are critical? Omega-3 and vitamin D are some of the most potent anti-inflammatory nutrients that help to dramatically improve insulin sensitivity. Supplementation of an omega-3 fatty acid at a dosage of 2 to 4 grams per day can increase insulin sensitivity. Vitamin D also plays an important role by decreasing the risk of developing insulin resistance and related conditions. Your levels of vitamin D will depend on a lot of factors, including your geographic location. We also need a lot of minerals, especially zinc and chromium. It's also very important to improve gut health by increasing probiotics and focusing on intestinal health and healing your digestive system.
Intermittent Fasting	Intermittent fasting is very beneficial for insulin sensitivity. You don't need to do it every day or for sixteen hours a day to have great results, either. Anything beyond twelve hours a day has been shown to be beneficial. It is very easy to stop eating at 7 PM and start again at 9 AM for a moderate fourteen-hour daily fast. See page 125 for more information.

HOW TO IMPROVE INSULIN SENSITIVITY

Exercise	Exercise is one of the greatest reducers of insulin, but in the case of insulin resistance, it's important to engage in more activities than slow walks. If you need to reverse your insulin resistance quickly, strength training like resistance training or high-intensity interval training (HIIT) is great. You want to engage in activities where you work very intensely and get your heart rate up, then allow it to return to normal. Stair climbing, sprints, skipping and HIIT workouts are all great options that will increase your growth hormone to dramatically improve your mitochondrial function and increase insulin sensitivity. We often think that thirty minutes of exercise three times a week is sufficient, but if you are someone with insulin resistance, you need to do up to sixty minutes of exercise every single day. I know that seems like a lot of exercise, but you can work up to that level. You don't need to pound your joints to get intensity of exercise. That's why I close my circles every day on my fitness tracker. I'm all about systems, and like to have that checkbox because it makes me feel so much better. Even when I'm sick, I do yoga in bed and count it as exercise.
Sleep Quality	Another important factor is sleep quality, and one-third of adults don't get enough sleep. Poor sleep is a cause of insulin resistance, but by improving sleep hygiene we dramatically increase our insulin sensitivity because we repair this important function in our sleep. Your stress hormones and appetite hormones increase so much when you don't sleep.
Lower Stress	You must reduce your stress with some everyday practices that will reduce your cortisol, as it is the driver of insulin resistance. What is your flavour of stress reduction? Some people colour, some use essential oils in a bath, others practise yoga, some journal, and others do Pilates or a workout or meditate. Check out our sugar-free program to be walked through many of these practices.

Breathing	You can change how you're breathing while reading this sentence. Breathe in deeply and exhale for twice as long. By extending your exhale, you will directly switch off your stress response.

Does the Off Switch on Your Appetite Feel Broken?

If you have tried in earnest to break up with sugar and continue to struggle with feeling full and satisfied, you may have to look deeper at your hormones. Leptin is the satiety hormone produced by your fat cells that reduces appetite and makes you feel full. Unfortunately, some people become leptin resistant, and the brain no longer gets the message to stop eating. Instead, it can feel like you are starving, so you're driven to eat even after a big meal. Fat cells produce leptin in proportion to one's body size, so people who are overweight have very high levels of leptin. When they become leptin resistant, it causes an insatiable appetite.

To make matters worse, there is another hormone called ghrelin that I like to call your weight loss gremlin because it messes with any attempt to restrict your food intake. Your stomach pumps out ghrelin when it is hungry. When you eat, ghrelin levels go down so that you feel full. Studies have also shown that if you are overweight, ghrelin will go down only slightly after eating a meal. Your hypothalamus won't get the message to stop eating, which can lead to overeating.

How do you reduce ghrelin and leptin resistance? One of the best things you can do to reduce ghrelin is to increase beta-hydroxybutyrate (BHB). People who take a ketone supplement known as BHB, or stick to a fat-fuelled diet called the keto diet, experience reduced brain inflammation and improved mental health. BHB enhances the expression of a molecule known as brain-derived neurotrophic factor (BDNF), which reduces depression and anxiety and also improves cognitive function. The anxiety reduction may come from the fact that BHB increases gamma-aminobutyric acid (GABA), the inhibitory neurotransmitter that works like a bouncer in the brain telling anxious thoughts to get lost!

Beyond enjoying the delicious meals in this book, alpha-lipoic acid and fish oil can help decrease leptin resistance. Giving up sugar and enjoying protein and fat at every meal has been shown to reduce ghrelin and promote a deep satisfaction that will help you reduce cravings naturally. For more amazing ideas, refer to Chapter 4.

HOW TO GET RID OF THE HIDDEN SUGAR LURKING IN YOUR FOOD

Sugar hides in all kinds of foods. It's not just about what's in the sugar bowl anymore. Consider this: You wake in the morning and have some yogurt with granola and a glass of orange juice. Most yogurt is sweetened with sugar, making it more like thawed ice cream, and the carbs in commercial granola immediately turn to sugar once they hit the tongue. And that glass of orange juice? It's been stripped of any fibre and is just sweet juice. This combination probably contributes 30 grams of sugar to your day. This high sugar intake in the morning is processed super-fast in the body, and around 10:30 AM you're craving something else. You go to the coffee shop and get a coffee (with sugar) and a muffin, thinking that the muffin is at least healthier than a doughnut or a cookie. But it's filled with sugar and refined flour, which contributes another 5 to 10 grams of sugar to your day, on top of the sugar in your coffee. You're already at more than 40 grams of sugar, and it's not even lunchtime. See how quickly that can add up? Throughout the day, your energy hits highs and lows, you feel cranky, you come home starving and raid the fridge before supper, and at the end of the day you feel disappointed with yourself.

Sources of Added Sugar in the Typical North American Diet

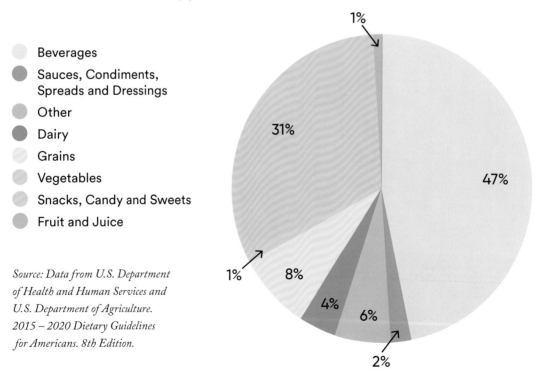

- Beverages
- Sauces, Condiments, Spreads and Dressings
- Other
- Dairy
- Grains
- Vegetables
- Snacks, Candy and Sweets
- Fruit and Juice

Source: Data from U.S. Department of Health and Human Services and U.S. Department of Agriculture. 2015 – 2020 Dietary Guidelines for Americans. 8th Edition.

1. **Dairy.** Many people do not realize that dairy naturally contains sugar and that many dairy products have added sugar even when they do not taste that sweet. It is not until you break down lactose into its simple sugars that you taste the sugar content. But beyond the naturally occurring sugar, we need to be aware that fruit-bottom yogurts often contain up to 30 grams of sugar. Ice cream is obvious, but many people make the mistake of thinking frozen yogurt is a good idea. I know that yogurt contains calcium, magnesium, protein and probiotics, which can seem like a better choice. However, yogurt is also high in sugar and if you are intolerant to it, it becomes inflammatory.

   Alternatives: Look for unsweetened coconut yogurt and add fruit and nuts for a great breakfast choice.

2. **Smoothies.** Did you know that the average smoothie can contain between 40 and 80 grams of sugar in a 20-ounce cup? When out, I like to check the breakdown of recipes and avoid high-sugar fruits in the base.

   Alternatives: Avoid all commercially made smoothies and make smoothies at home with frozen berries, coconut milk, coconut oil, high-quality collagen protein powder or a seed protein like pumpkin or hemp protein and maybe even an avocado to swap out the banana. I find that this keeps me satisfied and able to fight off hunger.

3. **Meal replacement bars.** You may think these products are healthy because they are called a meal replacement, but most bars are simply square cookies. They can contain high-fructose corn syrup, cane sugar and glucose syrup. I have seen them with 10 to 30 grams of added sugar. It is terrible that even bars marketed for weight loss have added sugars that cause inflammation and blood sugar imbalances.

   Alternatives: Look for low-carb protein bars sweetened with monk fruit or stevia. You can also eat sugar-free jerky (organic beef or turkey) or pack some guacamole in the bottom of a mason jar and then top it with chopped veggies for dipping.

4. **Juices and punches.** I watched my dad drink an entire litre of orange juice in one sitting, and it never dawned on me until I went to nutrition school that 1 cup of orange juice contains 22 grams of sugar. Watch out for commercially packed green juices because they often use fruit juice as a base, increasing the sugar content to as high as 30 grams a serving. Even if there are antioxidant-rich berries and powerful herbs in these drinks, that much sugar without fibre can cause a spike of inflammatory reaction. Be careful to avoid any punch because it often contains harmful artificial ingredients.

Alternatives: Our family makes sugar-free organic lemonade found on page 155. Consider sweetening things with monk fruit extract, which is two hundred times sweeter than sugar but is being researched for its anti-inflammatory properties. If you love juice, consider 1 ounce of juice for every 7 ounces of water. That way you have the flavour of juice with a lot of hydrating water.

5. **Sauces.** Most people love ketchup, and it is just as sugary as jam! Just 1 table-spoon of ketchup can contain 1 teaspoon of sugar. Barbecue sauce is an even larger source, containing up to 2 teaspoons of sugar per tablespoon.

   Alternatives: Use my Keto Ketchup (page 223) and Bold Barbecue Sauce (page 219). If you don't have time to make a sauce, use salsa! Grilling meat with sweet barbecue sauce is very unhealthy because it increases something called polycyclic aromatic hydrocarbons (PAHs). Most restaurants put commercial sauces on their various meat dishes to dress them up and give them unique and exotic flavours. Unfortunately, most of these sauces include high amounts of added sugars and corn starch, maltodextrin, glucose and high-fructose corn syrup. Avoid glazed foods because they are sure to contain added sugars. When eating at restaurants, order meat and fish grilled, baked or broiled and ask the serving staff to hold the extra sauces and glazes. Instead, add fresh or dried herbs, spices, unrefined vinegar, pesto, mustard or lemon juice and olive oil.

6. **Breads.** In his landmark book *Wheat Belly*, Dr. William Davis reported that eating two slices of whole wheat bread can increase blood sugar more than eating 2 tablespoons of pure sugar would. Even if you avoid white bread, brown bread is often coloured with molasses (from cane sugar). Even if you carefully read the labels to avoid sugar, remember that flour breaks down into sugar, and that process starts as soon as it enters your mouth. Many people think that if a bread is sprouted, it is healthy; although it doesn't appear to cause as drastic a blood sugar spike as whole grain or white breads, in some people it still spikes blood sugar because of the grain content.

   Alternatives: Look for commercially or homemade alternatives in the recipe section Bread, Chips and Crackers (page 183) that use nuts (almonds), seeds (coconut) and fibre (psyllium) as a replacement for grains. These are delicious options for your dips, veggies and sandwich ingredients.

7. **Dressings.** Salad dressing can be a minefield of sugars, corn syrup solids and starches that take away from all of the nutrition in the veggies you are enjoying. Check the label, and you may be shocked that a tablespoon of dressing can have as

many as 6 grams of sugar. Unfortunately, this is far too high, as most people use more than 1 tablespoon of dressing on their salad and this quickly adds up to about 12 grams of sugar.

Alternatives: A great way to keep things simple and delicious is to skip the fancy dressings and use olive oil with some apple cider vinegar or freshly squeezed lemon juice and a choice of dried herbs as your dressing. Try my Sunny Anti-Inflammatory Dressing (page 226).

8. **Nut and seed butters.** Nuts and seeds are very low in carbohydrates naturally, but most commercial nut and seed butters are spiked with sweeteners to enhance flavour and keep you coming back for more. Your typical peanut butter can contain up to 5 grams of added icing sugar per 2 tablespoon serving. Even health food brands use organic evaporated cane sugar as one of the top ingredients, so be very careful.

Alternatives: Stick with unsweetened nut and seed butters that are certified organic if your budget allows for it. Also shop for raw nuts and seeds that are free of added sugars and toxic oils.

9. **Cereals.** Commercial cereal is loaded with sugar and flour that sends your blood sugar soaring. The average breakfast cereal recommends serving only ¾ cup, which is such a small amount that most people double it. This larger serving can result in 30 grams of sugar before you even add milk. Popular granola brands use dried fruits that are sprayed with sugar or both sugar and flour to make up the oat clusters. A quarter-cup of sweetened dried cranberries contains 29 grams, nearly 6 teaspoons, of sugar.

Alternatives: I suggest you start the day out with protein and greens. I like to eat dinner leftovers for breakfast, but if you want something sweet, try my Chocolate Crunch Low-Carb Granola (page 176). By focusing on seeds for breakfast, you increase your cholecystokinin (CCK), the hormone responsible for feeling satisfied.

TIPS TO KICK CRAVINGS

Consider this alternative for a day without refined sugars. You wake in the morning and have a healing smoothie filled with fats or a couple of scrambled eggs with some sautéed spinach on the side. This leaves you feeling full, satisfied and with enough energy to make it to lunch without the need for a sugar rush. For lunch, enjoy some protein with some vegetables, then maybe have a snack of nuts and seeds in the afternoon. At supper, you again have warm veggies or a delicious soup or yummy stir-fry—all without sugar. You end the day feeling positive, uplifted, ready for tomorrow and proud of your decisions.

It's all about making choices—and you can start today. After you read through the ways to replace sugar in your life, you can explore the delicious recipes at the back of this book to help you get into a wholesome way of sugar-free eating. If you find yourself craving a sugar fix in this stage, there are a few things you can try to kick the craving:

1. **Eat a fibre-rich vegetable.** Before eating something sweet, enjoy fibre to reduce hunger and cravings. The best food for this is artichoke hearts packed in water or olive oil. They make everything taste sweeter, cleanse the liver and reduce hunger hormones.

2. **Enjoy something bitter to reduce sugar cravings.** A bitter herbal tincture, such as gentian root, works great as a wonderful stomach tonic, helping you to assimilate food. It also kills yeast in the body, which is behind a lot of cravings. You can also eat bitter vegetables such as endive and rapini.

3. **Enjoy something sour.** Acetic acid, the active ingredient in vinegar, helps keep food in the stomach for a longer period, delaying the release of the hunger hormone ghrelin. Vinegar also improves digestion, and it helps you feel full faster and for a longer period. Sour flavour also reduces the need for salt.

4. **Eat something rich in healthy fats.** Avocado contains epigallocatechin gallate (EGCG), which increases the hormone CCK that is responsible for creating the feeling of satiation. Feeling full between meals is the greatest weapon against the battle of the bulge. EGCG also stimulates your metabolism by activating thermogenesis, which means that your cells are burning energy—including fat.

5. **Go all-natural.** If all else fails, enjoy something with your new unrefined, natural sweetener options. There are many recipes at the end of this book for you to try out.

WHAT DOES IT FEEL LIKE TO REACT TO SUGAR?

I am in the middle of a sugar reaction while writing this section, so I thought I would take this opportunity to explain how it makes me feel. I have not intentionally eaten sugar for more than twelve years because the reaction I have is so negative. People naively say that a food is "sugar-free," and if I believe them but it does have sugar in it, I will have to batten down the hatches and wait out the storm.

The reaction starts with a subtle mood shift. I now know that my true nature is relaxed, connected, energetic, open and free. In less than an hour of consuming sucrose, such as cane sugar, beet sugar or maple sugar, I feel anxiety set in. An irritation with my surroundings comes next. All of a sudden, I don't feel safe. A strange level of insecurity comes next, and that is when I start to question whether sugar plays a role in this rapid shift.

For example, I was giving a public lecture tonight, and before I went on stage, I felt strange and could not put my finger on it. The audience was responding in all the right places; my family in the front row felt that the performance was great, but I kept feeling like I was off. I started to have repeated negative thoughts about myself that are not true: "Julie, you are dumb; you don't belong on this stage. You are off your game and can't get back on track." I started to have this sensation like I was crawling out of my skin. I felt like I had an itch that I couldn't scratch. The itch affected the inside of my ears, which was impossible to ignore. My belly felt bloated and I felt grief-stricken. I suffered on through my book signing and did my absolute best to smile for pictures and answer questions, but inside I just wanted to hide behind the stage curtain.

After the event, I traced back in my mind all the things I had eaten and, low and behold, I'd had a handmade chocolate square that a friend gave me an hour before the show. The waitress had told her it was sugar-free, but I called the restaurant and got them to check the actual ingredient list. On closer analysis with the chef, I discovered it did contain cane sugar. People often miss the other names for sugar, and this time it was disguised as cane juice crystals. It is a real issue with restaurants. I never have a problem with packaged foods because they have to disclose each ingredient, but you are taking someone for their word when you ingest food from an eatery.

I only have about two or three reactions a year now because I am so careful. The negative self-talk and the irritability is such a significant shift from my regular personality that my husband, Alan, can often notice it before I do. The trouble is that when I am within the reaction, the feelings of self-loathing seem so entirely real that I am hypnotized into thinking that the sky might be falling.

What if your anxiety, sadness or low self-esteem is actually caused by a reaction to sucrose? I know this is hard to imagine because the world is filled with so much sugar that you might live on an emotional roller coaster. Is it possible that you can't discern what is negative brain chemistry caused by a food reaction and what is in fact your true nature?

What do I do once I realize I have been accidentally "poisoned"? I actively tell myself over and over that this is just a temporary state and that it will pass the second my body recalibrates. It can take up to thirty-six hours for my sucrose reaction to completely dissipate. I now trust that I will feel as if a wet wool blanket has been lifted off of me mere hours from now! If I do a lot of yogic breathing, I can change my state even sooner. I look forward to my mind sharpening. I am excited to be able to laugh at Alan's goofy jokes and just feel comfortable in my own skin again.

Remember, you don't have to believe me, just try it on long enough to see for yourself. If you are suffering, what have you got to lose? Panic, self-doubt and unhappiness may be a few of the things that are not a figment of your imagination but instead a fabrication that starts with your brain chemistry.

Don't worry, you don't need to give up the sweet taste. Just keep reading to discover a world of tasty new sweets that keep you smiling while you eat them and even more the next day when you feel great.

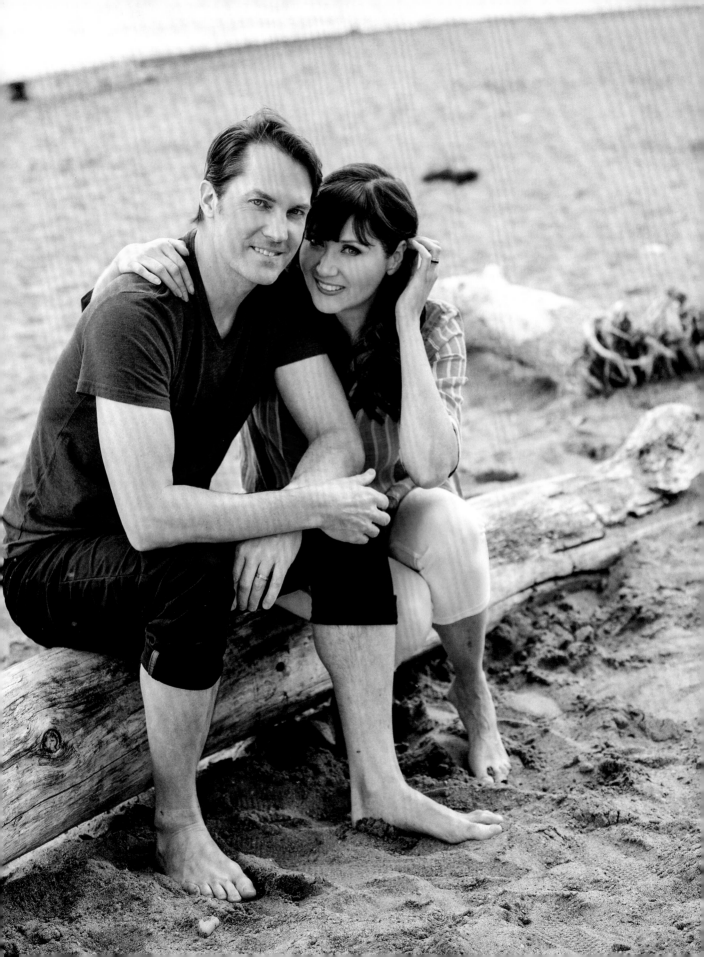

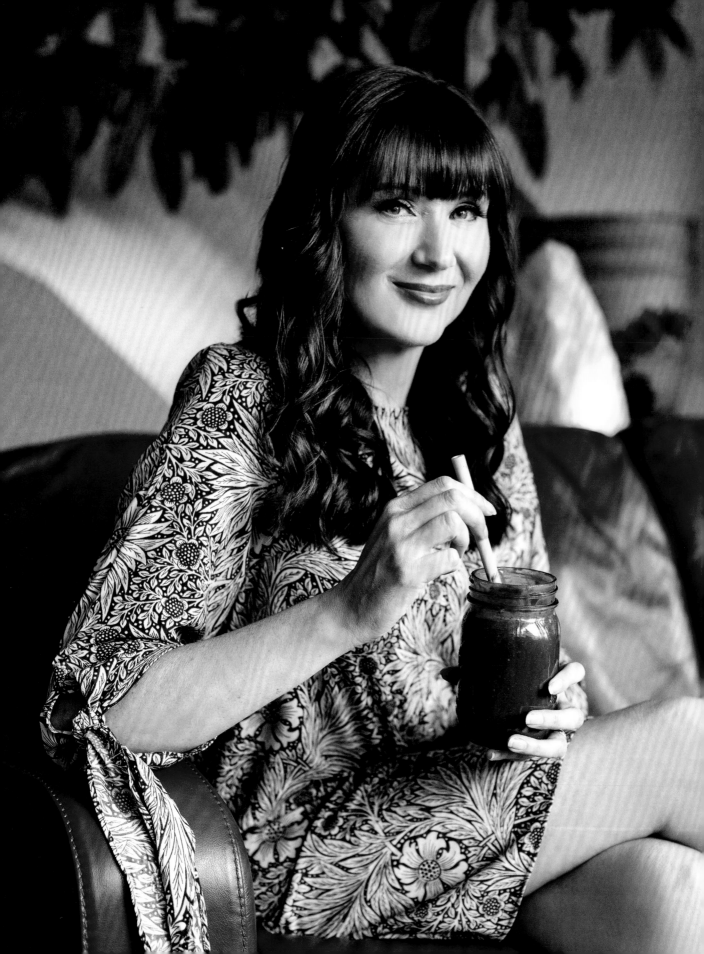

3

A Complete Guide to Natural Sweeteners and Sugar Alternatives

There's little doubt that everyone enjoys sweet-tasting foods—it's built into us. Humans have evolved to seek sweet flavours because they're an indication of a nutrient-dense, calorie-rich food source that isn't poisonous; toxic foods usually taste unbearably sour, bitter, or tart and astringent. We can't escape it. We love sugars! But as we've learned, refined sugars don't love us back. That's why we're kicking refined sugars to the curb and replacing them with real, whole, unrefined sweeteners and natural sugar-free solutions.

Now that we've walked through some of the reasons to give up sugar, let's take a look at a huge selection of natural sweeteners, their benefits, and how you might use them. Then you can enjoy the recipes at the end of the book to try out these nutrient-dense foods of nature. This chapter discusses some of the tastiest and most nutritious natural sweeteners available to provide you with a bounty of choices. Even so, you need to keep in mind that there may be pros and cons to any concentrated sweetener no matter how natural the source is. Make sure that you're not simply replacing a diet high in refined sugar with a diet high in another natural sweetener.

All of the alternative sweeteners I recommend in this book are safe and even beneficial for human consumption. You can purchase most of them at health food stores or online. Some of the sweeteners flavour smoothies nicely, whereas others sweeten your cooking and baking, although you may need to make some adjustments to original recipes. I suggest you explore these delicious sweeteners as a stepping stone on your journey to a sugar-free lifestyle. Find a few that you like best and experiment with making anti-inflammatory treats.

SWEETENERS FROM HERBS

Stevia

Stevia, honey yerba, sweet leaf and sugar leaf are the common names of an exceptionally sweet-tasting Paraguayan herb (*Stevia rebaudiana*). It has been used for centuries as flavouring and medicine by South American indigenous peoples and for more than forty years as an alternative sweetener in Japan, attesting to its safety. Recently, it has become quite popular across North America and Europe.

Stevia is antifungal and antibiotic, and thankfully the research doesn't seem to point toward it negatively affecting our intestinal microbiome. This makes it suitable for people trying to balance levels of candida (a type of yeast) or other microorganisms such as parasites or negative bacteria in the body. It also has anti-inflammatory and antioxidant properties, and it's safe for people who have diabetes or other metabolic disorders. Some studies suggest that stevia may also help prevent diabetes and may have anti-cancer benefits.

Unrefined stevia (which tastes about thirty times as sweet as the same amount of table sugar) is sold as a light green powder or liquid extract of the whole leaves. It has a strong anise or licorice flavour, which some people find delicious. Others may find that it clashes with the taste of other ingredients in a recipe. For baking and cooking, you may prefer to use refined stevia unless you like the full-flavoured overtones.

Like the whole leaf, refined stevia is also a calorie-free sweetener. It's sold in liquid or granular form. Refined stevia products are made by isolating the compounds that give stevia leaf its intensely sweet flavour, so refined stevia can taste 200 to up to 450 times sweeter than the same amount of table sugar! Be mindful to avoid using high doses.

The white granular stevia commonly found on grocery store shelves is usually refined stevia that has been highly diluted in a vegetable-based filler such as maltodextrin (often made from genetically modified corn). Some companies use inulin as filler, and these products may be more suitable for people who want to avoid maltodextrin. The filler is necessary because only very small doses of refined stevia are required to sweeten a beverage or food. It would be impossible to dose these minuscule amounts if you had a bottle of pure, isolated stevia compounds. If you want to use refined stevia extract, the healthiest choice is to buy it in a liquid form that is preserved with glycerin or with vitamin C in water.

Stevia extracts can also be suitable sweeteners, as long as the term *extract* refers to a process that draws out the full profile of naturally occurring plant compounds rather than one that purifies individual sweet-tasting compounds. Very refined sweeteners may cause insulin release simply because of their sweet taste.

Caution: Stevia is part of the Asteraceae/Compositae family, so you may want to avoid it if you're allergic to plants such as daisy, chamomile, goldenseal and ragweed. Recent research has confirmed that palatable doses of stevia extract are safe for consumption by people of all ages, including pregnant and lactating women. The plant and its purified compounds have been approved as dietary supplements in North America.

SWEETNERS FROM FRUITS

Monk Fruit

Monk fruit is known as *luo han guo* (*Siraitia grosvenorii*) in China and neighbouring countries. It is a natural sweetener made from the extract of a melon. In traditional Chinese medicine, monk fruit is revered for its anti-aging properties. It's used to promote bowel regularity, treat respiratory ailments and prevent or alleviate symptoms of diabetes. A recent study showed that the fruit is an effective antihistamine, and therefore it's a fabulous anti-inflammatory and anti-allergic sweetener.

Being rich in antioxidants, monk fruit helps prevent lipid peroxidation. Hence, it can protect low-density lipoprotein (LDL) in the blood from becoming oxidized. This reduces the incidence of arterial plaque and decreases the risk of developing cardiovascular disease. Research also indicates that monk fruit has anti-cancer and anti-inflammatory properties.

Monk fruit is 200 to 250 times sweeter than the same amount of table sugar and has no aftertaste. Though almost non-caloric (at only one calorie per gram), it has an amazing, natural sweetness and a low glycemic index. It's appropriate for people with diabetes and other metabolic disorders because it inhibits alpha-glucosidase.

Monk fruit can also help decrease the risk of non-insulin-dependent diabetes because it can stimulate insulin secretion and lower blood sugar levels. A single study in mice showed that monk fruit may stimulate Th2 cells, (T helper type 2 cells), a part of the immune system. Some nutrition experts say it should be used with caution if following a strict autoimmune diet until human trials confirm this effect on immunity. Use it moderately and in diluted doses if you suffer from a metabolic disorder such as insulin resistance or type 2 diabetes until your condition improves.

In China, whole monk fruit melons are sold in almost every supermarket. In North America, you can find them as whole dried fruits in Asian markets or as a liquid or powder in health food stores. In powdered form, this anti-inflammatory sweetener is sometimes mixed with erythritol to achieve a more familiar sweet flavour and a 1:1 granular ratio to sugar when used in baking.

You'll most likely be seeing much more of this fruit and its extracts as ingredients in various food products and beverages. In the United States, the Food and Drug Administration (FDA) has approved monk fruit (*luo han guo*) extract as GRAS (Generally

Regarded As Safe) for "use as a sweetener and flavour enhancer in foods . . . as well as use as a tabletop sweetener." In Canada, monk fruit is sold as a juice extract. It's my favourite sweetener, and I use it in many of the recipes in this book.

Lúcuma

Lúcuma (*Pouteria lucuma*), also known as eggfruit and lucmo, is a yellow-fleshed Peruvian fruit that has interesting anti-diabetic properties. It contains a substance that inhibits an intestinal enzyme known as alpha-glucosidase. This enzyme breaks down starches and complex sugars into simple sugars. When its activity is stopped, carbohydrates are not fully digested and glucose absorption from the intestines decreases. This is beneficial, as it decreases a sugar spike in the blood by decreasing its total absorption.

Does this sound a bit familiar to you? Unrefined sugars made from coconut and date palms do the same thing, although they inhibit different carbohydrate-digesting enzymes, thus helping to regulate blood sugar levels by preventing a spike.

Many popular anti-diabetic drugs contain synthetic chemicals that have a similar mechanism of action: they stop the activity of alpha-glucosidase. It's fabulous to know that you can get a similar blood sugar-regulating effect of a drug from a wholesome lúcuma fruit, which is a delicious, nutritious package.

Lúcuma also mildly inhibits an enzyme present in the blood (known as angiotensin-converting enzyme, or ACE) that increases blood pressure and water retention. Interestingly, some pharmaceutical drugs used to treat hypertension also work by inhibiting the function of this enzyme. Although lúcuma is less potent than these drugs, it's safe and lacks side effects. Hypertension increases inflammation in the circulatory system, which means that antihypertensive foods like lúcuma curb inflammation and can help prevent or alleviate cardiovascular diseases.

In Peru, lúcuma fruit is used fresh, mashed or juiced to flavour everything from main dishes to desserts (including ice cream). In North America, it's sold as a powder in health food stores, but you may also find it fresh as an exotic import in some urban markets. Some people describe the taste as a gentle blend of maple syrup and sweet potato.

Dates

Dates (*Phoenix dactylifera*) are the delectable fruits of the date palm, which is native to the Middle East. Dates are most commonly exported as dried fruits, but the fresh ones are just as delicious. As an alternative sweetener, the large and succulent Medjool variety is the best. You will find that savouring just one date stuffed with a few nuts or seeds can satisfy a sweet craving.

Date sugar is made by powdering the dried fruits. It's therefore packed with all of the nutrition and fibre of the whole fruit (but steer clear of white date sugar, which has been refined and stripped of all its goodness). Whole dates and unrefined date sugar are good sources of magnesium, manganese, iron, potassium, zinc and calcium.

If you can't find date sugar in the store, you can make your own moist sweetener by soaking dried dates in warm water until they are plump. Then purée them until smooth. Adjust the amount of water you include to reach your desired consistency. If any water remains, drink it as a refreshing sweet treat.

In the Middle East and India, dates have been used medicinally for thousands of years, and recent studies have validated the therapeutic applications of this fruit. Dates help improve digestion, cleanse the bowels and support liver detoxification. They also protect the liver and kidneys from toxins and support immune function. They're still used in some parts of Morocco to help treat type 2 diabetes and hypertension.

Their high fibre and polyphenol content mean they have a relatively lower glycemic index compared to other dried fruits. The glycemic index of dates differs across varieties but most commonly ranges from 31 to 58. This may make dates among the best whole food sweeteners. One study showed that in ten patients with type 2 diabetes, the glycemic index of five varieties of dates was lower or equal to the glycemic index observed in thirteen healthy patients. In the same study, subjects with diabetes remarkably ate a full serving of dried dates (70 grams, or seven to ten dates) without showing significant spikes in blood sugar. Similar to sugar made from the closely related coconut palm, date sugar can help inhibit certain enzymes that digest carbohydrates.

These tasty treats have also shown an impressive ability to protect nerve cells from various forms of damage or degeneration caused by stroke. Dates also may help people with anxiety or insomnia, as they contain melatonin and B vitamins. Check out the great date-sweetened T-Bars recipe on page 214.

MISCELLANEOUS FRESH AND DRIED FRUITS

You can use almost any fresh or dried fruit as a sweetener. Mashed bananas, apple or pear sauce, overripe peaches and mangoes, or figs and raisins soaked and puréed into a thick paste or syrup are all fantastic substitutes for refined sugar. You can use them in your cooking or make raw desserts with them. Some tropical fruits, such as mango, banana, papaya and pineapple, can be used fresh to sweetly thicken your recipes. Have fun and be creative with your experiments. For example, a fantastic Mango Gello Pudding is found on page 180.

SWEETENERS DERIVED FROM FLOWERS

Raw Honey

Raw honey is unrefined and unpasteurized—it's the healthiest honey to eat because it contains all of the nutrients bees collect during their forage. It's a source of vitamins B2 and B6, iron, manganese, amino acids, enzymes and phytonutrients. For thousands of years, honey has been used medicinally, and recent scientific research reveals how it helps heal and soothe inflammation.

Honey on the comb contains propolis, which is the antimicrobial and antifungal glue that bees use to seal the hive and protect it from harmful microorganisms. Honey is also high in hydrogen peroxide, a powerful antiseptic.

Packed with a punch of anti-inflammatory antioxidants, raw honey can reduce the damage to colon tissue afflicted by colitis. Similarly, raw honey can heal ulcerated tissues all along the gastrointestinal (GI) tract because it's a powerful wound healer of all epithelial tissues, including the skin. Honey derived from bees feeding on plants that have antiseptic properties (for example, manuka honey made from bees feeding on the tea tree) are especially effective as wound healers.

Honey contains carbohydrates from flowers that have been predigested by the bee, so people with an intolerance to disaccharides, such as those with inflammatory bowel disease or irritable bowel syndrome, benefit from the bees doing all the hard work for them.

Raw honey is also a source of anti-inflammatory, allergy-staving quercetin, which is a powerful antioxidant that prevents histamine release from mast cells. Research by Dr. Ezz El-Arab and others showed that honey protects the liver, kidneys and DNA from the harmful effects of various mycotoxins. They also found that honey is a nourishing prebiotic for *Bifidobacterium* spp. and *Lactobacillus* spp. intestinal bacteria, while at the same time it can inhibit the growth of intestinal pathogens such as fungi and yeasts, including *Candida* spp. Why can't all medicine taste so sweet?

Raw honey is an anti-inflammatory alternative to refined sugar because it doesn't cause a rapid spike in blood sugar levels. It has a glycemic index that ranges from low (about 35) to moderately high (up to 58), depending on the variety (which differs according to the bee's plant choices). Some studies suggest that it actually may help regulate blood sugar levels and therefore help prevent inflammatory reactions such as advanced glycation end products (AGEs) in the cardiovascular system.

Honey tastes 20 percent sweeter than sugar, so you need less of it to achieve the same level of sweetness. It's best to avoid heating raw honey so that you can retain its health benefits.

Some liquid honey products are adulterated with high-fructose corn syrup and/or sucrose syrup, so avoid cheap supermarket brands such as those sold in squeezable plastic bottles and honey from China. Large-scale apiaries may also feed these cheap syrups to their honeybees. This lowers the quality of the resulting honey products (while also negatively affecting the health of the honeybees) because the honey contains more fructose and sucrose than honey sourced from bees foraging on wildflowers. This may explain why some experts consider honey inflammatory, but it is important to remember that the source and method in which honey is processed can make all the difference. If you are following a low-carb or keto menu then you may want to use monk fruit or stevia instead of honey. You'll be pleasantly surprised by the difference in quality and taste when you purchase honey from a reputable source such as local apiaries and farmers' markets.

Caution: People with fructose malabsorption and/or fructose-sensitive liver disorders such as liver steatosis (also known as fatty liver) should limit or avoid liquid honey, as its sweetness derives from a high concentration of fructose and glucose. If you want to indulge in some honey for its health benefits, opt for moderate amounts of raw honey, replete with propolis and/or pollen, because it will contain greater amounts of amino acids.

If you ever see symptoms as a curse, try to reframe that to see them as simply the canary in the coal mine helping you know what's best for you. It's your body's way of telling you when something isn't right.

SWEETENERS DERIVED FROM ROOTS AND TUBERS

Licorice

The roots of *Glycyrrhiza* spp. plants (usually *G. glabra*, *G. lepidota* and *G. uralensis*) are an intensely sweet anti-inflammatory medicine. Syrup made from the roots can be used to sweeten tea and other beverages, but it goes without saying that it's appropriate only for those who enjoy the taste. Licorice has a strong, distinct flavour that not everyone appreciates. For those who do like it, licorice is an excellent option because it will add a rich flavour to your food. The good news is that you can adapt to enjoying this flavour over time. I now look forward to this remedy as a friendly morning ritual.

The medicinal properties of licorice are well documented and confirmed by years of scientific research. It's an integral part of the traditional medicines of North America, Europe and Asia. Licorice is an excellent adaptogen—it supports the adrenal glands and helps the body cope with stress. In appropriate doses, it also helps balance sex hormones, particularly in women, because healthy adrenals produce appropriate levels of sex hormones to complement those made by the ovaries and testes.

Licorice root is an energizing sweetener. Unlike caffeinated beverages, licorice doesn't lead to adrenal exhaustion or heart palpitations. Another plus is that licorice can help increase levels of dehydroepiandrosterone (DHEA), which is known as one of the body's "anti-aging hormones."

Licorice soothes the digestive tract and can decrease inflammation in even the most irritated guts. It has an antimicrobial effect, even against *Helicobacter pylori*, the bacterium that contributes to gastric ulcers. In the same way it can heal the tissue of your gut, licorice root can heal topical wounds and inflammatory skin conditions when it's applied topically as a poultice or rub.

This sweet root helps lower LDL levels in the blood, protect LDL from oxidation and prevent atherosclerosis. It's a powerful anti-diabetic medicinal herb that can help regulate blood sugar levels, prevent damage to the pancreas and protect cells from developing insulin resistance or pathological diabetic complications.

Caution: Licorice naturally causes an elevation in blood pressure because it can alter the regulation of potassium levels, leading to lower levels of potassium and higher levels of sodium. For people who suffer from adrenal fatigue or hypotension (low blood pressure), this is very beneficial. However, those who suffer from hypertension and/or who take antihypertensive drugs (including potassium-depleting diuretics) should consult their doctor before consuming any licorice products.

Glycyrrhizinic acid (also called glycyrrhizin or glycyrrhizic acid) is the major active compound that raises blood pressure (although other minor constituents also play a role). A process that removes this active substance from the plant yields deglycyrrhizinated (DGL) licorice, which is considered safer for people suffering from hypertension and other cardiovascular disorders. This type of licorice is fantastic for heartburn and gastroesophageal reflux disease (GERD). Make sure to source your licorice from sustainably grown sources. The harvesting of wild licorice in some parts of the world threatens the plant species and also causes environmental destruction.

Tiger Nut

Tiger nuts (*Cyperus esculentus*) aren't actually nuts at all. They're plant tubers, much like sweet potatoes. Because they tend to be small and round, they're sometimes called earth almonds, chufa tubers, yellow nuts, sedge nuts and zulu nuts. They're native to the Mediterranean regions of southern Europe and the Middle East, but also grown in North Africa and Central and South America for their sweet flavour and nutritious medicine.

They're used to treat digestive ailments, and they can help calm a bloated and inflamed belly. They help decrease the risk of diabetes because a small serving size satisfies sweet cravings without sending blood sugar levels out of control. The plant sterols, vitamin E and fibre they contain support healthy circulation by helping to lower blood cholesterol levels and prevent peroxidation of fats in the arteries.

Tiger nuts deeply satisfy cravings because they're rich in healing fats, including omega-9 oleic acid, omega-7 palmitic acid and omega-6 linoleic acid. Fat and sweet tastes always go well together.

The chromium and calcium in tiger nuts also help maintain stable blood sugar levels. Chromium is an essential nutrient that enhances insulin function and helps lower LDL, whereas calcium plays a role in moderating food intake, strengthening bone and improving fat metabolism.

You can find dried tiger nuts sold whole or powdered at most health food stores. They taste delicious on their own but can be added to almost any dish. They make smoothies rich and creamy, are excellent as a salad topper and add a subtle sweet surprise when added to soups and casseroles (see page 229).

Yacón

Refreshingly sweet and juicy, the Peruvian yacón (*Smallanthus sonchifolius*) tuber has a crunchy texture similar to water chestnuts and tastes like jicama root crossed with a crisp Red Delicious apple. It's common in South American and Asian cuisines as an ingredient in soups and raw salads. Milled as syrup, it can be used in equal amounts to replace other liquid sweeteners like honey or maple syrup in cooking and baking. The syrup tastes like caramel mixed with molasses and has a gentle cinnamon back note.

Yacón syrup isn't as well known as a sweetener yet, but it will probably catch on quickly because it's a great source of the prebiotic inulins. The high inulin content also means that yacón is naturally low in calories.

Yacón is rich in potassium, chromium, calcium, iron and B vitamins. Chromium and B vitamins promote healthy glucose metabolism, making yacón an ideal sweetener for people who suffer from metabolic conditions. It is also low in digestible carbs, making it perfect for those who want to reduce chronic inflammation.

Andean peoples have long used yacón as an anti-diabetic medicine, and this is probably because it satisfies your sweet tooth without sending your blood glucose levels soaring and crashing like a mad roller coaster ride. People with anxiety or insomnia will love this root because it's a modest source of tryptophan, the amino acid that the body uses to make the calming and mood-regulating neurotransmitter serotonin.

Caution: Yacón is part of the Asteraceae/Compositae family, so avoid it if you're allergic to plants such as daisy, chamomile, goldenseal and ragweed. In high doses, yacón may also cause some intestinal distress in people who are sensitive to the laxative effects of inulin.

TREE SAPS AND SYRUPS

Maple Syrup

Sugar maples (*Acer saccharum*) are the most common trees used to make syrup, but black and red maples (*A. nigrum* and *A. rubrum*, respectively), paper birch (*Betula papyrifera*), Alaskan birch (*B. neoalaskana*) and black walnut (*Juglans nigra*) trees also produce delicious mineral- and vitamin-rich sweet saps. Upon extraction from the tree, the raw sap is boiled into a syrup.

Tree syrups are far more concentrated in sugars and minerals than raw saps. Indigenous Peoples in North America traditionally drank the raw sap as a nutritive beverage, and recently this refreshment has regained popularity and is often sold as maple water.

Maple syrup contains an impressive amount of manganese (which means that it can help boost the levels of the antioxidant enzyme called manganese SOD, or superoxide dismutase). It also contains moderate amounts of calcium, potassium, magnesium, iron, zinc, vitamin B1 and antioxidants.

One of the most exciting features of maple syrup and other tree syrups is that they contain a phytonutrient called abscisic acid that has anti-inflammatory properties. Abscisic acid is one type of a naturally occurring substance that's a natural alternative to a class of anti-diabetic pharmaceutical drugs (such as thiazolidinediones) that affect the activity of peroxisome proliferator-activated receptors (PPARs).

The sweetness of tree syrups comes from sucrose. However, because tree syrups also contain vitamins, minerals, amino acids and water, they generally have a slightly lower glycemic index than refined sugar. Syrup made from late-season sap is higher in amino acids, including gut-healing glutamine and threonine, than syrup made from early-season sap. If you are following a low-carb or keto menu then you will want to use monk fruit or stevia instead of maple syrup. Because of its high level of sucrose, it is best to use maple syrup only occasionally if following Option 2 in the plan outline on page 124. All sucrose sources are a slippery gateway experience to eating more sugar.

If you are intolerant to sucrose, replace maple syrup with easy-to-digest raw honey or fibre-rich yacón syrup, or try my Faux Maple Syrup (page 225).

Coconut Sugar

Coconut (*Cocos nucifera*) trees and other palms from the Arecaceae family can be tapped for sap in much the same way maple and birch trees are. This is a popular tradition across tropical regions of Africa, Asia and South America. The unrefined sap is sometimes called toddy, but this is actually the name of the fermented, alcoholic drink made from coconut sap (neera is the correct term for raw coconut sap). It can be dried into a granular form, which is sometimes called jaggery. Be careful, because unrefined cane sugar is also called jaggery.

Unrefined coconut sugar is rich in antioxidants and phytonutrients that can help protect against diabetes and hypertension, which are two of the main causes of heart disease. For example, certain phytonutrients found in coconut sugar can inhibit the activity of some carbohydrate-digesting enzymes (namely alpha-glucuronidase and alpha-amylase), and therefore they help decrease the amount of glucose that's absorbed into the bloodstream from the intestines. Other phytonutrients inhibit an enzyme that's involved in increasing blood pressure.

Coconut sap is a good digestive and nutritive. It's a modest source of amino acids, iron, magnesium, vitamin C and vitamin A; contains traces of B vitamins; and has a neutral pH.

Coconut sap is sometimes commercially called coconut nectar because the most common technique for collecting this delectable sweetener is to extract the liquid sugar from the base of the inflorescence (which is the cluster of flowers that eventually mature into fruits after being pollinated). However, this sweet sap is not actually flower nectar, but rather the source of sugars that the flowers use to produce nectar. This practice, when done properly, is relatively sustainable because a single coconut palm can be tapped for more than twenty years without apparent damage to the tree.

Coconut sugar is a go-to for weaning people off white refined sugar because it's versatile, delicious and a great 1:1 substitute in recipes that call for refined sugar. Unfortunately, coconut sugar contains 75 percent sucrose, so it is not a good long-term solution for people looking to address metabolic issues or digestive trouble. If you don't digest disaccharides like sucrose, it is best avoided. If you are following a low-carb or keto menu then you will want to use monk fruit or stevia instead of coconut sap, coconut syrup or coconut sugar.

SWEETENERS DERIVED FROM GRASSES AND GRAINS

Brown Rice Malt and Syrup

Brown rice malt is made from sprouted varities of rice from the *Oryza sativa* family. It is air-heated and allowed to produce its own syrup naturally. No live yeasts or moulds are used to make the final malt syrup. The heat gently activates rice enzymes to digest starches into a sugar that sits at 98 on the glycemic index. This means that the sugar in the syrup elevates insulin quickly.

The only benefit of brown rice syrup is that it is free of fructose, so it's a popular option if you have a fructose intolerance. If it is pure glucose, it is also an option for certain athletes who need to elevate their blood sugar quickly for sporting events. Rice has recently come under fire because of elevated arsenic levels.

Sorghum syrup is made from the green juice of the sorghum bicolour plant, which is extracted from the crushed stalks and then heated to steam off the excess water, leaving the syrup behind. It is very similar to rice syrup.

Malt syrups are high in maltose, which is a simple sugar composed of two glucose molecules. Because it must be broken down before the glucose can be absorbed and it retains its complex of minerals and vitamins, it has a lower glycemic index than most refined sweeteners. This is not a good option for people who suffer from digestive trouble because it requires enzymes to break down maltose into glucose. If you are following a low-carb or keto menu then you will want to use monk fruit or stevia instead of brown rice or sorghum syrup.

The downside of grain syrups is that many people are sensitive to grain and these syrups have a high insulin response, so they are best avoided.

Unrefined Sugar Cane

Developed in India thousands of years ago, jaggery (also spelled jagerri or jaggeree) is a traditional type of granular sweetener that is made from the dehydrated, unrefined juice of the sugar cane plant (*Saccharum* spp.). You will now see unrefined sugar cane marketed as sugar cane juice crystals. Unrefined sugar cane is rich in nutrients, including vitamin C, vitamin B complex, zinc, chromium, magnesium, iron, silicon and boron.

A similar product is Sucanat™, which is sold in many food stores. Note that the evaporated cane juice listed in product ingredients may or may not be the same thing. The term is used loosely, and there are no regulations restricting its definition. Because it's so rich in nutrients, jaggery contains a little less sucrose than white sugar but tastes just as sweet. However, because of its high insulin response, I don't recommend using it. If you have an intolerance to sucrose or disaccharides, cane sugar (processed or unprocessed) has got to go. It is best to take a break from all cane sugar products to see if you feel happier without it. Consider a 30-day sugar-free challenge and journal how you feel if you reintroduce sugar. Many of my clients experience increased anxiety and brain fog when they eat sugar. If you are following a low-carb or keto menu then you will want to use monk fruit or stevia instead of unrefined sugar cane products.

SWEET-TASTING LEGUMES

Carob

Even beans can taste sweet. While carob (*Ceratonia siliqua*) isn't usually used as a sweetener on its own, it's a sweet-tasting bean that can enhance the flavour of your creations.

Carob powder is commonly used as a caffeine-free alternative to cacao because it has a mild chocolatey taste.

Carob isn't stimulating, so it won't exhaust your nervous system or adrenal glands. Instead, it may actually nourish your adrenals because this legume is a good source of vitamins B2, B3 and B6, plus calcium, copper, manganese and potassium. Manganese is a critical component of the powerful antioxidant enzyme manganese SOD, which is produced by the adrenal glands. B vitamins are also essential for coping with stress because they sustain the health of the adrenals and nervous system. Although copper is an essential mineral, it's possible to suffer from copper toxicity. If your water pipes are made of copper or if you have taken birth control pills or hormone replacement therapy, the chances are you have enough copper in your body and should reduce your intake of copper-rich foods.

Even though much of the sweetness of carob derives from sucrose, it's safe for diabetics because the sugar is bound in a fibre matrix, resulting in a low glycemic index. Pinitol (also known as D-chiro-inositol) is a unique molecule naturally present in several plants that traditionally have been used as natural anti-diabetic medicines. Pinitol has an insulin-like function, and so it can move glucose from the blood into the cells. Thus, pinitol can help improve glucose metabolism and prevent or treat inflammatory disorders such as insulin resistance and the formation of AGEs. Carob is rich in a soluble fibre known as galacto-mannan that is being studied for its ability to modulate the immune system and soothe an irritated GI tract.

Carob is an incredible bean because while its fibre content stimulates bowel movements and therefore helps to alleviate constipation, the bean is also rich in tannins, which help to prevent and heal diarrhea. Carob bean powder has been used as a traditional medicine in Arabian countries for treating a wide range of digestive disorders.

As with all other whole plant foods, carob beans are rich in antioxidants such as catechins and quercetin, helping to reduce the risk of kidney damage and GI diseases, including colon cancer. A study published in 2009 in the *Journal of Agricultural and Food Chemistry* showed that the gallic acid in carob beans is also effective at preventing mutations of the DNA in colon cells. Another interesting study published in 2007 suggested that carob consumption may increase fat metabolism by affecting two important metabolic hormones known as ghrelin and leptin.

Caution: Consume carob in moderate doses, especially if you have a sensitive GI tract. Some people are more prone to experiencing a laxative effect from carob consumption, whereas others may be more vulnerable to the relatively strong astringency of carob tannins. Carob is not acceptable if you have a sucrose intolerance or are intolerant to legumes, such as beans.

Mesquite

Mesquite (*Prosopis* spp.) trees thrive in arid soil across the southern Americas, Africa and Asia and produce sweet legumes. *Prosopis* has many common names, including mesquite, kiawe, huarango, American carob, bayahonda and algarrobo blanco, and the tree has been an important source of nutrition and medicine for indigenous peoples across the continents to which it's native.

The fibre-rich pod has been traditionally consumed as a powder or syrup. In all parts of the world, the tree has been used as a traditional medicine as well as a pleasant sweetener for juices and milk. Mesquite tastes like a sweet blend of cinnamon, cacao, carob and coffee—almost like a cinnamon mocha. It's absolutely delicious!

It has an excellent mineral profile, providing rich amounts of calcium, iron, manganese and zinc. It also contains a decent amount of protein, including all of the essential amino acids (in Africa it's used as a meat substitute), and it's high in fibre. These two macronutrients help keep the glycemic index of mesquite at a low 25. It's no wonder it's used as an energy booster for high-performance athletes and people under stress.

This sweetener may be good for people who are allergic to many foods because the immune system of a typical North American has likely never been exposed to it before. As a matter of fact, mesquite's plant sterols can actually help balance the immune system through their antioxidant and anti-inflammatory effects.

Mesquite is also an excellent choice for people who have diabetes or high blood pressure. It has the same properties as lúcuma: it can prevent the digestion of carbohydrates into glucose (and therefore decrease the amount of glucose that's absorbed by the intestines), and it helps lower blood pressure (by inhibiting the activity of ACE).

A study suggests that mesquite also has antibacterial properties. A study published in 2011 in the *International Journal of Pharma Sciences and Research* showed that *Klebsiella* spp. bacteria are the most susceptible to mesquite alkaloids. This finding is of particular interest to people who suffer from ankylosing spondylitis, because *Klebsiella* spp. bacteria have been implicated as a causative or exacerbating factor in this inflammatory condition.

Mesquite is usually sold as a dry powder, so you can use it as a substitute for grain flour or as a sweetener for smoothies. Because it's gluten-free and is suitable for making breads and cakes, mesquite flour can be used to replace a few tablespoons of nut or seed flour in a recipe. Mesquite is a legume that contains some sucrose and fructose, so test it and see if it's tolerated by your body. If intolerant, enjoy stevia or monk fruit instead.

INULIN

Inulin is a type of oligosaccharide called a fructan and passes almost fully untouched and unabsorbed through the small intestine. Most commercially available inulin is created by soaking chicory roots in hot water and extracting the inulin. It is a good sugar alternative, as it gives only 25 to 35 percent energy, but it has only about 10 percent the sweetness level of sucrose, so it often is combined with other low-carb sweeteners. It's considered to be a prebiotic (as it is digested by the bacteria that normalize your digestion) and can increase the number of good bacteria such as *Bifidobacteria* and *Lactobacilli*. It also seems to enhance mineral absorption, specifically absorption of calcium, magnesium and iron.

Since inulin contains high levels of fibre, it slows down transit time and keeps you feeling full for longer. In fact, its fermentation in the large intestine releases short-chain fatty acids that can help lower the hormone ghrelin and regulate your appetite. It also helps stabilize blood sugar levels, and research has shown that it can benefit people with prediabetes by decreasing insulin resistance. Because it is so high in fibre and considered to be a fermentable oligo-, di-, mono-saccharide and polyols (FODMAP), some people with a sensitive digestive tract have noticed abdominal discomfort, excessive flatulence or loose stools.

If you tolerate this sweetener, it can be of great benefit, but if it causes you digestive upset, then it is best to give it a miss and check back after you have balanced your digestive flora with your sugar-free lifestyle. Inulin can be used to sweeten puddings and smoothies and is a common ingredient in probiotic formations.

ALLULOSE

With increasing evidence that sugar is the culprit in health concerns, obesity and inflammation, the food industry is on the lookout for substitutes. Enter allulose, also known as D-psicose, a rare sugar naturally present in only a few foods, including wheat, figs, jackfruit and raisins. It's a monosaccharide (single sugar) that is absorbed in the small intestine but doesn't get used as fuel by the body, rendering it really low in calories because approximately 86 percent of it is excreted in urine unmetabolized.

Even though it is naturally derived from food sources, researchers are converting it from fructose; most of it is made from corn-derived fructose that is most likely genetically modified.

Let's look at the evidence. The main health claim is that allulose is very low in calories, doesn't trigger the usual blood sugar spike seen with sugars and other sweeteners and doesn't affect the insulin response. Evidence does show that it may be beneficial for blood sugar regulation. One study found that blood sugar was significantly lower at thirty and sixty minutes in participants who took 5 grams of allulose in comparison to those who took 0 grams of it. Another study found that consuming allulose with maltodextrin had the ability to suppress the glycemic response to maltodextrin. This implies that not only does it not trigger a blood sugar spike, but it has the ability to lower the glycemic impact of other foods. It also appears to help reduce abdominal fat, increase leptin release and significantly increase energy expenditure.

But is allulose safe? It appears to be well tolerated overall, with only a few side effects. A twelve-week human study found that one participant experienced digestive symptoms such as diarrhea and elevated liver enzymes. Animal studies found that it caused damage to the intestinal tract when consumed at levels that humans are unlikely to match, as well as enlargement of livers and kidneys. And when it comes to fat loss, it seems that although it is a positive finding that leptin levels increased significantly in the allulose group, we know that over time, high levels of leptin can lead to leptin resistance, diminishing satiety and causing cravings and weight gain.

Although allulose does seem to have benefits and is considered safe by the FDA, we don't yet have a lot of data on it, and most of what we do have comes from very small studies, animal studies or studies exclusively funded and conducted by the manufacturers themselves. I would suggest watching to see how this brand-new sweetener does in both the science lab and the real world. If you do want to explore using it, try small amounts, journal how you feel and push the manufacturer to offer a Non-GMO Project certified option, as much of it is genetically modified.

D-RIBOSE (MITOSWEET)

Have you heard of D-ribose? It's a sugar that makes up part of the structure of your DNA and RNA and is involved in producing energy in your body. Your body naturally produces D-ribose on a regular basis to be able to function.

There is research to support the use of D-ribose as a supplement in the diet in certain conditions where energy production in the mitochondria would be beneficial. For instance, in cardiovascular conditions such as heart failure, it seems that adding D-ribose supports the mitochondria's production of energy, known as adenosine triphosphate (ATP), to support the heart muscle. It also seems to be beneficial for those with chronic fatigue syndrome or fibromyalgia and to improve athletic performance and reduce symptoms of pain following exercise.

For athletes, the evidence seems to point toward recovering stores of ATP in muscle cells a few days after intense exercise in comparison to placebo. This is important because a depletion of ATP can cause a lot of muscle soreness, cramps and pain after exercise.

D-ribose seems to also improve pain intensity, energy levels and sleep at a dosage of

15 grams per day in people with fibromyalgia and chronic fatigue syndrome, though there aren't a lot of studies.

Small amounts of D-ribose are best added to beverages, as it cannot be heated.

INOSITOL

Inositol, or more precisely myo-inositol, is a unique carbohydrate that was once considered vitamin B8. It is an integral part of the actions of many of our bodily processes and can have a therapeutic impact on general health. Though not considered a sweetener, it has a lovely sweet taste, approximately half the sweetness of table sugar.

One of the most powerful ways in which inositol is beneficial is through supporting mental health. It appears to help decrease symptoms associated with depression, premenstrual syndrome (PMS), premenstrual dysphoric disorder (PMDD) and anxiety. In fact, in those with a panic disorder, it can help reduce the number of panic attacks from 4 to 2.4 attacks per week.

Interestingly, it can also support blood sugar regulation even though it is considered a carbohydrate. It is naturally found in oranges and cantaloupes, and when used as a supplement it can support metabolic syndrome and decrease triglycerides, cholesterol, serum glucose and insulin. Who knew that something so sweet could actually be beneficial for the body and the mind?

Small amounts of inositol are best added to beverages, as it cannot be heated. Enjoy it as a booster in many of the beverage recipes in this book.

SUGAR ALCOHOLS

Sugar alcohols are a group of relatively small and diverse molecules. They tend to share certain characteristics, such as being indigestible by human enzymes, low calorie, low glycemic index, low insulinemic index and non-glycating, meaning that they don't form AGEs. They have a laxative effect to varying degrees, so this can be a problem over time.

Although all sugar alcohols have the potential to cause GI side effects such as bloating, flatulence and osmotic diarrhea, it's common to develop a tolerance so that you can safely and comfortably consume slightly greater doses over time. The one exception may be erythritol, which is very unlikely to produce digestive upsets even at high doses. However, combinations of different sugar alcohols in the same product, meal or day may have synergistic or compound effects on the digestive system. The bottom line is to be mindful of (and moderate in) the amount and type of sugar alcohols you consume. They are a form of alcohol, after all. Here, we discuss only naturally occurring sugar alcohols. Other sugar alcohols such as maltitol, isomalt and lactitol aren't naturally present in foods or the environment and are instead produced by various laboratory methods and best avoided.

Erythritol

Erythritol (also known as erythrite and food additive E968) has a sweetness level of 60 to 80 percent that of sucrose. It's naturally present in small amounts in various fruits (especially grapes, peaches, pears, watermelons and other melons), mushrooms, sea vegetables, algae and fermented liquids (especially beer, cheese, miso, sake, soy sauce and wine). Out of all the sugar alcohols used presently, it is the best tolerated.

Erythritol is an attractive sugar alternative because it isn't metabolized by oral bacteria, and studies show that it helps prevent cavities. It may also help promote remineralization of teeth, including teeth affected by cavities. Erythritol is an antioxidant, and it may even protect tissues—especially the cardiovascular system—from free radical damage.

In humans, 60 to more than 90 percent of dietary erythritol is quickly absorbed by the small intestine. Therefore, very small amounts reach the colon and so this sweetener isn't fermented by colonic bacteria. As a result, moderate doses of erythritol rarely, if ever, cause flatulence, bloating or osmotic diarrhea. Any erythritol that is fermented by colonic bacteria is converted to short-chain fatty acids, which nourish the cells of the intestinal mucosa.

Erythritol is well tolerated, even by infants, people with a sensitive GI tract and those suffering from imbalanced gut flora such as an overgrowth of *Candida albicans*. In humans, GI tolerance for laxation ranges from 0.5 to 1.0 grams erythritol per kilogram body weight per day. For example, a 150-pound person could consume up to 150 grams of erythritol a day, which equals 37 teaspoons or ¾ cup, before it would cause a laxative effect. Having said that, some people who are intolerant to alcohol can tolerate very little erythritol before experiencing negative effects.

Human digestive enzymes don't metabolize erythritol very well, so it's a low-calorie sweetener that yields a mere 0.2 calories per gram. It's rapidly filtered by the kidneys and excreted in the urine. Erythritol has a glycemic index of 0 and an insulinemic index of 2 because it doesn't affect blood concentrations of glucose or insulin. Therefore, erythritol is safe for people with diabetes, liver diseases, obesity and other metabolic disorders, and it helps protect against cardiovascular damage caused by high blood glucose levels (for example, AGEs).

Research has shown that moderate doses of erythritol do not cause any acute side effects or long-term detriment. No carcinogenic or reproductive effects have been observed in animals or humans. Erythritol is most commonly commercially synthesized from wheat or corn, so people with allergies to these grains may want to avoid this sugar alcohol. I hope that a Non-GMO Project verified product is available soon. Because of its benefits, you will find recipes using this sweetener in the recipe section of this book.

Glycerin

You probably don't think of glycerin as an alternative to sugar because it comes from fats, either animals or vegetables. Typically, it is derived from coconut, palm or soybean oil but can sometimes be synthetically made from corn syrup, sugar cane or a petroleum derivative called propylene.

Although it is an alternative to sugar, it actually contains more calories than sugar and is only about 60 percent as sweet, which means that you might need slightly more glycerin to get the equivalent sweetness as sugar. Classified as a sugar alcohol, it may have a laxative and diuretic effect if you eat a lot of it. Older sugar-free cookbooks may offer it as a sweetener choice, and it sweetens and preserves many flavour extracts such as vanilla and peppermint extracts. Alcohol-free herbal preparations use it as a preservative and carrier because it gently extracts herbs and keeps them fresh for up to a year. In small amounts, it is quite harmless as long as it is naturally derived from coconut or palm. It is not the best liquid sweetener for baking because it is expensive and can be a laxative in the amount needed to sweeten baked goods.

Xylitol

Xylitol (also known as food additive E967) is a naturally occurring sugar alcohol found in small amounts in berries, stone fruits such as plums, lettuces and various mushrooms. The sugar was discovered in 1891. However, it wasn't until sugar cane was scarce in Europe during the Second World War that xylitol was widely used as an alternative sweetener. Since the 1970s, its popularity has been increasing because it's a low-calorie, low-carbohydrate sweetener that has some interesting health properties.

Xylitol is widely heralded as an anti-cavity sweetener. Numerous studies have shown that xylitol reduces the number of cavity-forming bacteria in the mouth, reduces plaque buildup, prevents some types of cavity-causing bacteria from adhering to tooth enamel and stimulates saliva secretion, which naturally promotes tooth remineralization and prevents cavities. Xylitol seems to have stronger anti-cavity effects than fluoride. Over the long term, xylitol can help promote the remineralization of teeth.

Research suggests that the ideal dose for preventing cavities is 5 to 10 grams of xylitol per day. Generally, one piece of gum contains 1 gram of xylitol, so chew one to three pieces of gum for five to ten minutes, three to five times per day if you want to help prevent tooth decay. Xylitol is most commonly used to sweeten chewing gum, oral care products such as toothpaste and mouthwash, various candies, cookies, desserts, diabetic-friendly sweets and even children's vitamins.

Xylitol has a glycemic index of approximately 7, and it is considered safe for diabetics and children over the age of one.

Some studies suggest that xylitol may help slow osteoporosis (experiments in older rats suggest that xylitol increases bone calcification, and this is likely because xylitol doesn't stimulate excessive secretion of insulin in the way other refined sweeteners do). In addition to preventing oral cavities, xylitol can also help prevent inner ear and throat (otolaryngeal) infections, and it may help boost the body's own bacteria-fighting immune response. In vitro, xylitol prevents the adhesion of macrophages, which suggests that the sweetener may have anti-inflammatory and immune-modulating properties.

Despite its benefits, high or daily doses of xylitol may not be suitable for people who suffer from certain conditions such as some food allergies, GI inflammation (IBD and IBS) and/or kidney disorders. The commercial synthesis of xylitol may make it an unsuitable sweetener for those who suffer from certain food allergies because the most efficient methods of large-scale production of xylitol involve yeast fermentation of corncobs, wheat, oat straw or sugar cane pulp using various yeasts. If you want to try this sweetener, be sure to buy one that is sourced from birch or beech tree bark.

Xylitol tends to be very well tolerated by healthy people, but the most common side effect in sensitive people is GI upset. Consuming more than 40 to 130 grams of xylitol per day (as little as ⅓ cup) can cause diarrhea, depending on a person's digestive health.

However, it's important to note that some people who tend toward GI sensitivities and/or inflammation may experience bloating, flatulence and/or diarrhea at moderate doses. Xylitol can also increase levels of uric acid and oxalic acid, and it should be avoided by people who suffer from gout, kidney stones or bipolar disorder.

Caution: Xylitol is toxic to dogs. It can cause extreme hypoglycemia and acute liver toxicity in canines. If your dog has eaten xylitol, rush him or her to a veterinarian.

Mannitol

Mannitol (also known as food additive E421) is naturally abundant. It's found in various species of herbs, trees, fungi, sea vegetables, algae, lichens, yeasts and bacteria. Chemically and structurally, it's very similar to sorbitol. Mannitol tastes about 50 percent as sweet as the same amount of sucrose. It ranks as 0 on both the glycemic and the insulinemic indices, and it yields 1.6 to 2.4 calories per gram.

Mannitol is poorly absorbed by the cells of the small intestine (up to 75 percent passes through the gut undigested by human digestive enzymes). Consuming more than 5 teaspoons (20 grams) can lead to intestinal discomforts such as bloating, flatulence and diarrhea. However, people with a sensitive digestive system may not be able to tolerate even small amounts of mannitol well.

It's fermented into acid by oral bacteria, so it doesn't have the same antibiotic properties against cariogenic bacteria as do erythritol and xylitol.

Mannitol doesn't absorb water very readily and crystallizes easily, so it's very useful as a binder in tablets for drugs and nutritional supplements. If you have an intolerance to mannitol, be sure to check the labels of non-food items in case it's an unexpected ingredient.

Mannitol is made from seaweeds (as is popular in China), chemical hydrogenation of fructose (derived from sucrose or starches) and microbial fermentation of starches such as corn, wheat or tapioca by organisms such as yeasts (for example, *Candida magnoliae*), lactic acid bacteria or fungi. Mannitol has a stronger laxative effect and is not as well tolerated as other options, so avoid using it.

Sorbitol

Sorbitol (also known as food additive E420) is naturally found in some fruits, particularly those of the family Rosaceae (prune, plum, apple, pear, cherry, peach, apricot), and in algae. It tastes about 60 percent as sweet as the same amount of sucrose. It has a very low glycemic index value of 9 and an insulin index value of 11. It yields 2.4 to 3 calories per gram. The laxation threshold of sorbitol is approximately 50 grams a day. Like mannitol, it's fermented into acid by oral bacteria.

Sorbitol is very soluble and is therefore more commonly used in syrups, beverages and baked goods.

Sorbitol is commercially produced by enzymatic hydrolysis of starch or dextrose sourced from various foods such as corn, wheat or tapioca. People who have sensitivities to any of these foods may want to avoid consumption of sorbitol for this reason.

Sorbitol can be particularly troublesome for diabetics. People with diabetes don't metabolize sorbitol as efficiently as non-diabetics. If sorbitol accumulates in the body, it may lead to macular degeneration, cataracts, kidney inflammation, peripheral neuropathy and tissue damage from oxidative stress.

In people who have diabetes, glucose and sorbitol metabolism can deplete vitamin B3 (niacin), because this nutrient is required for the conversion of these sugars. As a result, the body lacks sufficient vitamin B3 for regenerating the powerful antioxidant enzyme known as glutathione.

Sorbitol also poses a problem for people who suffer from liver diseases such as non-alcoholic fatty liver disease (NAFLD). When blood and tissue levels of glucose and/or sorbitol are high in people with impaired glucose metabolism and liver disorders, sorbitol is metabolized into fructose. This contributes to the impairment of liver function because fructose increases lipogenesis, which further congests the liver and leads to inflammation in liver cells. Sorbitol has a laxative effect and is not as well tolerated as other sweetener options, so it is best avoided.

ALTERNATIVE SWEETENERS TO CONSUME CAUTIOUSLY OR AVOID ALTOGETHER

Agave Nectar or Syrup

Agaves (*Agave* spp.) are succulent plants that grow abundantly throughout tropical regions around the world. There are more than 250 species that produce a sweet sap that has been enjoyed by indigenous peoples for hundreds of years.

Cheap agave syrup is an industrially refined product that may be processed with black mould, spiked with corn syrup and/or be much higher in fructose than is safe for consumption by people with diabetes or liver diseases.

Although high-quality agave nectars may contain iron, calcium, potassium and magnesium, they still tend to be high in fructose, even if they haven't been contaminated with corn syrup. All agave farming poses a threat to four endangered bat species that rely on agave for food. With that said, use organic agave only sparingly or avoid it altogether.

Caution: Agave sweeteners may cause problems for those who have bowel intolerance to fructose, and they may cause gas or bloating. A high-fructose diet can also exacerbate or lead to insulin resistance and NAFLD. If you are following a low-carb or keto menu then you will want to use monk fruit or stevia instead of agave syrup. Note that agave manufacturers use the words *syrup* and *nectar* interchangeably because there's no legal standard distinguishing the quality of agave products.

Tapioca Syrup

Tapioca is a starch extracted from the root of the cassava plant (*Manihot esculenta*), which is also known as manioc and yuca (note that yucca is actually a type of agave and not related to tapioca). Cassava is well tolerated by people who have autoimmune issues, so it has become very popular in healthy recipes. The cassava plant itself doesn't produce sweet syrup, but its root starches yield a sugary mixture when they're broken down by various amylases (naturally occurring enzymes that digest starches). Similar to beets, the whole food is healthy and healing, but the refined sugar made from it can cause nutritional imbalances.

This sweetener is unsuitable for people who suffer from poor fructose absorption or metabolism. It is mentioned here because people may use it as an occasional option if they're allergic to sugar cane. Tapioca syrup can be used as a starting material for producing high-fructose syrups, which can be just as inflammatory as refined sugar cane and beet sugars.

Caution: Tapioca syrup is usually made with enzymes derived from yeasts, most commonly *Saccharomyces cereviseae* (commonly known as baker's yeast). However, some companies may use black mould (*Aspergillus niger*) or other yeasts. Although this alternative sweetener is a popular option, it is best avoided if possible. If you are following a low-carb or keto menu then you will want to use monk fruit or stevia instead of tapioca syrup.

DON'T BE FOOLED BY FAKE!

Now that you have an idea of all of the alternative sweeteners, what about artificial sweeteners? These were created to give people the sweetness they crave without the caloric impact. Food labs got to work creating artificial sweeteners (although some were discovered accidentally) with the intention of alleviating the problems associated with consumption of refined sugars. Unfortunately, you will quickly realize that these synthetic chemicals aren't without harmful side effects.

Artificial sweeteners are touted as zero-calorie, guilt-free flavourings that are safe for diabetics. The general belief was that because the body didn't metabolize artificial sweeteners, they wouldn't increase the risk of developing metabolic diseases. With the increasing awareness of the damaging health effects of artificial sweeteners, people have been exploring various natural sources of unrefined alternative sweeteners that won't promote inflammatory diseases.

Artificial sweeteners are not an option. In truth, there are plenty of healthy alternatives to refined sugar that taste delicious, are not manufactured in a lab and are anti-inflammatory. The best part is that when eaten in moderation, all of these natural sweeteners can help minimize or even prevent and heal inflammation. For example, recent studies have shown that natural, unrefined sweeteners retain their natural anti-inflammatory antioxidants, which are key nutrients in healing and helping to prevent chronic diseases.

Globally, most artificial sweeteners have gained widespread approval. However, their safety remains a controversial and unresolved issue because data are contradictory. Please avoid all artificial sweeteners.

Aspartame (NutraSweet®)

Aspartame is probably one of the most notorious artificial sweeteners on the market. It's an amino acid–based sweetener that tastes 1500 to 2000 percent sweeter than the same amount of sucrose. It was discovered accidentally in 1965 by researchers at the Searle & Company laboratories (bought by Monsanto, which is now owned by Bayer). Aspartame is used as the primary or adjunctive sweetener in a wide range of products, most notably in diet foods and beverages, some pharmaceutical products such as mineral-vitamin supplements, gum and sugar-free candies.

The toxicity of aspartame is due not to the molecule itself but to its metabolites. In the GI mucosal cells, aspartame is broken down into two amino acids, aspartic acid and phenylalanine, plus the alcohol methanol. These metabolites are then absorbed into the bloodstream. Under normal metabolic conditions, aspartic acid is rapidly metabolized and is nontoxic. However, when phenylalanine is present in high concentrations relative to other amino acids (especially tyrosine), it can significantly affect brain chemistry by decreasing the production of catecholamines. Because aspartame appears to selectively increase brain levels of phenylalanine, this sweetener could cause side effects in healthy people as well as in those who suffer from mental disorders. Moreover, people who have a congenital condition known as phenylketonuria (PKU) aren't able to metabolize phenylalanine, and so aspartame is toxic and potentially fatal for these individuals.

In addition to these adverse effects, the other primary concerns associated with aspartame are the following:

- The potential excitatory effects of aspartame on the nervous system, including the brain

- The potential interaction and synergistic effects of ingesting aspartame together with other neuroexcitatory substances such as monosodium glutamate (MSG)

- The potential impacts of aspartame on brain biochemistry and daily (circadian) body rhythms

- The toxicity of methanol, which is converted into formaldehyde and then into formic acid. Formaldehyde is a cellular toxin that can mutate DNA and accumulate in tissues. Formic acid is toxic to the kidneys and irritating to the eyes, skin and mucous membranes. Approximately 10 percent (by weight) of ingested aspartame is converted into absorbable methanol.

Proponents who claim that aspartame is safe point out that methanol, formaldehyde and formic acid are also naturally present in the environment. However, neutralizing and eliminating these toxins—regardless of their origin—from the body requires antioxidants such as the body's own glutathione and/or dietary phytonutrients as well as essential nutrients (such as vitamin B9). If ingested in large quantities, aspartame could contribute to the load of toxins in the body, and people with compromised metabolic or detoxifying mechanisms may be more sensitive to aspartame than healthy individuals are.

Several studies have shown correlations between aspartame consumption and

- Incidence of cancer

- Declines in dopamine levels in the brain

- Increased inflammation and angiogenesis

- Increased free radical production

People who should be particularly cautious about aspartame ingestion include those with PKU, multiple food and/or chemical allergies and sensitivities, asthma, compromised blood-brain barrier integrity (also known as leaky brain), hyperintestinal permeability (also known as leaky gut) and behavioural or cognitive disorders, as well as pregnant and lactating women, children and the elderly. Please avoid aspartame in all processed foods and beverages (for example, diet soda and chewing gum).

Sucralose (Splenda™)

Sucralose is a disaccharide derived from sucrose, but it is by no means a natural sweetener. In a process involving microbial cultures and/or enzymes, chlorine atoms are added to sucrose molecules to yield a synthetic sucralose that tastes 450 to 650 times sweeter than table sugar. Human digestive enzymes don't break down sucralose, and it is therefore classified as a calorie-free sweetener.

Sucralose is most often sold commercially as Splenda, which contains sucralose together with the fillers maltodextrose and glucose. When combined with other sweeteners, the taste of sucralose synergizes with fructose, acesulfame K, cyclamate and saccharin, but not with aspartame and sucrose. Sucralose has a sweet, lingering aftertaste, and it retains its sweetness over a wide range of conditions, making it a preferred sweetener for the food industry.

Most ingested sucralose is excreted via the stool, but approximately 11 to 27 percent (average of 15 percent in humans) is absorbed into the bloodstream. The absorbed sucralose may be metabolized by metabolic enzymes in the body's tissues, or it's filtered by the kidneys and then eliminated through the urine. Despite the rapid clearance of sucralose from the body, it can still affect physiology.

Even though mammals lack the enzymes to digest sucralose in the gut, a study on mice and on human intestinal cells in vitro showed that sucralose does indirectly stimulate the release of insulin by activating sweet taste receptors in the small intestine. However, it remains unclear whether sucralose has a similar insulin-stimulating effect in humans in vitro because various studies have yielded contradicting results. Sucralose has been shown to increase the absorption of glucose from the small intestine in rats, and it may temporarily increase blood pressure and heart rate in humans.

The toxicity and safety of sucralose and of its major metabolites are controversial. Despite the global acceptance of this artificial sweetener, it's important to note that a large proportion of safety and toxicological studies on sucralose have been conducted by the companies that produce and sell sucralose, and therefore the reliability of these data may be questionable.

Multiple studies show that sucralose (in the form of Splenda) fed in various doses to rats for twelve weeks led to a decline in beneficial intestinal bacteria (namely *Bifidobacteria* spp., *Lactobacillus* spp., and *Bacteroides* spp.), an increase in fecal pH, alterations in the physiology of intestinal absorption and aberrant changes to intestinal cells, all of which increase the risk of developing colorectal cancer. Rats given Splenda also experienced weight gain. At the lowest dose administered (100 mg Splenda per kilogram body weight per day, which translates to approximately 1 mg sucralose per kilogram body weight per day), probiotics decreased by 50 percent relative to the control, whereas at the highest dose administered (1000 mg Splenda per kilogram body weight per day) decreases of up to 80 percent of the resident intestinal microflora occurred. After the treatment period, microflora did not replenish, suggesting that the treated rats didn't recover from the loss of flora. The doses of sucralose used in this study are comparable to the acceptable daily intake (ADI) for humans, and it would be prudent for people who suffer from any intestinal imbalance to avoid or limit the intake of this artificial sweetener. Sucralose has been implicated as a potential trigger for migraine headaches.

A major concern regarding sucralose is that, because it's a chlorinated sugar, it may be as toxic as other chlorinated compounds (for example, some pesticides and environmental toxins). However, companies that produce sucralose claim that, unlike other chlorine-containing toxins, sucralose is not fat-soluble, and it doesn't accumulate in tissues. Industry-funded research also contends that under normal physiological conditions, sucralose appears to be stable and doesn't break down (dechlorinate) to release free chlorine atoms, which can be irritating in high doses.

Sucralose is often marketed as one of the safest artificial sweeteners, but it is best avoided. The unbiased data on this sweetener are insufficient to determine whether sucralose is suitable for consumption. Besides, there's certainly no shortage of deliciously natural anti-inflammatory sweeteners for you to choose from, so replacing sucralose in your recipes will be easy.

Saccharin

Saccharin was one of the first artificial sweeteners to be discovered, made by oxidizing the chemical o-toluenesulfonamide or phthalic anhydride, and it is approximately 200 to 700 times sweeter than sucrose.

It is almost completely absorbed in the GI tract (only about 3 percent is recovered in the feces) and is eliminated unchanged in the urine. It doesn't appear to have the same satiating effects as other sweeteners and can increase hunger, food intake and weight gain when consumed on a regular basis. Perhaps another reason it can lead to these changes is by increasing blood sugar levels despite being a zero-calorie artificial sweetener, indicating glucose intolerance. This metallic-tasting artificial sweetener causes gut microbiome dysregulation and is best avoided. There appears to be an increase in the total number of aerobic microbes in the GI tract and a decrease in total bacterial enzymes after the consumption of saccharin. Since our gut microbiome is crucial for wellness, any changes in its composition can have a drastic effect on overall health.

Acesulfame K

Acesulfame K, also known as Ace-K, is another zero-calorie sweetener that is, on average, 200 times sweeter than table sugar. It's one of the major artificial sweeteners used in the modern diet and is derived from acetoacetic acid and fluorosulfonyl isocyanate. It's commonly used with other sweeteners to help the blends retain their sweetness over time because it is highly stable.

Although it is a zero-calorie sweetener, it appears that Ace-K increases glucose uptake in the small intestines of animals at high concentrations. This can mean that blood sugar levels may be higher when Ace-K is consumed with naturally occurring sugars.

Ace-K also alters gut microbiome, body weight and metabolism profiles in a gender-specific way. It increased body weight in male but not female mice and induced different gut bacterial composition changes in male and female mice. It also supports the fact that long-term ingestion alters cognitive memory function. Ace-K is a popular sweetener in protein powders and diet products and is best avoided.

THE FUTURE OF SWEETENERS

There are many amazing plants from exotic locations that could be developed into the next sweetener, but to avoid having you wish for products that are not yet on the market, I will leave you with only one exciting example.

Oubli

Oubli (*Pentadiplandra brazzeana*) is an African climbing shrub that contains two intensely sweet proteins, pentadin and brazzein. By weight, pentadin tastes 500 times sweeter than sucrose, whereas brazzein tastes approximately 2000 times sweeter.

Brazzein is very resilient to high temperatures and so is suitable for cooking and baking. Brazzein is one of the smallest and sweetest-tasting proteins yet discovered, and it has no bitter, salty, sweet or astringent overtones or aftertastes. Locally, oubli fruit has been used for centuries. It's consumed raw or cooked to sweeten various dishes and beverages. The leaves are used as an anti-diarrheal and the root is used medicinally as a treatment for peptic ulcers and to increase male and female fertility. I hope that this sweetener is available soon to provide another option for a natural low-carb sweetener.

THE ULTIMATE SWEETENER CONVERSION CHART

This chart presents the healthiest sweeteners in green, sweeteners with cautions in yellow and inflammatory sweeteners in red. This will help you choose the best option for you, based on your needs. All sweeteners have different qualities. Many are not direct substitutes that work in classic recipes (that is, some sweeteners contain more liquid than others) and adjustments must be made.

SWEETENER	GLYCEMIC INDEX	HOW TO USE	1 CUP SUGAR =	CAUTIONS
Green Light				
Dates	31 to 58	**Uses:** Fresh, dried or softened to create a paste that can be used to sweeten and thicken recipes for baking. **Tip:** Fruit increases moisture and thins recipes, so you may have to scale back liquid.	N/A	Generally well tolerated. Avoid if intolerant to fructose. Reduce if following a low-carb menu.
Fruit	20 to 60	**Uses:** Raw, dried or the sauce version of fruit can be used to sweeten and thicken recipes for baking. Figs and raisins are popular examples. **Tip:** Fruit increases moisture and thins recipes, so you may have to scale back liquid.	N/A	Generally well tolerated. Avoid if intolerant to fructose. Reduce if following a low-carb menu.
Inositol	0	Powder form. Formerly known as vitamin B8. It is not considered a sweetener, but it has a lovely sweet taste. Reduces anxiety attacks and improves blood sugar balance.	1 teaspoon = ½ teaspoon sugar	Can cause digestive upsets and diarrhea in some people.

SWEETENER	GLYCEMIC INDEX	HOW TO USE	1 CUP SUGAR =	CAUTIONS
Green Light				
Inositol (continued)		**Uses:** It can only be used in cool beverages. Reduce other sweeteners if using. **Tip:** Small amounts of inositol are best added to beverages, as it cannot be heated.		
Licorice Root	0	Liquid or powder form. An herbal remedy that heals the stomach lining. Contains substances with an anti-diabetic effect and might serve as an effective aid in the treatment of type 2 diabetes. **Uses:** Root sweetens tea and the extract can be used as a booster in elixirs and smoothies.	N/A	Glycyrrhizic acid found in licorice can raise blood pressure, so avoid if you have high blood pressure.
Lúcuma	25	Powder form. Sweet flavour that's often likened to a mix of sweet potato and butterscotch with a hint of maple. **Uses:** Beverages, smoothies, yogurt, granola, puddings, pastry. **Tip:** Ideal for making frozen desserts, drinks and smoothies because it helps combine and emulsify fats and oils with sugars and polysaccharides.	50 percent as sweet as sugar but experiment, as it does not work well in all recipes.	Lúcuma is a fruit, so it is not tolerated on a low-carb menu or by those with a fructose intolerance.

SWEETENER	GLYCEMIC INDEX	HOW TO USE	1 CUP SUGAR =	CAUTIONS
Green Light				
Mesquite	25	Powder form. Naturally sweet and nutty flavour with a hint of caramel. Often used as a sweet flour instead of a primary sweetener. **Uses:** Smoothies, baked foods, frozen desserts, breakfast dishes.	Varies	Mesquite is a legume, so not tolerated by people avoiding beans.
Monk Fruit, 100% Pure	0	Liquid or powder form. 150 to 200 times sweeter than sugar with no aftertaste. **Uses:** Cold and warm drinks, baking, dressings, sauces. It is not possible to substitute more than 1 teaspoon at a time because doing so changes the recipe chemistry.	1 teaspoon = ½ cup sugar	Generally well tolerated. Monk fruit may stimulate Th2 cells (immune cells). Use with caution if following a strict autoimmune diet
Raw Honey	35 to 58	Distinct flavour with subtle characteristics from the flower nectar. **Uses:** Warm beverages, desserts, dressings, sauces. **Tip:** Reduce other liquids in recipe by one-third, increase baking temperature by 25 degrees and add a few more minutes to the timer.	¾ cup	Well suited if following a carbohydrate-specific diet. It is high in natural sugars, so avoid if following a low-carb menu.

SWEETENER	GLYCEMIC INDEX	HOW TO USE	1 CUP SUGAR =	CAUTIONS
Green Light				
Stevia Leaf, 100% Pure	0	Powder form. A green powder with a strong licorice taste. **Uses:** Best used in small amounts in beverages.	N/A	Generally well tolerated. Not recommended during pregnancy.
Stevia Liquid Extract	0	Liquid form. 200 to 450 times sweeter than sugar and can have a slight licorice-like aftertaste. **Uses:** Baked goods, drinks, sauces, dressings. **Tip:** Combine with lemon, cranberry or chocolate-based recipes to cut the aftertaste.	½ teaspoon = ½ cup sugar	Generally well tolerated. May affect hormones in high doses and is not recommended for some versions of the autoimmune diet.
Stevia Powder **Mixed with a Small Amount of Inulin to Create a Powder**	0	Granulated or powder form. Often sold in packets. Can have a slight licorice-like aftertaste. **Use:** To sweeten beverages.	½ teaspoon packet = 1 teaspoon sugar	Inulin can cause digestive stress in some people.
Tiger Nut	N/A	Whole, sliced or powdered. It is not a nut at all but instead a tuber. **Uses:** Enjoy whole or ground into a powder and used in baked goods and smoothies. It can replace part of the amount of flour in recipes. (Reduce other sweeteners if using as a flour.)	N/A	Well tolerated but, because of resistant starch, it can cause digestive issues in sensitive people. Does contain some natural sugars, so not acceptable for low-carb menu.

SWEETENER	GLYCEMIC INDEX	HOW TO USE	1 CUP SUGAR =	CAUTIONS
Green Light				
Yacón Syrup	36 to 40	Similar consistency and colour to dark molasses with a delicious caramel taste. **Uses:** Beverages and food. **Tip:** One-third the calories of honey or sugar.	¾ cup	High in fructo-oligosaccharides (inulin fibre) that can cause digestive issues in sensitive people.
Yellow Light				
Allulose	0	Granulated form. Taste and texture of white sugar. **Uses:** Baked goods, beverages, dressings, sauces.	1⅓ cups	Seems well tolerated. This sweetener may be ranked higher in the green category once proper human trials show long-term benefit.
Birch Syrup	50	Distinct mineral-rich and caramel-like taste (similar to molasses). Very different from maple syrup and can be used like vanilla extract. **Uses:** Marinades, sauces, dressings, baked beans, baked goods, frozen desserts.	¾ cup	Not well tolerated by those sensitive to sucrose.
Carob	40	Powder form. **Uses:** Can be used as a chocolate substitute and in a smoothie.	N/A	Carob is a legume rich in sucrose, so best avoided if intolerant. Use caution if allergic to legumes (for example, peanuts).

SWEETENER	GLYCEMIC INDEX	HOW TO USE	1 CUP SUGAR =	CAUTIONS
Yellow Light				
Coconut Sugar and Nectar	35 to 42	Liquid or granulated form. Sugar: Similar texture, appearance and taste to brown sugar. Nectar: Thicker texture than maple syrup. **Uses:** Baking and for drizzling on food.	1 cup	Popular and well tolerated because it is low on the glycemic index but does contain sucrose, so avoid if intolerant.
Erythritol	0	Granulated or powder form. 70 percent as sweet as sugar. **Uses:** Warm beverages and baked goods.	1⅓ cups	Generally well tolerated compared to the other sugar alcohols, however avoid if intolerant.
Fruit Juice Concentrates	Varies	**Uses:** Homemade lemonade, hot breakfast cereals, non-dairy drinks, yogurt. **Tip:** Works well in most baked goods except chocolate recipes, where flavours can clash.	Varies	Well tolerated by most people but high in fructose. Avoid if fructose intolerant.
Glycerin	0	Liquid form (derived from coconut or palm). 60 percent as sweet as sugar. **Uses:** Avoid corn-based sources.	1 teaspoon = ⅔ teaspoon sugar	A laxative if taken in large amounts. In small amounts it is quite harmless as long as it is naturally derived from coconut.

SWEETENER	GLYCEMIC INDEX	HOW TO USE	1 CUP SUGAR =	CAUTIONS
Yellow Light				
Inulin	0	Powder form. Typically used in healthy prepared products, such as probiotics, smoothies, packaged chocolate and meal replacement bars. Watch for this ingredient and make sure your digestive system can tolerate it.	N/A	It is a laxative and not suitable as a sugar replacement. Maximum tolerance is approximately 30 grams per day.
Maple Syrup	54	Sweet and has a distinct flavour. **Uses:** Pancakes, smoothies, and any recipe calling for liquid sweetener.	¾ cup	Not well tolerated by those sensitive to sucrose.
Maple Syrup Crystals	54	Granulated form. Sweet and has a distinct flavour. **Uses:** Substitute for granulated sugar in baking.	1 cup	Not well tolerated by those sensitive to sucrose.
Monk Fruit with Erythritol	0	Granulated or powder form. Powder is 2 times sweeter than sugar with no aftertaste. **Uses:** Cold and warm drinks, baking, dressings, sauces.	1 cup (granulated) but some powdered products claim 2 times sweet	Monk fruit is well tolerated, but when mixed with a sugar alcohol, the combination may cause digestive issues in some people.

SWEETENER	GLYCEMIC INDEX	HOW TO USE	1 CUP SUGAR =	CAUTIONS
Yellow Light				
Stevia with Erythritol	0	Granulated or powder form. **Tip:** Combine with lemon to cut the aftertaste.	½ teaspoon = 1 teaspoon sugar	Stevia is well tolerated, but when mixed with a sugar alcohol, some people will be sensitive.
Xylitol	7 to 12	Granulated or powder form. **Uses:** Beverages, baked goods, gum, mouthwash. **Note:** Xylitol is toxic to dogs and can be fatal if they ingest it.	1⅓ cups	Can cause a laxative effect or rashes in people sensitive to sugar alcohols.
Red Light				
All Artificial Sweeteners	0	• Acesulfame K aka Ace-K, ACE and acesulfame potassium. • Aspartame, APM, aspartyl-phenylalanine methyl ester and related sweeteners called Advantame, Alitame and Neotame. Brand names: NutraSweet, Equal, Spoonful, Equal Measure, Canderel, Benevia, AminoSweet, NatraTaste.	Varies	Caution, as these may contain harmful neuro-toxins. Avoid completely. Artificial sweeteners have many safety concerns, including elevated risk of cancer and seizures, and have been implicated in neurological and immune disorders.

SWEETENER	GLYCEMIC INDEX	HOW TO USE	1 CUP SUGAR =	CAUTIONS
Red Light				
All Artificial Sweeteners (continued)		• Saccharin aka sodium saccharin, calcium saccharin, and potassium saccharin. Brand names: Sweet'N Low, Necta Sweet, Cologran, Hermesetas, Sucaryl, Sucron, Sugar Twin, Sweet 10. • Cyclamate aka calcium cyclamate, cyclamic acid, sodium cyclamate. Brand names: Sucaryl, Cologran. • Sucralose aka 4,1′,6′-trichlorogalactosucrose. Brand names: Splenda, Nevella.		Several of the artificial sweeteners have been known to alter our gut microbiome and impact the beneficial bacteria that inhabit our GI tract. They also raise insulin levels, which may lead to cravings and weight gain.
Brown Sugar (aka brown cane sugar), **Turbinado Sugar** (aka sugar in the raw), **Jaggery**	65 to 88	Granulated form. Distinct caramel flavour and wet, sandy texture. **Uses:** Baked goods and savoury dishes.	1 cup	Refined table sugar with molasses added. Best avoided.
Corn Syrup and High-Fructose Corn Syrup	73 to 80	Liquid and powder form. **Uses:** Soda pop, candy, baked goods.	¾ cup	Caution, as it may contain harmful neurotoxins and when consumed in high amounts, has been linked to an increased risk of the non-alcoholic fatty liver disease.

SWEETENER	GLYCEMIC INDEX	HOW TO USE	1 CUP SUGAR =	CAUTIONS
Red Light				
Corn Syrup and High-Fructose Corn Syrup (continued)				The body digests fructose differently than glucose. It increases appetite and may create excess body fat.
Demerara Sugar, Rapadura Sugar (aka Barbados sugar), **Muscovado Sugar**	43 to 65	Granulated form (crunchier than white sugar). Toffee flavour. **Uses:** Baked goods, beverages, dressings, sauces.	1 cup	Varying degree of cane sugar refinement that results in high glycemic index. Best avoided.
Dextrose	100	Liquid and granulated form. It is similar to maltodextrin and has a very sweet taste. **Uses:** Made from corn sugar and used in food as a filler and sweetener, especially in baked goods. Packaged food also commonly contains dextrose.	1⅓ cups	Avoid any products with dextrose, as it is very high on the glycemic index. Made from corn that is genetically modified.
Evaporated Cane Juice (aka dehydrated cane juice, granulated sugar cane juice, unrefined cane juice)	43	Liquid or granulated form. Slight to strong molasses flavour depending on brand. **Uses:** Baked goods, beverages, dressings, sauces.	¾ to 1 cup	Sugar cane is rich in minerals but poorly tolerated by those with digestive and mental health concerns.

SWEETENER	GLYCEMIC INDEX	HOW TO USE	1 CUP SUGAR =	CAUTIONS
Red Light				
Grain Syrups and Malts (rice syrup, oat syrup/malt, brown rice syrup/malt, barley syrup/malt, sorghum)	25 to 85	Liquid form. **Uses:** Baked goods, raw desserts, barbecue sauces, baked beans, candied vegetables.	1¼ cups	Can cause allergic reactions and may contain mould. Some products are high on the glycemic index.
Honey, Pasteurized	50 to 80	Liquid form. Heated at high temperatures, which destroy beneficial properties. **Uses:** Anywhere a liquid sweetener is needed.	¾ cup	Well tolerated but heating damages structure and kills beneficial effects. Cheap honey is often cut with high-fructose corn syrup.
Inverted Sugar	60	A modified and processed sugar. Sweeter than sucrose.	¾ cup	May cause a high insulin response, so best avoided.
Maltitol	35	Granulated form. **Uses:** Baked goods, toothpaste, candy.	1¼ cups	Strong laxative effect and best avoided. People with diabetes should remember that it's a carbo-hydrate.

SWEETENER	GLYCEMIC INDEX	HOW TO USE	1 CUP SUGAR =	CAUTIONS
Red Light				
Maltodextrin	110	Fine white powder. **Uses:** Often used as a thickener, filler or preservative.	N/A	High insulin and allergy response, so best avoided. If you must use maltodextrin, make sure it is sourced from cassava (tapioca) root.
Mannitol	0	Granulated form. Tastes about 50 percent as sweet as the same amount of sucrose. **Uses:** Not used as a sweetner; used in coating tablets.	2 cups	Strong laxative, so best avoided.
Molasses (blackstrap, dark, light and granulated)	55	Liquid form. 65 percent as sweet as sugar and has a distinctly rich flavour. Comes in a range of flavours, including light, dark and blackstrap. **Uses:** Pancake syrup, natural remedies, baked goods, marinade, rubs, sauces.	½ to ¾ cup	The highest in nutrition of the sugar cane–based sweeteners. Many brands are high in the toxin acryamide. Will cause a reaction if sensitive to cane sugar.

SWEETENER	GLYCEMIC INDEX	HOW TO USE	1 CUP SUGAR =	CAUTIONS
Red Light				
Refined Date Sugar	103	Granulated form. Very sweet and has a caramel taste. **Uses:** Hot cereal and crumble on pies.	⅔ cup	Very high on the glycemic index with a strong insulin response.
Refined Fructose	25	Granulated or powder form. Crystalline fructose increases the viscosity of glazes and dairy products. **Uses:** Baked goods, beverages, dressings, sauces.	¾ cup	Similar to corn syrup. Damaging to the liver and best avoided.
Sorbitol	11	Granulated form. **Use:** A popular choice for sugar-free candy.	1⅔ cups	Strong laxative effect, so best avoided. Dangerous for diabetics, see page 73.
Sucanat	65	Granulated form. Strong molasses flavour. **Uses:** Baked goods, beverages, dressings, sauces.	1 cup	Sugar cane is rich in minerals but poorly tolerated by those with digestive and mental health concerns.

SWEETENER	GLYCEMIC INDEX	HOW TO USE	1 CUP SUGAR =	CAUTIONS
Red Light				
Tapioca Syrup	85	Liquid form. Interchangeable with rice syrup. **Uses:** Beverages, baked foods, table syrups, frozen desserts, candies.	1 cup	Well tolerated by people with allergies. Caution for those following the Autoimmune protocol menu. Can be high in glucose, which can cause an elevated insulin response.
White Sugar, Table Sugar (aka cane sugar), **Beet Sugar**	65 to 80	Granulated form. **Uses:** Warm beverages, baked goods, and sprinkled on foods.	1 cup	Very high in sucrose, which breaks down into fructose and glucose quickly.

SWEET ENDING

The best part about giving up sugar and other refined sweeteners is knowing that there is no shortage of alternative, deliciously natural anti-inflammatory sweeteners you can choose. Remember that it's important not only to replace inflammatory refined sugar and artificial sweeteners with whole, natural sweeteners, but also to moderate your intake of sweet-tasting foods. By enhancing sour and bitter foods, you can actually alter your cravings for sweets.

The good news is that when consumed in moderate amounts, the alternative sweeteners outlined in this book won't spike your blood levels of glucose or insulin, so you won't suffer "sugar crashes" that leave you craving more sweets and refined carbohydrates. How wonderful it is that even delicious foods can help you prevent and heal inflammation! Keep reading to find out how you can enjoy the deliciousness of natural sweeteners in real, whole food recipes.

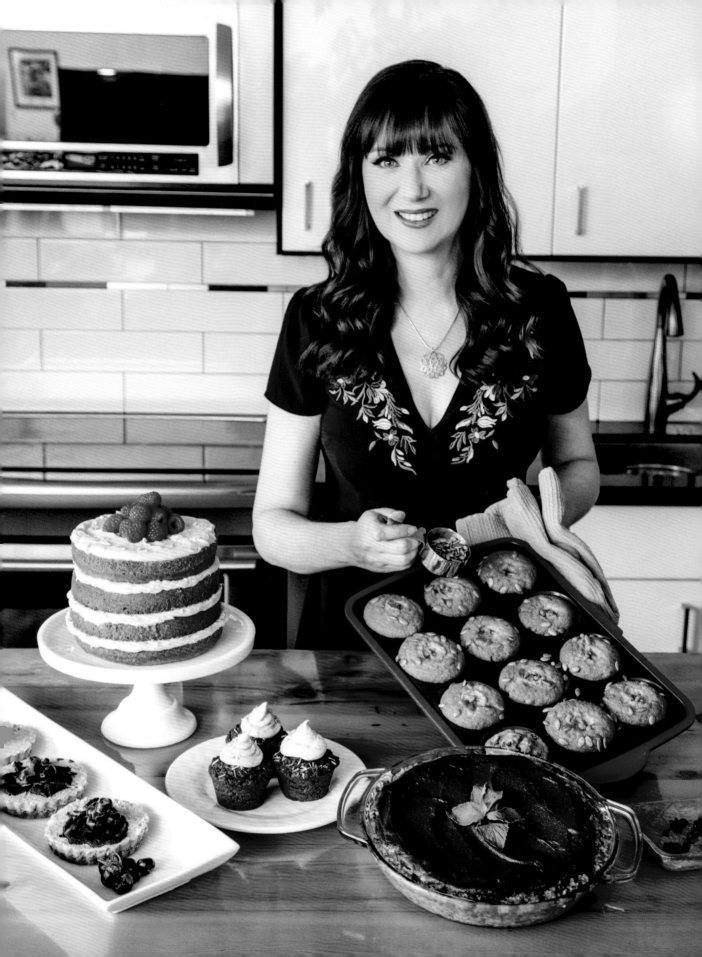

4
How to Break Up with Sugar

Do you want to let go of emotional eating for good? Then we need to close the gap between what you *know* and what you *do*. How many people know to avoid sugar, but they just keep eating it? As a nutritionist and a coach of Dynamic Eating Psychology, it is my job to help you close the gap and get you into action.

When you begin, avoiding sugar seems like a huge shift, but it eventually becomes your new normal. When I went off sugar, there was an adjustment phase, and now I can't imagine living any other way. People ask me, "How do you have such iron-clad will-power?" But willpower has nothing to do with it! I developed strong habits that carried me through the difficult moments. Many people fall back into their former crummy diet or unhealthy habits when difficulties arise, but it doesn't have to be that way for you. My community and I are living proof that you can get off sugar and thrive. If I can go sugar-free and teach others to do the same, I am confident that you can do it too.

MY SUGAR ADDICTION

I wish I'd had the tools outlined in this chapter at my fingertips when I was struggling with my sugar addiction. Do you agree that they should be taught in school? Before I fell in love with yoga and nutrition, I used to be addicted to sugar and flour. I finally figured out how to break up with my refined food habit for good by using a blend of the therapies I describe in this chapter. Let me disclose just how powerfully sugar ruled my life.

In one sitting, I once ate a whole loaf of bread with sugar, cinnamon and salted butter on each slice. I estimate that binge at 3222 calories. The danger was not only the sugar. Most "complex" carbohydrates we consume, such as bread (including whole wheat), bagels and pasta, aren't really complex at all. They contain starches that break down into sugars right in your mouth. Next, I would start into a box of cookies and not be able to stop. Pirate Oatmeal Peanut Butter Cookies and I had a dangerous love affair! I could eat all 20 cookies in a box (that's 3400 calories) served with a tall glass of milk (156 calories) for a whopping 3556-calorie binge.

Then there were the celebration binges for special occasions: a pint of mint chip ice cream (600 calories); Rice Krispies squares with chocolate topping (18 squares × 171 calories = 3078 calories); or my favourite "happy" binge, a large bag of Fritos corn chips (1280 calories). The "lonely" binge skulked out when I was at the movies by myself: one large popcorn with butter (1234 calories) and a caramel pecan cinnamon bun with extra frosting (1210 calories). That's almost 2500 calories while barely moving a muscle.

You get the picture. Things were out of control! I decided to not just take control, but truly heal my relationship with food. Have you ever considered how we personify food to fill emotional gaps that are unfulfilled? Let's call it out for what it is: sugar and refined starch are like being in a bad relationship. You get knocked around but keep coming back for more. It's time to find a loving relationship that edifies, protects and makes us feel secure. Keep reading to learn how to find a new partnership today.

HOW DO WE CLOSE THE GAP?

The first step in closing the gap is acknowledging that there are two "brains" at work inside of you: there's your higher brain, which is conscious, loving and smart; which knows what to do and has the world's best interest at heart and which wants to make a contribution, to love and be loved. Then there's your lower brain, which is reactive and indulgent, the one that is running the show when you go into fight or flight. In happy, easy times, it's easy to listen to your higher brain because your basic needs are being met, and you can focus on connection and contribution. When you're upset, triggered or threatened, your lower brain is activated and you enter fight or flight mode.

Many years ago, the threat could have been a bear, and your fight or flight response would have saved your life. In the modern world, the threat may manifest as a stressful boss, and since you can't leave work or fight your employer, you cope with your stress by numbing yourself with food, typically food that delivers a hit of dopamine or increases serotonin. The food acts to block your feelings of wanting to run away or express anger.

To create a breakthrough in this behaviour, we need to reconcile the higher brain with the lower brain, so that instead of reacting, we cope by applying healthy eating tools. We start by recognizing that there is no true emergency, then choose and apply the tools outlined in this chapter to take you out of fight or flight. The techniques of vagus nerve stimulation on page 110 will help snap you out of the feeling that the sky is falling, the feeling that you're standing on the edge of a cliff, about to jump off into a sugar and flour binge. It creates a moment of choice. You can choose to binge, to run away and lose control, or you can choose to stimulate the vagus nerve, calming you down and helping you cope with the stressor.

It's not your fault that there are automatic patterns you've learned to follow under stress. Stop placing blame on yourself. You are not weak, and you don't have faulty willpower. These key patterns may have been ingrained in you since childhood. Placing blame on yourself only makes you a victim of circumstance and leaves you in fight or flight mode.

The good news is that you now have the tools and the power to make new choices. When you put yourself in the driver's seat and apply the tools outlined in this book to calm yourself and feel good, everything changes. You are in control of the rest of your life. You may have felt like a victim in the past, but in the present you get to choose the rest of your story.

IDENTIFY SYMPTOMS AS WARNING SIGNS

Once we identify the foods or lifestyle patterns that aren't serving you, how do you correct the course? Many people don't realize that they are functioning in a state of fight or flight and anxiety until the symptoms disappear. Once you eliminate refined sugar, I feel confident that you will notice some positive changes. My clients report that their pain fades, brain fog lifts, mood lightens, headaches disappear, weight drops without strict dieting and energy comes back. Once you know you can feel that good, it's easy to keep going. This positive outlook also makes dealing with crises and tough situations much easier. Many people, when they face a challenge or crisis, eat the crave foods that used to make them feel good: refined sugar, carbohydrates such as refined flour, chips, cookies and cakes. Then they experience the negative symptoms associated with these foods and finally make the connection that they don't want to eat these foods anymore. They simply cannot pretend that eating sugar is benign and does not cause these negative symptoms.

Imagine the flip side: facing a crisis without sugar and all of the negative implications of eating it. Imagine how much more focused, calm, collected and capable you would be to deal with that crisis. Your body wouldn't stay in fight or flight. It would be centred and relaxed. With your body less focused on dealing with refined sugar, it will be more able to see you through the crisis and learn from it. If you lean into your healthy habits instead of sugar as a way to cope with a crisis, it will forever change your ability to be the healthy first responder—the person who can come to your own and other people's aid.

This is why I am so committed to this book and why I was moved to write it. I remember when my dad had a heart attack and we discovered multiple blood clots in his lungs that could potentially kill most men much younger than him. In the past, I would have chewed through dozens of chocolate bars and gummy candy. Instead, my husband, Alan, and my sister, Lynn, and I took turns cooking real food and carrying it into the hospital not only to nourish ourselves but also to speed my dad's recovery. I managed to avoid eating even 1 gram of refined sugar, and doing so kept my head clear, my stress reduced and my heart open.

DO YOU FEEL YOU HAVE TOO MANY DECISIONS TO MAKE?

Let's go back to my story of the moment I decided I was giving up refined sugar and flour for good. That choice may come across to some people as limiting, but it actually freed up thousands of decisions that I no longer had to make in my day-to-day life. A modern adult can make up to 35,000 decisions each day. Cornell University reported that we make 227 decisions a day just on the foods we eat.

The trouble is that the brain has a limited capacity for making decisions before it can fall prey to decision fatigue. That means your brain could already be overwhelmed before making food decisions, never mind the many other decisions you will make in the span of twenty-four hours. If you have a firm boundary in your mind that you don't eat sugar, that automates a whole bunch of choices, giving you more bandwidth to make other decisions. I don't have to consider the white sugar breakfast cereal or find the willpower to turn down the chocolate-covered croissant at lunch. I have developed healthy habits, such as sticking to the outside aisles of a grocery store to pick up produce, fridge and freezer items. It prevents me from making comparison shopping decisions and saves me a tremendous amount of time.

Another great example of how a boundary can create greater freedom is the concept of having a cheat day. Many people think that they can eat healthfully for six days and then have a day where anything goes. The problem I have with a cheat day is that it can be moved around to suit a person's schedule, and the next thing you know a cheat day becomes a cheat weekend or even a cheat week. A simple reframing makes it easier. What if you plan to have a treat each day instead of a cheat day each week? It doesn't become about restriction, but rather a method of eating enjoyment that can lead to greater freedom and happiness. This concept removes the stress about what to eat and will empower you with your food choices.

Believe it or not, this is a far easier way to operate than the 80/20 rule (eating clean during the week and "cheating" on the weekend). This one decision allows you room for play: we do not eat refined sugar food. There is no menu plan or complicated plan to follow or calories to count. You simply need to commit so that you can experience how freeing and delicious food can be. Once you learn how to use sugar substitutions in your favourite dishes, you won't even miss it. Get rid of the bad sugar lover and embrace something that makes you feel great in the moment and the next day. Break up with it and move on to something better!

This new way of eating opens up new opportunities to enjoy life, such as visiting a healthy restaurant with a friend or making sugar-free treats you can enjoy anytime. I like to make a batch of Avocado Keto Brownies (page 199) and keep them in my freezer for a delicious hit of dopamine around 2 PM. When you do the same, you may find that there are more fun things to eat than you ever thought possible.

INTUITIVE EATING TOOLS

If you find yourself regularly eating in response to your emotions, try to break the habit with some of the strategies outlined below.

1. **Retrain Your Taste Buds.** Mindful eating is becoming very popular around the world to create food consciousness. Book fifteen minutes in your schedule to try this exercise. Grab an apple (or fresh berries), sit somewhere quiet with no interruptions and follow these steps:

    a. Set your apple in front of you and really look at it. Look at it closely to see its uniqueness.

    b. Smell your apple. What else does it smell like? What emotion do you connect with this smell? What memories come up?

    c. Put your apple up to your mouth. Feel the skin against your lips. Roll it around a bit, feeling the texture. Bite into it. Notice what happens to your taste buds. Chew it slowly, thirty times or until it's a liquid. Does the taste change as you chew?

    d. Swallow the apple piece and repeat, taking fifteen minutes to eat your apple.

    e. Journal your experience:
    -   What did you notice?
    -   What emotions came up?
    -   How did it feel to slow down?
    -   Who can you share this exercise with?
    -   Where would this exercise be helpful in your life?
    -   Did you notice any change in the apple's sweetness?

By eliminating refined sweeteners for thirty days, you will be wonderfully surprised at how the complex sweetness of yams, beets, fruit, squash and red sweet peppers is highlighted and your cravings for refined sugar are reduced.

2. **Learn to Recognize Your Hunger.** Eat two to three meals and allow for healthy snacks throughout the day if needed. Calorie-restricted diets are proven to fail over time, and skipping nutritious foods may make you feel uncontrollably "hangry." It is best to stay aware and solve low blood sugar issues before you hit the snack bar or vending machine. Try a non-caffeinated herbal tea or a bowl of soup or broth. Before you go for a snack, drink a glass of your favourite sugar-free drink, then decide if you really need that snack.

Before you automatically pop something into your mouth, rate your hunger on a scale of 1 to 10, and make every effort to avoid eating when you're an 8, 9 or 10.

THE HUNGER SCALE

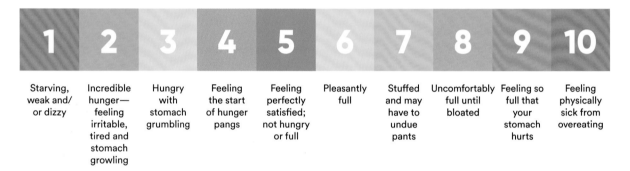

1	2	3	4	5	6	7	8	9	10
Starving, weak and/ or dizzy	Incredible hunger— feeling irritable, tired and stomach growling	Hungry with stomach grumbling	Feeling the start of hunger pangs	Feeling perfectly satisfied; not hungry or full	Pleasantly full	Stuffed and may have to undue pants	Uncomfortably full until bloated	Feeling so full that your stomach hurts	Feeling physically sick from overeating

Understanding the Hunger Scale

1. **Starving, Weak and/or Dizzy.** It's gone too far. You are so hungry that you may experience dizziness and headaches. You are completely sapped of energy and may lose coordination.

2. **Incredible Hunger.** The classic "hangry" situation where you get cranky and irritable. You are intensely hungry, have low energy and may even feel nauseous.

3. **Hungry with Stomach Grumbling.** You really want to eat and feel a pit of hunger in your stomach.

4. **Feeling the Start of Hunger Pangs.** You are getting hunger signals from your body that you may want to eat soon.

5. **Feeling Perfectly Satisfied.** You feel energized and balanced mentally and physically.

6. **Pleasantly Full.** You feel full and satisfied.

7. **Stuffed.** You are totally full but feel you can have "just one more bite." It is a mental game now, as your body is telling you to stop.

8. **Uncomfortably Full.** You have eaten so much that your stomach is stressed.

9. **So Full That Your Stomach Hurts.** You are uncomfortable and perhaps feel like napping. Your body feels heavy and bloated.

10. **Feeling Physically Sick.** You are busting a gut and promise yourself you will never overeat again. You might fast to overcompensate for overeating.

How to Use the Hunger Scale to Become an Intuitive Eater

1. Ask yourself before each meal where you are on the hunger scale. Try to eat when you are between 3 and 4 instead of waiting until you are starving. By getting ahead of your hunger, you avoid cravings.

2. Put your fork down between bites and breathe deeply. Ask again where you are on the hunger scale, with the understanding that it takes twenty minutes for your stomach to tell your brain you are full.

3. When you hit 5 or 6 on the hunger scale, you are done eating. Switch to a cup of digestive tea and focus on your journal or friendly conversation.

   After trying this exercise for a few days, check in if you don't have normal hunger or fullness cues. Check in with a few more questions:

   • Do I feel like I have regular and healthy eating cues?

   • Do I skip meals and snacks even when I am hungry?

   • Do I graze all day on food and never feel hungry?

If you don't listen to your body—feeding it when it's hungry, stopping when it's not—you can mess up your hormonal hunger and fullness cues. The big lesson is to listen to the whispers so that your body does not have to scream.

CONQUERING EMOTIONAL EATING

Emotional eating occurs when you eat in response to feelings instead of hunger. Sadness, anger, boredom, isolation, poor relationships, lack of self-confidence and stress can lead to emotional eating.

The first step in getting off of refined sugar is to accept that it has a firmer grip on our taste buds and mind than nature intended. For me, it was a substance I felt powerless over, and I decided that it was time for me to take back my power. This is the biggest step. You don't have to do it alone: pray, tap into your higher power, seek counselling, attend a support group and be honest with your partner, family or friends who come with you on your journey. When you talk to someone about your emotional feelings about sugar and flour, the weight starts to lift, and you begin to feel less alone.

Once you've admitted you have a problem with sugar and have created a support system, you're ready to jump into the sugar-free life.

Why Do We Engage in Emotional Eating?

I believe that every action we take, even a negative one, has a payoff tied to it or a hidden motive that drives it. If we can uncover the conscious or unconscious agenda that's pushing your behaviours, we can change your actions radically. Many of your actions could be attributed to learned behaviours that were established when you were young. Take eating behaviour, for example. If you were rewarded with food, if you were punished with food, if you hid in your room and soothed yourself with food, if you had scary experiences with food (for example, food poisoning or allergies), all of these experiences dramatically shaped your personal preferences, your choices at every meal and even your appetite.

I was trained in eating psychology with Marc David at the Institute for the Psychology of Eating. I have also studied life coaching with therapist Cloe Mandanes and Tony Robbins, and this training has made a considerable difference in my ability to help people close the gap between knowing intellectually that they need to stop eating sugar and taking the leap of actually letting go of sugar for good.

You may have heard of Maslow's Hierarchy of Needs, which describes a person's drive to fulfill the needs of physiology, safety, love and belonging, esteem and self-actualization. Cloe Madanes went on to expand this area of research, which has been popularized by Tony Robbins. I agree that all human needs can be organized into six categories. If two or more of these needs are not fulfilled, we can become discontented with our life. We may even unconsciously fulfill a need in a negative way, because we have to satisfy one need more than another that is rooted in a healthy behaviour. That said, you can choose to change your behaviour at any time, and I have witnessed miracles with my coaching clients. What follows is a brief outline to inspire you to investigate why you may be overeating. If you want to learn more about this, check out my support programs at www.JulieDaniluk.com.

BREAK THE CRAVING CYCLE BY FULFILLING YOUR SIX HUMAN NEEDS

The Six Human Needs	Actions You Can Take to Heal
Certainty Certainty makes us feel secure and ready for any emergency. When crisis strikes, it is natural to want to hoard, store, eat too much, collect and share food for our family and loved ones. Remember how people responded to the COVID-19 virus pandemic? Whether it was overeating or hoarding food, each of these behaviours stems from a need for food security, which connects to our basic human need for certainty.	Prepping meals and having snacks readily available keeps anxiety at bay about issues of food security. The key is to ensure that the food you are preparing or keeping in good supply is nourishing your body instead of breaking it down. Pack healthy, ready-to-eat bars in your purse or place a small bag of trail mix in your computer bag. If you have a deeper trauma from being undernourished in the past, work with a qualified therapist to be de-triggered for memories that may be locking you into unhealthy eating patterns (see How Does EMDR Work? on page 106).
Variety Variety is the need for uncertainty or to be surprised, as it provides the spice of life. This need is fulfilled when you have variety in what you're eating. Variety restriction is the number one reason why I dislike rigid menu plans and don't believe in harsh dieting. When we restrict the variety of our food, eat monochromatically, or have a boring menu, your brain and body eventually rebel and fall back into the world of your comfort foods. Severe restriction actually heightens your brain's awareness of the foods you're trying not to eat. Inversely, allowing yourself to eat a variety of wholesome, healthy foods keeps your appetite at bay and meals from getting boring. Variety is the best way to ensure that you succeed with any dietary shift.	Keep exploring new tastes to ensure variety in your food choice. For example, look at new dishes outside of your usual patterns. Try Ethiopian food, a new Asian restaurant or unique Latin American recipes . . . they are all delicious! On each shopping trip, allow $5 to $10 to buy a produce or grocery item you've not tried before and then seek out a fun way to prepare it. I enjoy visiting farmers' markets and trying a new variety of medicinal mushroom, an artisanal nut-based cheese or a heritage variety of vegetable that inspires me. By prioritizing eating a variety of healthy foods, you continuously expand your palate and stay excited about the culinary surprises you discover.

The Six Human Needs	Actions You Can Take to Heal

Significance

Significance drives the need to feel wanted, important or that we're indispensable in the world. In the food realm, lack of feeling significant may manifest in becoming sick through overeating or eating foods to which we are allergic or intolerant. This behaviour creates a situation that needs emergency help, which results in us getting the attention and significance we crave. If you overeat to the point where you can't go to work, it gives you permission to take a sick day. For people who overwork, who are overachievers, and who overgive, becoming sick gives them a moment to allow themselves to become significant by actually slowing down.

Look for areas in life where you can build significance in positive ways. Get in tune with yourself and allow yourself time, without becoming ill, to be significant. What makes you feel good? Is there a hobby you could begin or get back to? As long as these things come from positive behaviours, they are great sources of significance. Never underestimate the power of self-care. Take thirty minutes for yourself, whether it's doing yoga, taking a bath, or going for a walk—these things build the significance of you just as you are. If you feel that you don't have enough sources of positive significance, read about the need for contribution.

Love and Connection

Love and connection are the key to thriving. We are pack animals, and many people are shown love through food. This is one of the biggest challenges to overcome when we are trying to make a healthy change. Consider a grandmother who shows love by feeding her grandchildren cinnamon buns or a mother who rewards a job well done with an ice cream cone. These may have been expressions of love and kindness, but potentially have negatively ingrained in us that a sugary or starchy food is connected to love and reward. When this happens, or if you are feeling disconnected or lonely, you will often run, not walk, to the comfort foods of your childhood to remember the love you received in the past by eating that food again.

Make a list of all the ways you give and receive love. We often teach others our personal love language by demonstrating the actions we yearn for. Can you offer more words of encouragement, touch and gratitude to boost oxytocin (the love hormone)? If you show love with food, my sincere hope is that this book will provide you with substitutions and healthier low-carb or sugar-free options that remind you of the comfort foods from your childhood. If you share these treats with your friends and family in a blind taste test, I'd bet my last chocolate chip cookie that they will be enrolled in the healthier version. The desired outcome in this case is that you can feed your need for love and connection while feeding your body the nutrients it needs to thrive.

The Six Human Needs	Actions You Can Take to Heal
Growth Growth is key to happiness. I'm going to go out on a limb here and say that we're either growing or we're dying. That's a big statement, but when you think about it, living things are either blossoming or starting to wilt. As humans, we need to grow in a myriad of ways (mentally, physically, emotionally, spiritually), and when we're not exploring new horizons or learning new skills, we start to stagnate. When this happens, some people will start to grow physically because they're not growing in other ways. People are happiest when they are making progress.	Challenge yourself to find new hobbies and avenues of education that excite you. Choose to eat foods that grow your body in a positive way, such as eating more clean sources of protein to grow more muscle. Become more agile and capable by embracing movement practices such as dancing, juggling and playing with children. Also explore artistic projects because you will be surprised how much easier it is to put a cookie down when your hands are full of knitting! Start to journal about your eating patterns. Connect your problematic choices to times when you feel stuck or bored. When you try a few of the techniques found on page 37, you may experience growth and fulfilment in a new way.
Contribution We must go beyond ourselves and give back to humankind. If we feel that we are not a contribution to the planet, we can become despondent or depressed. How can there be a negative realm of contribution? A lot of people think they are making a contribution by pushing sugar cookies and lollipops on other people. Do you know someone in your life who says: *"Just have it! Come on! I made this whole tray of treats for you, aren't you going to have some while I watch you?"*	Look for where you can build your legacy. What are your hobbies, accomplishments and passions? Is it through children and grandchildren? Is it through your art? Where can you pay it forward? Who can you mentor or assist? What can you do to better the world around you? Consider how you can nourish people's relationship with food in a positive way. Sharing the contribution of healthy food has now become my focus, and it's a gift that gives back!

DO YOU NEED THERAPY?

A number of popular methods are helpful in the fight against sugar, including neuro-linguistic programming and hypnosis, but the one that has provided me with life-changing results is Eye Movement Desensitization and Reprocessing, or EMDR. It was developed in 1989 by Francine Shapiro, who noticed that her negative emotions were reduced when her eyes darted from side to side to mimic rapid eye movement (REM) sleep. She decided to try it with her patients and had such positive results that she nurtured it into a full technique that is now endorsed by the American Psychiatric Association.

How Does EMDR Work?

You process life events over time. Normally, your brain learns to store appropriate and useful emotions and dump inappropriate ones. However, with the shock of a sudden or repeated distress, your brain can become overloaded, leaving the event unprocessed and filed incorrectly. Similar to your body experiencing indigestion from a big meal, your brain simply cannot digest the massive chunks of tough emotional meat.

An everyday life moment might trigger your mind to pull up an old memory file that is still "raw and unprocessed" with every sound, sight and feeling that is attached to it. Even a seemingly mild, unconnected moment can evoke a traumatic event because it is possibly unconscious and trapped in your nervous system. Negative behaviour in adults can often be a result of unresolved earlier experiences in childhood that have locked them in a reactive state. EMDR work allows unresolved emotions and memories to become unlocked and gently processed.

EMDR therapists are trained to reduce the pain connected to old memories, leaving clients with a rewritten version of the past that allows them to experience old memories in a new way. Resolving traumatic memories can free you from reactivity. After Alan and I both had treatments of EMDR, our arguments dropped by 95 percent. It is empowering to calmly choose how I react to my life. Because many memories are interconnected, multiple EMDR sessions are often recommended, but making the time and money investment has been worth it for us. By freeing myself of trauma, I now have the ability to create quality relationships that fulfill me and keep me away from sugar. My cravings for refined sugar and flour have completely disappeared.

Need More Help Changing Your Behaviour?

Cognitive behavioural therapy (CBT) is a type of mental health counselling founded in the 1960s by Dr. Aaron T. Beck, a psychiatrist at the University of Pennsylvania. Many people who struggle with addiction have been helped by CBT techniques when addressing challenging thoughts and feelings, and it has been shown to reduce symptoms of anxiety, eating disorders and post-traumatic stress disorder (PTSD).

CBT flushes out harmful behaviour and emotions caused by core beliefs that people hold about themselves, others and the world. Therapists help patients identify these automatic thoughts that no longer serve their best interests. By revisiting and reducing the pain of old memories, it is possible to wire new positive behaviour that helps the person heal. Unlike talk therapy, which can go on for years, CBT can achieve good results in as few as sixteen sessions.

Some powerful exercises are helpful in sugar addiction recovery, including examining your automatic thoughts, planning pleasant activities and working through emotions when exposed to triggers.

HOW TO SWITCH OFF YOUR STRESS RESPONSE: THE VAGUS NERVE

Did you know that there's a way to take yourself out of that panicked state and return to a state of calm? The vagus nerve is the longest nerve in the body, and it runs from your brain into your lungs, heart and belly. When stimulated, it shifts you from fight or flight (sympathetic nervous system) to rest, repair and relax (parasympathetic nervous system). It's like a master switch, so it's important that you learn what it is and how to control the switch.

When you experience a shock or stressful situation, your body goes into fight or flight mode, engaging your sympathetic nervous system. When this happens, you experience all of the classic signs and symptoms that happen when you're stressed out. What's interesting is that this reaction happens regardless of what produces that shock or stress, good or bad. It could be when someone cuts you off in traffic or when your child stomps their muddy feet on your white carpet. Going into fight or flight can even happen because of a trauma that has occurred in the past. For example, if you were attacked by a dog as a child, you might go into fight or flight as an adult whenever you see a dog. On top of those constant states of living in fight or flight, you have dozens of stressors in everyday life—traffic jams, work projects, child or elder care. In addition, we do things to ourselves to make our stressed-out state even worse. Did you drink coffee today? Did you invent emergencies that don't really exist? Did you hype yourself up on sugar? All of these things can contribute to a heightened fight or flight state. It's no wonder that so many people find it so hard to calm down and relax.

To understand how to move forward, it is helpful to visit the past for just a minute to understand that this problem has not always been this way.

WHAT HAPPENS IN VAGUS, STAYS IN VAGUS

Toning the vagus nerve helps to switch off the flight or fight response (sympathetic) and return it to the rest and digest mode (parasympathetic).

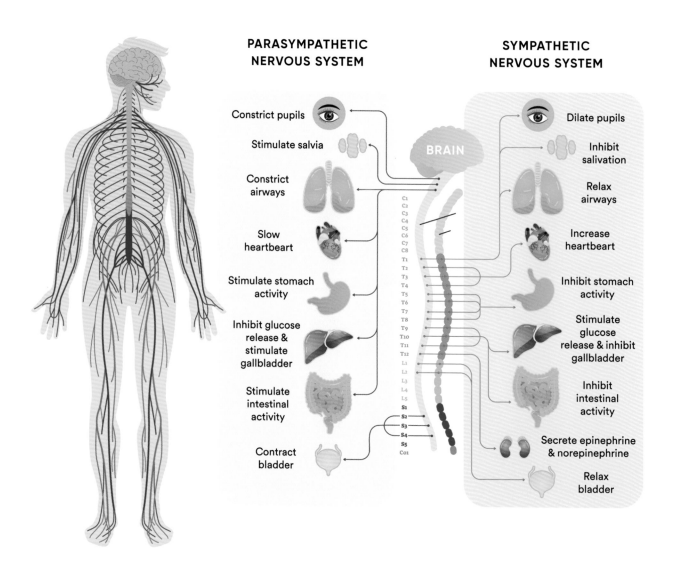

Improving vagal tone (activity of the vagus nerve) improves the function of the organs featured above. Improve vagal tone by gargling, humming, singing, acupuncture, osteopathy, deep breathing, yoga, tai chi, alternating hot and cold water, hugs, and enjoying more prebiotic fibres, probiotic foods and healthy oils.

The Body Reactions During Fight or Flight

The fight or flight response was very necessary in our evolutionary history. It helped us run faster, see in the dark and escape predators. It kept us away from dangerous situations so that we could live longer, survive and thrive. In the present day, it's much different. Although we do still need these reactions from time to time during truly dangerous situations, most of the things that trigger the fight or flight response are not actually life-threatening dangers.

Let's take a look at what happens in our body during stress.

1. One of the first reactions is that your eyes dilate, and you become very sensitive to light.

2. Your salivary glands stop producing saliva. Because you don't need to digest food when you are running away from a bear, your body economizes resources to focus on energy to the muscles.

3. Then, your heart rate accelerates, and you might experience palpitations, anxiety or a racing heart. In fight or flight mode, your heart needs to get more oxygen to the muscles so that you can run.

4. Your lungs start to expand to bring in extra oxygen.

5. Your stomach stops digesting your food because your body thinks it's in an emergency. If you're running from a bear, you don't need to digest food but instead need to conserve all of your energy so that you can run away. If we shut down our digestion repeatedly, it may cause issues like heartburn, irritable bowel syndrome (IBS) or, worse, the slowing down of peristalsis. In fact, a genuine reason why so many people are constipated may be because they're constantly living in a fight or flight state, and their body has turned off their digestive function so often in order to deal with other stressors. It's like the body is saying, "I'll let you go to the bathroom when the emergency is over."

6. Your liver liberates stored glucose, causing blood sugar levels to soar. Insulin is released from the pancreas to shuttle the sugar into cells to be turned into energy. But if you don't use the sugar, the cells become resistant to insulin, creating all kinds of inflammation and hormonal imbalance. This is important to understand, as you may be eating healthy foods, but if you're stressed all the time, your blood sugar and insulin levels still can be dangerously high.

7. Finally, your adrenal glands, which sit on top of your kidneys, start pumping out stress hormones (epinephrine, norepinephrine and cortisol) that ramp up the hormonal chaos raging inside your body.

This all sounds exhausting, doesn't it? It's no wonder the world is sick and tired all the time. Our bodies are constantly trying to fight off monsters that, most of the time, don't even exist. So, what's the solution?

Take a fascinating journey into the techniques that stimulate your vagus nerve to switch off your automatic anxiety and fear response. Overcome painful inflammation, reduce autoimmunity and embrace more joy and contentment with techniques that take just minutes a day.

The parasympathetic mode is the rest and repair mode of the nervous system, making you feel calm and relaxed. If you move from sympathetic to parasympathetic mode, the negative reactions described above reverse. Your heart rate slows, your digestion works correctly, your liver detoxes and releases more bile, your adrenals calm down, your bowels move and your bladder works better.

SEVEN METHODS TO STIMULATE THE VAGUS NERVE

1. **Manual Stimulation.** The number one thing that helps flip the switch from sympathetic to parasympathetic is to manually stimulate the vagus nerve.

   a. **Gargle for two minutes.** Take a large sip of water and gargle for two minutes, which vibrates the vagus nerve.

   b. **Hum like a bee!** This yoga technique works in the same way as gargling, as the vibration of the buzzing stimulates the vagus nerve and calms you down. To do this, plug your ears and hum like a kid trying to ignore the people around you. I actively used this technique the first time I was on *The Dr. Oz Show*. I was terrified before my first appearance, and I couldn't get my words out in the right order during dress rehearsal. I was panicking. I called my brother, Yogi Shambu, and asked for one technique to help my stage fright, and he asked me to focus as if bees were buzzing in the centre of my brain. It quickly shut off my stress response and, within two minutes, I had found peace and privacy. The stage fright was gone, and I was able to speak clearly and enjoy meeting Dr. Oz. Bee humming also helps shut off your negative self-talk—there is simply no room for it when you're buzzing loudy.

   c. **Chant or sing a hymn.** Pick a tune that connects with you. The act of prayer or saying "amen" or "ohm" loudly in a wonderful tone of voice are also good techniques. Anything that allows you to raise your voice in song or chanting a positive mantra will stimulate the vagus nerve.

d. **Laughter.** When I was depressed, after losing five family members in one year, I developed a habit of watching funny YouTube clips to change my attitude. Laughter releases feel-good hormones and stimulates the vagus nerve.

e. **Osteopathy.** This is a type of complementary medicine that emphasizes physical manipulation of muscle tissue and bones. Practitioners of osteopathy are referred to as osteopaths and are trained in special manual techniques that help downregulate the sympathetic nervous system. If you're constantly in sympathetic mode, consider seeing an osteopath to help you relieve stress. My osteopath helped balance my low blood pressure beautifully.

f. **Acupuncture.** We can unblock stagnant energy in the body using acupuncture. Some people who have overstimulated nervous systems and elevated adrenaline can be helped by a well-trained traditional Chinese medicine practitioner. Request a tuina massage after the needles are inserted for a one-two punch against stress.

2. **Deep Breathing and Meditation.** Both of these techniques are other ways to stimulate the vagus nerve. For deep breathing, try exhaling twice as long as you inhale (for example, in for five seconds, out for ten). By doubling your exhale, you're sending a message to your body that you are not in an emergency. When you're in an emergency, you start to hyperventilate. When you manually exhale twice as long, you're giving your body a signal to relax, because if you can exhale that deeply, you must not be in danger. Meditating can help us achieve a relaxed state by focusing on breathing in this way.

3. **Yoga, Tai Chi or Any Slow Movement.** These techniques take us to a state of relaxation. It's a moving meditation. Taking up swimming, tai chi, Pilates, yoga or other slow-moving exercises can help calm you down. People with chronic stress should stay away from extreme sports and boot camps that put you deeper into a stressed-out and exhausted state. Do you need to play a sport where people hit or injure you? It's ideal to upgrade to a form of movement that repairs your nervous system while still keeping you in shape.

4. **Hot and Cold Hydrotherapy.** Moving ourselves from hot to cold and back again can be both exciting and soothing. This is also good for you if you're angry or triggered to help move you into a consciousness where you can be clear headed. Warm therapies such as sauna can elicit heat shock proteins that are good for the body. Heat shock proteins are shown to help us live longer. When you expose yourself to heat, you have an incredible ability to empower the immune system to destroy old cells, which helps clear out plaque in the brain that causes cognitive issues like dementia. Dr. Rhonda Patrick summarized a study that found that frequency of sauna use was associated with a decreased risk of death. Using the sauna two to three times per week was associated with 24 percent lower all-cause mortality, and using it four to seven times per week decreased all-cause mortality by 40 percent.

5. **Pressure.** Compression has been proven to turn off the fight or flight response and calm the central nervous system. You can create this sensation of being held by buying a weighted blanket or putting some heavy pillows on top of your bedsheet. This discovery is credited in part to Temple Grandin, an autism advocate who invented the "hug machine" after observing how cattle calmed down when moving through squeeze shoots. Just like animals, human beings can be calmed by compression. Hugs also work as long as both parties are enrolled in the hug!

6. **Healthy Oils.** Healthy oils include good-quality omega-3 fats found in seeds, fish and algae. This type of oil helps nourish the digestive lining, sending calming messages to the brain via the vagus nerve. Our brain contains 8 percent omega-3 fat, but less than 1 percent of the modern menu is composed of omega-3. It's also one of the great remedies to reduce anxiety and depression, as it helps make serotonin when paired with vitamin D.

7. **Probiotic Fermented Foods.** Consider consuming more sauerkraut, pickles and olives, as they can be naturally fermented, helping to nurture the more than one thousand trillion bacteria that live in our microbiome. I have a problem with people drinking a lot of beer, wine and kombucha, because the yeast strains these products contain grow on sugars. Instead, focus on ferments that grow on vegetables, as they are the perfect prebiotic food that the good bacteria eat. Healthy bacteria promote more serotonin production, which makes us happy. A great study from McMaster University looked at the microbiome of mice and its connection to their emotional well-being. The digestive tracts of baby mice were kept sterile (they didn't have a microbiome), and half were given a probiotic supplement. While they were nursing, the mice were pulled away from their mother, and their cortisol levels were measured. The group given the probiotic had a dramatic reduction in their stress response because the probiotics helped reduce the impact of stress via the vagus nerve.

    Probiotic microbes are being shown in research studies to have a beneficial impact on mental health. Strains of *Lactobacillus* help improve our stress resilience and alleviate anxiety, memory loss and symptoms of cognitive impairment. The bacteria to look for include *L. paracasei, L. acidophilus, L. plantarum, L. fermentum* and *L. rhamnosus.* A 2017 study showed that patients with IBS who suffer depression saw a marked reduction in symptoms by supplementing *Bifidobacterium longum.* So, eat your vegetables and enjoy more fermented foods that are rich in healthy bacteria to make sure you balance your microbiome. You will be happy that you did!

BECOMING SUGAR-FREE CREED

Many support groups have a creed, a set of beliefs that help influence the way you live. I hope you might be inspired to post this list on your vision board or fridge to assist you in your transformation.

1. I once had an insatiable craving for sugar,* and it negatively affected my life

1. I now choose to take charge of my health and accept responsibility for my food choices.

2. I once ate down my feelings and avoided letting people know how I really felt.

2. I now express my feelings, ask for help and work on reducing my triggers in a healthy way.

3. I once used sugar as a substance to feel momentary happiness.

3. I now understand that I can create my own true joy, and it is a habit that I am nurturing.

4. I once used sugar as a way to isolate and would "lone wolf" my attempts to make better choices.

4. I now consciously reach out for community and get support to address my cravings and resolve self-sabotage.

5. I once let other people define me.

5. I now generate myself as a powerful, positive, connected person who loves life.

6. I once worried that life was better for other people.

6. I now see that comparison is the thief of joy. I consciously choose to be the superhero in my own adventure.

*All refined carbohydrates break down to sugar in your mouth. Your cravings may be for bread, corn, potato and other starches, but they all become sugar within minutes; for simplicity, this creed focuses on sugar.

7. I once let my problems overwhelm me.	7. I now understand that my problems can only bother me as much as I allow them to and choose to conserve energy. I actively reduce anxiety and worry with all the tools available. I am giving up "crazy busy" and embracing "happily engaged."
8. I once lived in the past and let my trauma define me.	8. I now choose to live in the present and let go of being a victim. I put my emotional healing in the spotlight and let forgiveness and compassion be my guiding light.
9. I once let the sadness, anger and pain eclipse my life.	9. I now choose to focus on the love, compassion and hope that can change the course of reality.
10. I once killed time and indulged distraction.	10. I now have gratitude for every breath and every moment I get to enjoy. I use my time to be a contribution because that brings me deep fulfillment.
11. I once kept score of all the hurts and gifts exchanged.	11. I now choose to believe that the love you take is equal to the love you make. I am a loving person who is deeply loved.
12. I once focused on my insecurities and faults.	12. Now I complement my gifts and acknowledge how strong I am in important areas of life. I take full responsibility to generate my new actions. I declare: I am committed to having a beautiful life.

50 WAYS TO LEAVE YOUR SWEET LOVER

By being conscious of these simple changes, you can empower yourself to take control of your cravings, reduce your stress and turn your day around. Keep this list close at hand so that you can stay relaxed, connected, energetic, empowered and free.

1. Admit that you have a problem.
2. Get counselling to address the root of your emotional eating.
3. Break up with the big trigger foods through journaling.
4. Get an accountability partner.
5. Seek out beautiful, delicious and colourful vegetables.
6. Read labels and learn how to identify hidden sources of sugar.
7. Find healthy substitutions that compare to your favourite crave foods.
8. Run an experiment in which you relish in the reasons why you love sugar. Write sugar a big love letter, and you may find it a bit like breaking up with that intimate person who you love but is not right for you anymore. This can uncover the true payoff for the habit and, with this realization, the habit is easier to release.
9. Say a prayer and practise self-love with the food you eat.
10. Try three-food interference, a technique where you eat three buffer foods to reduce consuming the crave food. For example, eat some protein (pumpkin seeds), good fat (avocado) and fibre (celery) and you might find you have more ability to resist the chocolate lava cake.
11. Overhaul your menu and cupboards and get rid of sugar-laden foods.
12. Eat protein at each meal.
13. Post a glycemic index chart (measures how fast a food raises your blood sugar) on your refrigerator.
14. Prepare healthy snacks and place them in your computer bag, purse, glove box and office desk drawer.
15. Slow down and chew your food well.
16. Change your routine to reduce habitual eating (for example, take up knitting while watching TV).
17. Make simple switches such as adding stevia or monk fruit instead of sugar to sweeten your lemonade.
18. Practise hydrotherapy and self-massage to reduce stress.

19. Close your ears and buzz like a bee to induce a sense of relaxation and inner peace.

20. Make a positive affirmation to build your confidence (for example, "I am energetic and joyful with everyone I meet.").

21. Join a solid support system that you can connect with (for example, join our sugar-free support group).

22. Let go of the circumstances that are out of your control (for example, through prayer or yoga).

23. Increase your magnesium foods (for example, leafy greens and seeds) to help reduce your reaction to stress.

24. Drink bitter-tasting juices and herbal tonics (for example, vegetable juice or herbal tea) to reduce sugar cravings.

25. Eat breakfast to balance your blood sugar and bust cravings.

26. Eat some olives to reduce salt cravings and cortisol.

27. Enjoy some green tea or yerba mate if craving caffeine to increase focus and energy.

28. Smell vanilla to shift brain chemistry.

29. Dance to naturally suppress your appetite.

30. Get eight hours of sleep each night to reduce cravings for carbohydrates.

31. Avoid artificial sweeteners.

32. Spice up your food to increase flavour and enjoyment.

33. Enjoy more omega-3 fats to improve insulin sensitivity.

34. Ask which of your six needs are fulfilled when you eat sugar (see page 103). Every action we make serves a purpose, so figure out the true payoff for your sugar habit.

35. Boost your fibre to feel full faster and help reduce anxiety.

36. Create a power move, such as Wonder Woman or Victory pose, that you can do when you need to change your emotional state.

37. Boost apple cider vinegar intake to reduce cravings.

38. Eat nuts and seeds to reduce feelings of hunger.

39. Volunteer at a food charity where you have the opportunity to eat with strangers.

40. Avoid eating after sunset and aim to eat within an eight- to ten-hour window.

41. Take an afternoon power nap.

42. Brush your teeth and gargle with a mint flavour.

43. Avoid monosodium glutamate (MSG) and artificial colours and flavours.

44. Avoid alcohol. It is fermented sugar, after all.

45. Drink more water, adding natural flavours if you need to.

46. Choose sugar-free dark chocolate.

47. Look for non-food rewards to stimulate dopamine.

48. Try acupuncture to reduce stress and cravings.

49. Plan fun activities that you can look forward to.

50. Be gentle with and kind to yourself.

Which of these strategies will you take on today, this week or this month? Remember to reward yourself with a lot of praise, high-fives and pats on the back.

I would love to share more amazing tools of transformation with you. Check out our sugar-free support program at www.JulieDaniluk.com. As you will read in next in The Sugar-Free Plan, I am a big fan of flexibility to reduce tension around food. You choose whether to go slow or fast; it depends on how fast you like to travel. All that matters is that you start the journey.

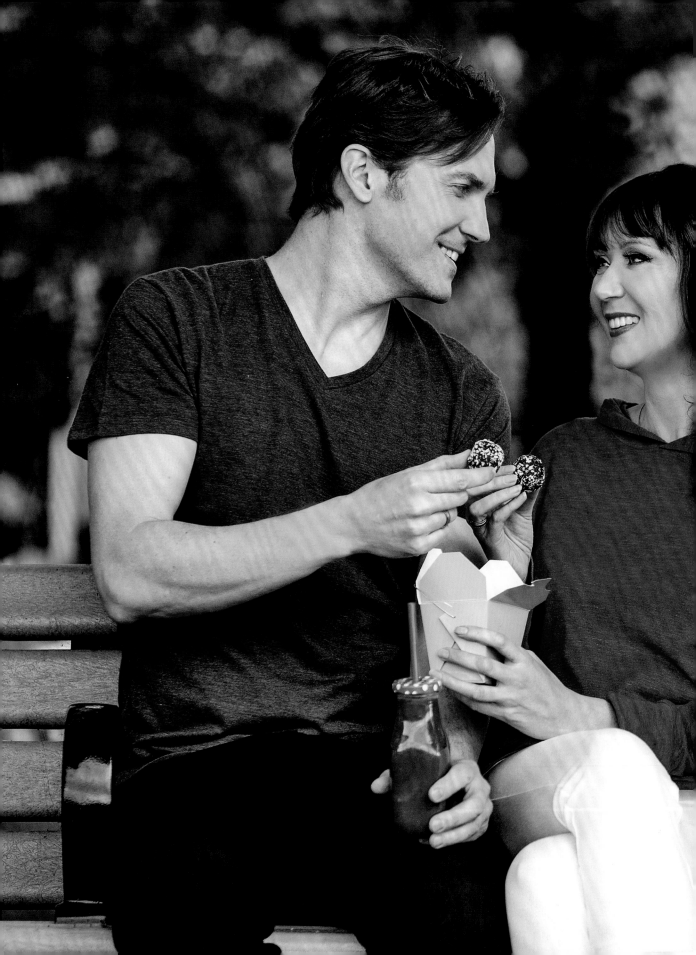

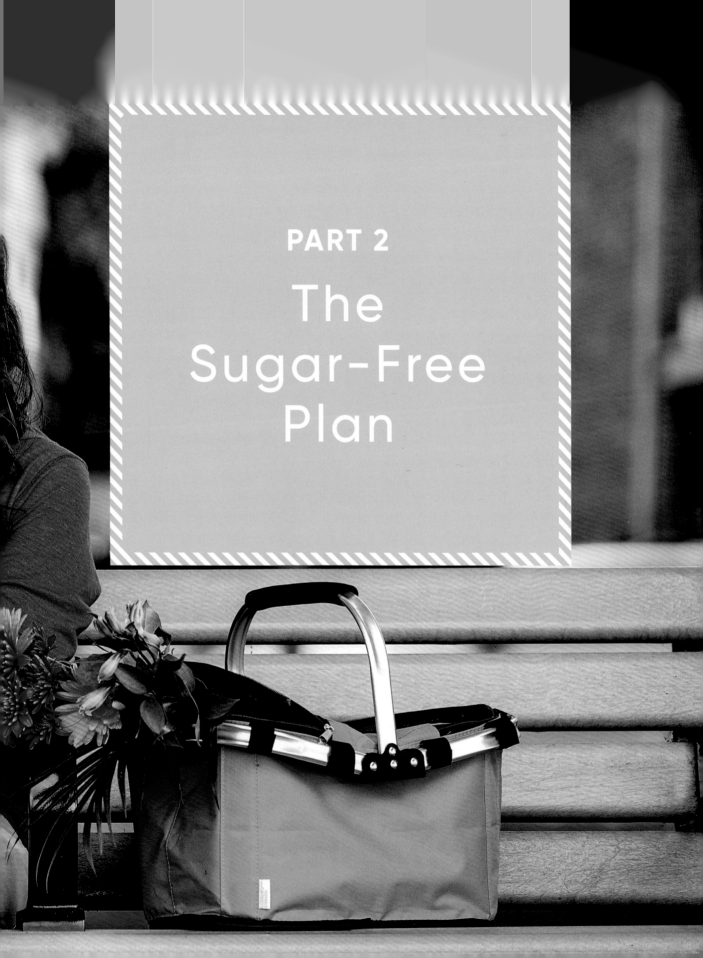

PART 2

The Sugar-Free Plan

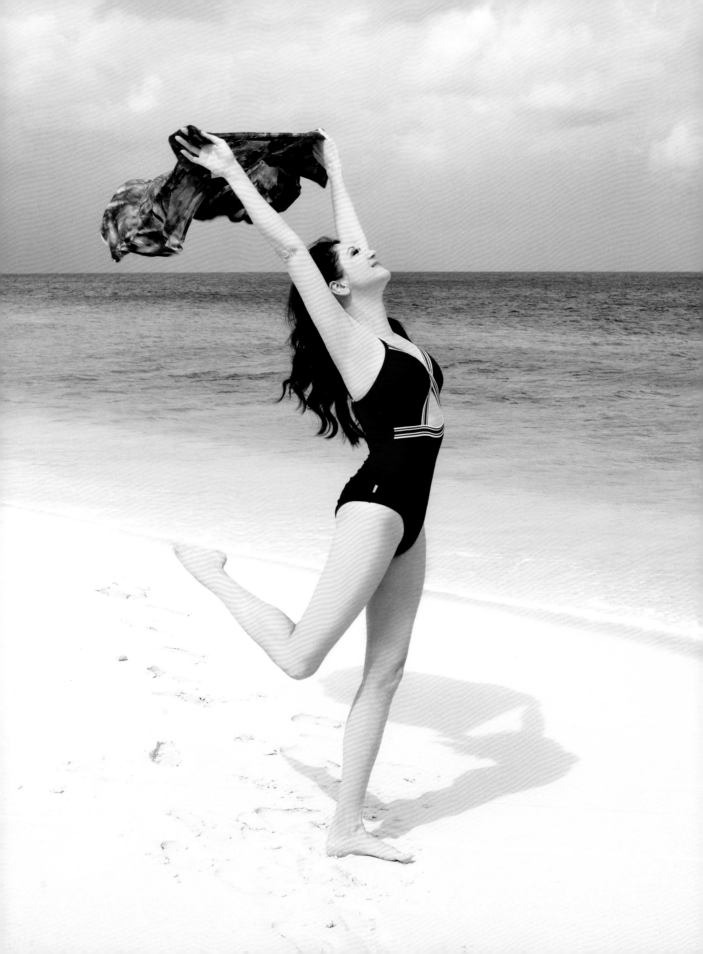

5

The Different Stages of Going Sugar-Free

It is time to put what you've learned into practice and make your plan a reality. To get started on your sugar-free life, you first should decide whether you are the type of person who sticks your toe in, who eases in slowly, or the type of person who likes to jump right in and get going. With the sugar-free life, you have two ways to move forward: go fast and advanced or go slow and easy. By choosing your own pace, you will feel empowered and in control. That way, you will be more likely to succeed. If you decide at any point that going fast is too much, instead of giving up entirely, you can slip back into the slower route and still feel like you're making progress. Likewise, if you choose the slow-and-steady route and feel ready to pursue the fast track, you can speed up results. Either way, you're taking a step forward and making progress, and you should celebrate that. People's happiness is not tied to their grandiose plans of success; their happiness is tied to their progress. Even if you take two steps forward and one step back, you are dancing.

Going sugar-free will mean something different for everybody. There are different levels of sugar-free living, and you have the opportunity to choose the best one for you. You can find your sweet spot at any of these levels and thrive.

OPTION 1: THE FAST BREAKUP: ELIMINATE ALL ADDED SUGARS AND ENJOY NATURAL SWEETNESS

Are you someone who wants to explore diving into the deep end and letting go of all sources of added sugar, even calorically dense alternative sweeteners? If you are curious about what happens when you let go of all sweeteners that contain excess calories, refined or alternative, this is the right track for you. Let's focus instead on naturally occurring sweetness in plants. Your palate will recalibrate, and healthy foods will start to taste amazing. Your mind can focus on big, important tasks, and you may notice a more joyous mood set in.

If you are ready for the fast track, then it is time to move away from all added sugars and instead focus on natural sugar-free replacements like monk fruit and stevia. You may also enjoy the naturally occurring sweetness of fruit and vegetables, such as dates, pineapples, mangoes, beets, carrots, sweet potatoes and more.

If you started on the slow track and want to go deeper, now is the time to try eliminating the alternative sweeteners that are rich in calories. If you are happy with natural unrefined sweeteners, that's fine too. Listen to your body and consider this option if you need a health boost or if you are ready to experience a true sugar-free lifestyle.

Optional Bonus: Letting Go of High Glycemic Carbohydrates

The most advanced (and optional) phase of going sugar-free is experimenting with a lower carb menu. This improves your metabolism and brainpower. If you have assessed with your medical team that you are insulin resistant or intolerant to carbohydrates, you may decide that you want to eliminate any and all sweeteners that contain calories—including honey and other unrefined natural sweeteners. In the sugar-free plan, we focus our attention on monk fruit and stevia, as they are easy to find and great zero-calorie options. These plant-based sweeteners contribute low or no carbohydrates to your menu and are super easy on the digestive system. In this phase, only use alcohol sweeteners for special occasions because they can cause digestive issues at higher doses. If you're going to use an alcohol sweetener, choose erythritol when possible, as it is the best tolerated.

Why Slow Down on Carbs?

Some people who are following a sugar-free lifestyle may feel that they need to adhere to a period of time when they eat a low-carb menu to help reset their metabolism and increase their insulin sensitivity. For those who struggle with their metabolism—for example, those with type 2 diabetes, metabolic syndrome and obesity—going lower carb helps improve insulin sensitivity so that they don't get completely derailed when they do eat a carb. By becoming fat adapted (able to fuel ourselves with healthy fat), insulin receptors can start to work correctly. When we rest our cells from insulin, we adapt and start to liberate fat stores.

Do You Need to Go Keto?

The classic ketogenic (keto) diet involves eating very few carbs (5 percent or less of your calories), moderate protein (25 percent), and high fat (70 percent). This can be very challenging to follow, but you may want to cycle in and out of a fat-fuelled, lower carb menu to get the results you are seeking. It can be challenging to forgo fruit, starchy vegetables and all grains, but for certain conditions, it is worth the effort.

Ketosis, where our liver makes ketones in the absence of carbohydrates, was never intended to be a permanent state because humans are metabolically flexible. We evolved to flip our fuel from carbs to fats and back again, depending on what we had available to us. In the deep winters of old, we could survive on a fat-fuelled menu because carbs were less readily available to us, so we would rely on preserved meats and fats that we could store like nuts and seeds. Instead of seeing the keto diet as a hard and rigid plan, we could see ourselves as cycling in and out of the keto state, depending on our personal needs.

If you have any neurological condition, such as mood disorders, any sort of epilepsy, brain injury or concussion, being on a keto or fat-fuelled menu is truly anti-inflammatory for the brain. In these conditions, it would be okay to extend the time you're on the keto plan with just the occasional experiment with carbs to keep your hormones and your family happy.

Limiting your sugar intake to follow a more ketogenic diet has immune and weight balancing benefits. It is used for people who suffer from autoimmunity and is being researched for its ability to reduce cancer cell growth.

Remember when we said sugar is the most common source of fuel for the body—but not the best? Ketones, which are produced when you're in ketosis, are an anti-inflammatory form of fuel. Ketones are produced when you don't take in any glucose. Ketones are made by your own liver and do not cause the metabolic issues that refined sugar does. Your liver takes them out of fat storage and uses them to fuel your body and brain, thereby burning body fat as fuel. This is much smoother than burning carbohydrates as fuel, which is why you don't have the mood imbalances or the highs and lows of energy when you're in ketosis. For a deep dive into the pros and cons of going ketogenic, visit www.JulieDaniluk.com for my special report.

My advice is to try a fat-fuelled, slow-releasing carbohydrate diet for a set amount of time, and if you feel great, jump further into the benefits of ketones. Many people are exploring the use of extra therapeutic ketones, aka exogenous ketone supplements such as BHB (beta-hydroxybutyrate), that allow you to use both carbs and ketones as fuel. Supplemental ketones can provide the body with a secondary fuel source that allows for greater energy and performance without a harsh restriction in carbohydrates.

It's up to you to choose whether to stay away from any added sweeteners or rich sources of carbohydrates in order to see the benefit of ketosis. I encourage you to let go of strict dogma and labels and allow yourself to be the metabolically flexible human you are meant to be. In that way, you have the greatest grace, ease and joy in your approach to your menu.

OPTION 2: THE SLOW BREAKUP: CUT OUT REFINED SUGAR AND EMBRACE HEALTHY ALTERNATIVES

Many people want to just break up with refined sugar. Where do we start? Sugar can hide under different names, as well. Avoid all added refined sugars, and that means don't add it to your food and don't eat foods with refined sugar listed in the ingredients. Check the list of different names for sugar on page 132. Refer to the list of the most common foods that sugar hides in on page 44.

The slow breakup focuses on eliminating refined sweeteners—for example, white sugar and corn syrup. First, let's talk about going slow. When we go slow, we go wide, because we are making changes that translate across many areas of our health. We are approaching this sugar-free life with a lot of substitutions that will make the journey easier and allow you to adapt to better alternative sweeteners in a lovely way. It's the alternative to cutting out all sweeteners cold turkey. By going slow, you're able to enjoy the alternative sweeteners that we know are healthier and that will be kinder to your blood sugar and your body.

It is time for you to let go of the refined sweeteners that are derailing your health efforts, as well as any sweeteners, even healthier alternatives, to which you may be sensitive. For example, I am intolerant to cane sugar; it's like my kryptonite. I need to avoid not only refined sugar, but also molasses, jaggery, cane syrup, maple syrup, dried cane juice and even coconut sugar because, like cane sugar, they contain sucrose and make me feel poorly. I can feel myself react to them quite quickly, so even though they're healthier options, I still need to avoid them. As you start out by replacing the refined sweeteners with healthier alternatives, test the waters a bit. See how you may or may not react differently to different sweeteners. Does maple syrup feel good, or does it cause your blood sugar to crash? Do you feel bloated or cranky after molasses? Does coconut sugar irritate your tummy? You'll be able to find out pretty quickly which alternative sweeteners are right for you. Kick any that cause you adverse reactions to the curb along with the refined sugar.

To play it safe with the best alternative sweeteners, I recommend avoiding those related to cane sugar because many of my clients are intolerant or sensitive to them. Instead of cane juice crystals or molasses, lean toward some of the new and dynamic choices outlined in Chapter 3, so that you can see if they feel better in your system. You'll know it feels better when your blood sugar stays more balanced. You may also notice that your mood stays elevated, you have more focus at work or school, your energy is more consistent and you don't have as many digestive issues.

Which calorically dense sweetener do I suggest if you want to go slow with a change? My personal favourite is raw honey. As humans, we have evolved to enjoy honey, and it helps heal the gut lining. It's easier for our bodies to handle because it's already been predigested by bees and it has the ability to kill off candida (when consumed raw). It doesn't elevate your insulin levels in the same way as refined sugar, and it's the go-to sweetener for autoimmune problems, anxiety, mental health issues, Crohn's disease, colitis and other inflammatory conditions.

To get started, review the complete guide to alternative sweeteners on page 53. You'll notice that there are ones to avoid and ones to include in your sugar-free lifestyle, as well as my favourite ones to enjoy. Again, to be safe, start with raw honey and buy monk fruit as soon as you can to enjoy many of the truly sugar-free recipes in Part 3 of this book.

If you feel good about where you're at in this option, enjoy it! If you want to try the faster, truly sugar-free option, we'll be right there with you.

INTERMITTENT FASTING (TIME-RESTRICTED EATING)

Intermittent fasting (IF), also known as time-restricted eating, refers to a meal schedule that reduces the eating window to eight to ten hours per day to increase detoxification and weight loss. It is a powerful tool in the fight against sugar because it helps you avoid overeating at night and improves insulin sensitivity. An overnight fast of eight to ten hours is normal for most people. With IF, you simply expand the amount of time you avoid food to twelve, fourteen or even sixteen hours. If you are new to IF, or time-restricted eating, I suggest you start slow and enjoy food from 8 AM to 8 PM. When you are ready, you can cut time off as desired. For example, if you want to fast for fourteen hours, you would stop eating at 7 PM and then eat again at 9 AM the following day. I don't suggest extensive fasting in the morning for women, as it can impact their thyroid hormones.

Intermittent fasting (or time-restricted eating) has a number of amazing benefits, including:

1. It increases insulin sensitivity and reduces carb cravings. IF reduces the risk of type 2 diabetes. It shuttles the sugar into your cells more effectively, reducing the inflammatory effects of advanced glycation end products (AGEs). When insulin is reduced, your metabolism burns more body fat as fuel.

2. It balances leptin sensitivity. If your leptin signalling is working properly, a surge in your leptin level will signal your brain that you are full. Your hunger and cravings go down without the need for forced willpower.

3. It promotes human growth hormone (HGH) production. Research has shown that fasting can raise HGH by as much as 1300 percent in women and 2000 percent in men, which plays an essential role in health, fitness and slowing the aging process. HGH is also a fat-burning hormone, which helps explain why fasting is so effective for weight loss.

4. It helps lower triglyceride levels and improves other biomarkers of disease for example, hypertension.

5. It reduces oxidative stress. By eating in smaller windows, your body does not use precious antioxidants to decrease the accumulation of oxidative radicals from food. It can focus on the repair of our cells, reducing aging at a cellular level.

6. It has proposed benefits such as reduced risk of cancer, improved blood sugar control and increased longevity as shown in animal studies.

7. It promotes weight loss. In the January 1998 issue of the journal *Diabetes Care*, a group of researchers investigated the effect of IF on type 2 diabetics. After treatment, the fasting group lost more weight than the control group.

Does Intermittent Fasting Reduce Inflammation?

The answer is a definite yes. One study published in the journal *Nutrition Research* revealed that men and women who practised fasting had lower levels of circulating proinflammatory markers (that is, cytokines like IL-1β, IL-6 and TNF-α). Furthermore, their systolic and diastolic blood pressures, body weight and body fat percentage were significantly lower.

Before starting intermittent fasting, talk to your health care practitioner to ensure that it would be safe for you to do.

THE SUGAR-FREE PLAN SUMMARY TABLE

Remember that one option is not better than the other. Relax, breathe and decide on your own path without the pressure to do it perfectly or right. I have swung in and out of both of these options for fourteen years now. Both options have advantages. The fast breakup gets rapid and great results, but the slow breakup works better with family life and a travel schedule—and let's face it . . . carbs are delicious!

OPTION 1: THE FAST BREAKUP

Foods to Avoid

Sugar: Look for hidden sugar in packaged foods: agave nectar, barley malt, brown sugar, cane sugar, caramel, castor sugar, confectioners powdered sugar, corn syrup or high-fructose corn syrup, date sugar, demerara sugar, dextrin and maltodextrin, dextrose or crystal dextrose, evaporated cane juice or fruit juice, evaporated corn sweetener, fructose, glucose, lactose, maltodextrin, maltose, mannose, maple syrup, molasses, r=aw sugar, rice syrup, simple syrup, succanat, sucrose, sweet sorghum, tapioca syrup and turbinado sugar. See a complete list on page 132.

Refined Flour: Avoid all forms of refined flour because they quickly become sugar in your mouth. For example, avoid conventional bread, pasta, pastry and cereals (see alternative on the following pages). Also consider reducing or eliminating other gluten grass grains, including spelt, kamut, barley, oats and rye.

Alcohol: Alcoholic beverages such as wine, beer, hard cider, rum and mixed drinks are loaded with sugar and yeast and are very hard on the brain and liver.

Dairy: Avoid conventionally processed cheeses (that is, boxed macaroni and cheese). Dairy is high in lactose sugar and can feed infections and inflammation if you are sensitive, allergic or intolerant. If you are of African or Asian heritage, you have a much higher chance of being lactose intolerant.

Carbonated Beverages: Soda contains 9 teaspoons of sugar per can and is very inflammatory. Artificial sweeteners are dangerous and best avoided. Sparkling mineral water is permitted.

Pickled and Smoked Meats: Hot dogs, corned beef, smoked fish and luncheon meat contain nitrates and sugars that are dangerous to human health.

Other Carbs That Convert to Sugar Easily: Potatoes, corn, white rice, popcorn, chips, corn chips and so on.

Allowed Alternatives
(Balance Insulin and Blood Sugar with Lower Carb Choices)

Sweeteners: The only sweeteners to use freely are monk fruit or stevia extract, as they are calorie-free and make the transition to natural sweetness possible. Other low-calorie options (that is, erythritol) can be used for special occasions.

Fruit: Low-sugar fruit can be enjoyed. Focus on berries, avocado, pomegranate, apples, plums, peaches, citrus fruits, kiwi fruit and cranberries (sugar-free).

Note: If you are feeling fragile and close to bingeing on sugar, the safest choices are dates or raw honey because they are easy to digest and do not cause as much digestive or brain inflammation. Before you eat them, try to get to the root of why you feel you want to binge. Do you feel sad, angry or lonely? Reach out for help and eat whole foods to prevent a slip.

Foods to Focus On

Hydration: Drink eight to twelve glasses of healthy fluids a day such as pure water, green juice, stevia-sweetened lemonade or herbal tea. Dilute veggie juices higher in natural sugars, such as beet and carrot, with pure water to maintain smooth blood sugar levels.

Vegetables: Make 50 percent of your diet brightly coloured and dark green vegetables and aim to eat ten servings a day. Eat as many low-starch greens as possible, such as kale, broccoli, cabbage, chard, celery and dandelion. If you have irritable bowel syndrome (IBS) or a sensitive stomach, it is best to steam vegetables until tender. Enjoy all green vegetables, red onions, red cabbage, garlic, spinach, kale, broccoli, cauliflower, parsley, cilantro, artichoke and Brussels sprouts. Only eat red sweet pepper, eggplant or tomato if tolerant to nightshades.

Dairy Alternatives: Use unsweetened almond, cashew, sunflower, coconut or hemp milk or beverage as desired.

Grains: Eliminate grain consumption if you want to lose weight or suffer from heavy inflammation, as they are high in carbs and lectins. If you must eat grains, rotate the choice of gluten-free grain (wild rice, quinoa, amaranth, buckwheat and teff) to avoid developing an allergy. Soak grains in spring water before cooking to increase digestibility.

Meat: Free-range or organic chicken, turkey, lamb, wild game, emu and eco-friendly fish such as arctic char, spring trout, wild line-caught Pacific salmon, sardines and halibut are good options.

OPTION 1: THE FAST BREAKUP

Allowed Alternatives
(Balance Insulin and Blood Sugar with Lower Carb Choices)

Raw and Freshly Roasted Nuts and Seeds: Brazil nuts, filberts, pumpkin seeds, hemp seeds, sunflower seeds, sesame seeds, flax or chia seeds and nut butters made from these options.

Beans: Navy, adzuki, kidney, black, turtle, lima, red, white and mung beans, chickpeas, split peas and lentils are a good source of protein and fibre when sprouted and/or cooked well. Limit intake if you suffer from inflammatory bowel disease (IBD). Eliminate bean consumption if you suffer from substantial inflammation, as they are high in carbs and lectins.

Snacks: Nuts and seeds, kale chips, fresh coconut slices, seasoned seaweed and many of the sugar-free recipes featured in this book, such as Tummy Gummies (page 261) and Keto Seed Crackers (page 191).

Salad Dressing: Make your own using lemon or lime juice and good-quality olive oil. Enjoy the liquid from fermented veggies as a good substitute for white vinegar. When using restaurant or health food store dressings, the least harmful vinegar is apple cider vinegar. Avoid cheap balsamic vinegar, as it contains sugar. Use garlic for its antifungal qualities.

Spices and Herbs: Cloves, oregano, cinnamon, ginger, turmeric, rosemary, sage, curry, basil, cilantro, cumin, caraway, thyme, nutmeg, allspice, star anise, tarragon and parsley.

Eat Slow Carbs in Moderation: Yams and sweet potatoes, carrots, red beets, celeriac root, rutabaga and pumpkin can be enjoyed unless following the low-carb plan.

OPTION 2: THE SLOW BREAKUP

Foods to Avoid

Sugar: Look for hidden sugar in packaged foods: agave nectar, barley malt, brown sugar, cane sugar, caramel, castor sugar, confectioners powdered sugar, corn syrup or high-fructose corn syrup, demerara sugar, dextrin and maltodextrin, dextrose or crystal dextrose, evaporated cane juice or fruit juice, evaporated corn sweetener, fructose, glucose, lactose, maltodextrin, maltose, mannose, raw sugar, rice syrup, simple syrup, succanat, sucrose, sweet sorghum and turbinado sugar. These are all forms of sugar that can cause brain inflammation.

Refined flour: Avoid all forms of refined flour, such as bread, pasta, pastry and cereals, as they quickly become sugar in your mouth. Reduce other gluten-containing grass grains, including spelt, kamut, barley, oats and rye, as best as you can.

Alcohol: Alcoholic beverages such as wine, beer, hard cider, rum and mixed drinks are loaded with sugar and yeast and are very hard on the brain and liver.

Dairy: Avoid milk, cheese, ice cream, etc. Use unsweetened almond, cashew, sunflower, coconut or hemp milk or beverage as desired. If you must eat dairy, sheep and goat milk are easier to digest, or look for lactose-free cheese.

Carbonated beverages: Soda contains 9 teaspoons of sugar per can and is very inflammatory. Artificial sweeteners are dangerous and best avoided. Sparkling mineral water with added fruit is permitted.

Pickled and smoked meats: Hot dogs, corned beef, smoked fish and luncheon meat contain nitrates and sugars that are dangerous to human health.

Reduce carbs that convert to sugar easily: Potatoes, corn, white rice, popcorn, chips, corn chips and so on.

Allowed Alternatives

Sweeteners: When necessary, use small amounts of honey and dates, but remember that this is a type of sugar and will slow down weight loss efforts. Explore all of the green and yellow alternatives in the Ultimate Sweetener Conversion Chart on page 80. Limit the use of coconut nectar, maple products and molasses to emergencies only, because they are also sources of sucrose. The only sweeteners to use freely are monk fruit or stevia extract, as they are low calorie

Allowed Alternatives

and make the transition to natural sweetness possible. Yacón syrup is permitted, but it is high in prebiotic fibres, so reduce intake if it causes gas.

Fruit: Raw fruit, dry fruit and fruit sauces can be used as sweeteners and thickeners in baking. Focus on berries, avocado, pomegranate, apples, plums, peaches, citrus fruits, pineapple, kiwi fruit, cherries and sugar-free cranberries. For those with digestive troubles, turn to easy-to-digest sweeteners. Although the sweeteners in option 2 are natural and unrefined and come with beneficial minerals and vitamins, some of them may still be difficult to digest for some people. If you have a bowel problem like diarrhea, IBS, constipation, Crohn's disease and so on, your body may not break down disaccharides well because they have double bonds that require enzymes that might be in short supply. In this case, you would want to eliminate maple syrup, molasses, coconut sugar and the other sweeteners listed above, except for honey. Raw honey is a safe, easy-to-digest sweetener that most people with bowel issues can tolerate. Enjoy raw honey in place of the unrefined sweeteners listed above and you should find that your digestive problems start to clear up. Fruit nectars or juice (for example, pear nectar) are permitted in moderation if well tolerated.

No matter what phase you land in, you're doing your body a favour by kicking refined sugar to the curb. Find your comfort zone and enjoy it. And remember that your comfort zone today might be different from your comfort zone six months from now. Explore the sugar-free continuum and relish the authentic joy it brings.

THE MANY NAMES FOR SUGAR

Here is a list of all refined sugars. Keep a copy in your wallet to hand to waiters and chefs. If you are sensitive to gluten or dairy, it is good to make a list for those items as well.

Avoid

- Agave nectar
- Agave syrup
- Barbados sugar
- Barley malt (or barley malt syrup)
- Beet sugar
- Brown sugar
- Buttered syrup
- Cane juice crystals (light)
- Cane sugar
- Caramel
- Castor sugar
- Confectioners powdered sugar
- Corn sweetener
- Corn syrup or high-fructose corn syrup (aka HFCS)
- Demerara sugar
- Dextrin and maltodextrin
- Dextrose or crystal dextrose
- Evaporated corn sweetener
- Fructose (aka fructose solids)
- Glucose (aka glucose solids)
- Golden sugar
- Golden syrup
- Golden treacle
- Grape sugar
- Icing sugar
- Invert sugar
- Lactose
- Maltodextrin
- Maltose
- Malt syrup
- Mannose
- Muscovado (light or golden)
- Panocha
- Powdered sugar
- Raw sugar
- Refiner's syrup
- Rice syrup
- Saccharose
- Simple syrup (aka syrup)
- Sucrose
- Sugar (granulated sugar)
- Sweet sorghum (sorghum syrup)
- Tapioca syrup
- Turbinado sugar
- Yellow sugar

Unrefined Sugars That Are Not Ideal Because of High Insulin Response and High Glycemic Index

- Maple syrup (maple sugar)
- Black treacle
- Molasses
- Jaggery
- Succanant
- Cane juice
- Dark muscovado
- Dehydrated cane juice
- Evaporated cane juice

Well-Tolerated Alternative Sweeteners Permitted in Option 2, The Slow Breakup (Use in Small Amounts Because of Moderate Insulin Response)

- Coconut palm sugar (aka palm sugar)
- Coconut nectar
- Raw honey
- Dates and other fruit

Remember to Cut All Artificial Sweeteners Because They Have Side Effects and Spike Cravings

- Acesulfame K (aka Ace-K, ACE, and acesulfame potassium).
- Aspartame, APM, aspartyl-phenylalanine methyl ester and related sweeteners called Advantame and Alitame, and Neotame brand names: NutraSweet, Equal, Spoonful, Equal Measure, Canderel, Benevia, AminoSweet, NatraTaste.

- Saccharin (aka sodium saccharin, calcium saccharin and potassium saccharin). Brand names: Sweet'N Low, Necta Sweet, Cologran, Hermesetas, Sucaryl, Sucron, Sugar Twin, Sweet 10.
- Cyclamate (aka calcium cyclamate, cyclamic acid and sodium cyclamate). Brand names: Sucaryl, Cologran.

- Isomalt brand names: DiabetiSweet, ClearCut, Decomalt.
- Sucralose (aka 4,1′,6′-trichlorogal-actosucrose). Brand names: Splenda, Nevella.

SUPPLEMENTS THAT BUST CARB CRAVINGS AND BALANCE BLOOD SUGAR

Berberine	A compound that can be extracted from many different plants, such as goldenseal (*Hydrastis canadensis*), Oregon grape (*Berberis aquifolium*), barberry (*Berberis vulgaris*), Chinese goldthread (*Coptis chinensis*), Californian poppy (*Eschscholzia californica*) and tree turmeric (*Berberis aristata*). Many studies show that berberine can decrease blood sugar levels in people with type 2 diabetes. It works by decreasing insulin resistance, making the insulin more effective and responsive to blood sugar, decreasing sugar production in the liver and slowing the break-down of carbohydrates in the gastrointestinal (GI) tract.
Zinc	A mineral commonly used for the immune system. There are many studies to support its use in people with diabetes or poor blood sugar regulation. It can decrease blood sugar levels two hours after a meal and decrease hemoglobin A1C. There also seems to have been a reduction in total cholesterol and low-density lipoprotein (LDL) in those who took zinc compared to placebo.

SUPPLEMENTS THAT BUST CARB CRAVINGS AND BALANCE BLOOD SUGAR

Chromium	An essential trace mineral that can augment the actions of insulin. Studies show that the use of chromium helps maintain healthy glucose levels for people with blood sugar concerns. It helps insulin regulate blood sugar, and it enhances insulin absorption, resulting in a reduction of blood sugar. Because of this effect, it also seems to decrease cravings for carbohydrates.
Alpha-Lipoic Acid	An antioxidant that helps our mitochondria produce energy. Studies have shown that it can improve blood sugar metabolism, reduce insulin resistance and lower fasting blood glucose and hemoglobin A1C. Because of its strong antioxidant action, it can help support nerves and treat diabetic neuropathy by decreasing oxidative stress and supporting nerve regeneration.
Bitter Melon (*Momordica charantia*)	A vegetable that contains constituents shown to improve glycemic control by improving insulin signalling pathways and improving glucose tolerance. The evidence shows that bitter melon affects blood sugar levels by decreasing it in both a fasting state and after a meal.
Holy Basil (*Ocimum tenuiflorum*)	Holy basil supplement, not the culinary basil you find in the kitchen, has been shown to help decrease fasting blood glucose and glucose levels following a meal. In addition, research suggests that holy basil can be used in conjunction with diet and drug therapy in the treatment of mild to moderate type 2 diabetes and can significantly decrease hemoglobin A1C when added as adjunctive therapy to diabetes medications compared to medication alone.
Globe Artichokes	A flower bud that has a long history of use as a digestive and liver tonic, but its properties in helping weight loss have only recently been discovered. Artichoke can have some rather unusual effects on your appetite, causing an alteration in taste perception; this is called "the artichoke effect" and is caused by some chemical components the plant contains. Along with altering taste, artichokes can also decrease the craving for

SUPPLEMENTS THAT BUST CARB CRAVINGS AND BALANCE BLOOD SUGAR

Globe Artichokes (continued)	some foods and make them less desirable during meals, leading to weight loss. Cynarin and chlorogenic acid are the main components found in artichokes that inhibit taste buds. For people who are concerned about gallstones, the active compounds in artichoke reduce the accumulation of bile salts that crystallize into stones. Their high fibre content can help you feel full.
Fenugreek (*Trigonella foenum-graecum*)	Excellent for blood sugar balance. Studies have shown that participants with type 2 diabetes had significantly lower blood sugar levels after consuming fenugreek seeds. These effects can take a few months, but fenugreek works well at decreasing both fasting blood sugar and hemoglobin A1C by slowing down digestion and absorption of carbohydrates. Fenugreek is also beneficial for improving blood cholesterol levels by decreasing circulating LDL and increasing high-density lipoprotein (HDL). It also has shown an ability to significantly decrease triglycerides and total cholesterol.
Bilberries (*Vaccinium myrtillus*) and blueberries (*Vaccinium angustifolium*)	Contain anthocyanins, which are antioxidants that help improve circulation and can enhance the strength of capillaries and artery walls through enhancing collagen integrity and stabilizing capillary permeability. Bilberry extract may reduce inflammation and is useful in the treatment of conditions such as rheumatoid arthritis and circulation problems that have been linked to heart disease. Bilberry and blueberry extract also contains a substance called glucoquinine, a type of anthocyanin that can stimulate the secretion of insulin and prevent the breakdown and absorption of carbs in your GI tract.
Turmeric	Contains curcumin, an active component credited with providing many health benefits. We know how great it is for inflammation. A systematic review has found that it can help decrease blood sugar levels and hemoglobin A1C and improve insulin sensitivity. It also helps decrease complications associated with diabetes, such as liver dysfunction and neuropathies (damage or dysfunction of one or more nerves that typically results in numbness, tingling, muscle weakness and pain in the affected area).

SUPPLEMENTS THAT BUST CARB CRAVINGS AND BALANCE BLOOD SUGAR

Ashwagandha Root	An adaptogen (stress-reducing herb) that can be added to nut butter or smoothies. Its many benefits include decreased hyperglycemia, reduction of corticosterone, decreased incidence of gastric ulcers, alleviated symptoms of depression, prevention of loss of libido, prevention of decreases in cognitive function and reduced incidence and reversal of immunosuppression.
B Vitamins	Important because of their synergistic effect, but it is particularly important to increase vitamin B6, as it is a precursor to serotonin. When serotonin is low, we crave more food. By consuming more avocados, chicken, green peas and other foods high in vitamin B6, we can reduce our emotional food cravings. If you still struggle, supplementing vitamin B6 (100 mg/day) has shown some beneficial effects on cravings. B vitamins are involved in converting carbohydrates into energy and the metabolism of proteins and fats. Vitamin B6 is also involved in the metabolism of estrogens, leading to greater hormonal balance, which can reduce cravings caused by premenstrual syndrome (PMS).
L-carnitine	Helpful in the absence of glucose when the body switches to producing energy from fat stores. Amino acids, such as L-carnitine, play a crucial role in the production of energy by transporting fatty acids into your cells' mitochondria. There are several types of carnitine: D-carnitine, acetyl-L-carnitine, L-carnitine and L-tartrate, to name just a few. Acetyl-L-carnitine seems to be the most effective and better used by the body. Another great benefit of L-carnitine is that it increases a key enzyme called AMPK (5' AMP-activated protein kinase), which improves your ability to use up carbs by increasing your muscle's sensitivity to insulin. In fact, it seems to decrease insulin release as well as improve overall blood sugar levels after drinking a glucose solution.
Ubiquinol	The active form of coenzyme Q10 (CoQ10) is an antioxidant produced naturally in your body that can help with a wide range of health benefits, including energy production, as it is stored in the mitochondria. Because heart muscle cells have more mitochondria than other cells, ubiquinol is well known for its cardiovascular benefits. It also helps with glucose metabolism,

SUPPLEMENTS THAT BUST CARB CRAVINGS AND BALANCE BLOOD SUGAR

Ubiquinol (continued)	lipid profiles and reduces oxidative stress. In people who have diabetes, CoQ10 can significantly improve insulin sensitivity, helping with sugar metabolism even though blood sugar levels remained unchanged.
Supplemental Ketones	Recently, scientists discovered in a laboratory how to make a supplement called Beta-Hydroxybutarate (BHB), an exogenous ketone that assists weight loss in three ways. Ketones (BHB) fuel the brain as an alternative fuel source, reducing hunger stress and helping to tell the body, "You are safe." Because you feel safe and "not starving," BHB helps reduce carb cravings directly, as your body is not needing glucose to fuel the brain. Moreover, when you balance your energy needs, you prime insulin receptors to shuttle any glucose in your blood into your cells to be burned as energy instead of it lingering outside the cells, which can create inflammation and trigger fat storage. Because ketones (BHB) fuel the brain and vital organs, any glucose can be used to create glycogen—energy for your muscles. This allows for maximum muscle performance, which leads to larger muscles, which can translate to a faster metabolism. You can burn more calories per hour with more muscle with the side benefit of greater mobility as you age. Studies show that a great way in which ketones (BHB) help with natural weight loss is that they can reduce anxiety by up to 30 percent. Since many people eat carbs in response to stress, by reducing anxiety, people report more willpower in combating their cravings. Research also suggests that ketones (BHB) may help increase brown fat in the body; this is a healthy type of fat that is metabolically active and keeps your hormones well adjusted. Ketones (BHB) also reduce inflammation, a key culprit in weight gain. Using ketone supplements can reduce excess sodium in your system, so you may be able to enjoy more unrefined pink salt if you have low blood pressure.

Let go of the rigid meal plan! I have been a nutritionist for more than twenty years, and one thing I have learned is that no one follows a rigid meal plan for long because it does not fit into their lifestyle. Ninety-five percent of people will fall off a diet with a restricted meal plan, so let's forgo the meal plan and instead embrace delicious and satisfying recipes as part of a sustainable eating plan that I like to call the Live-It.

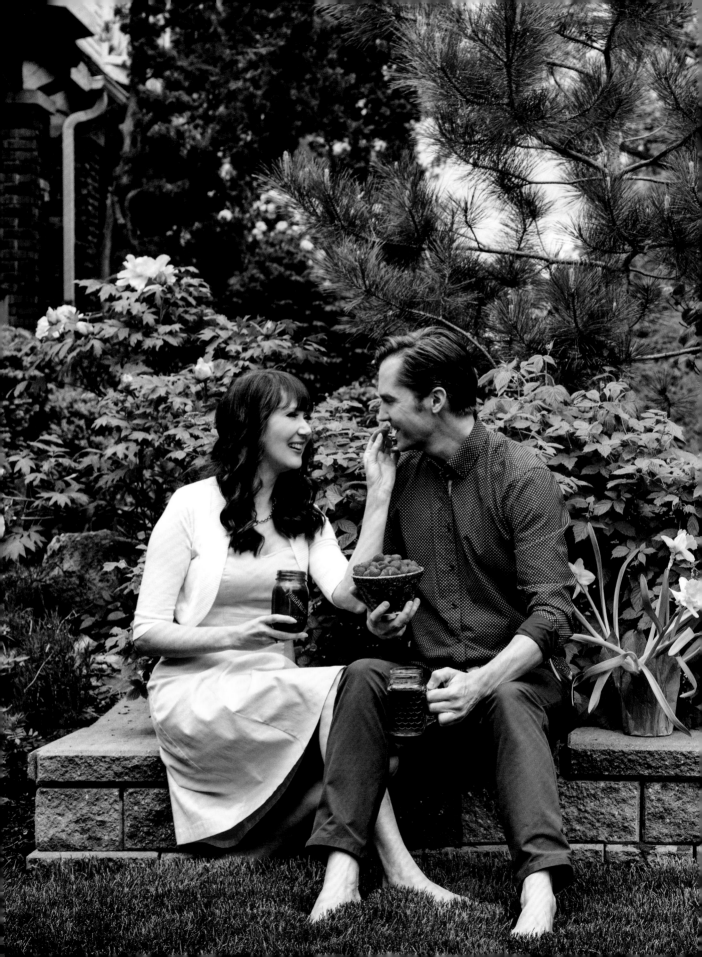

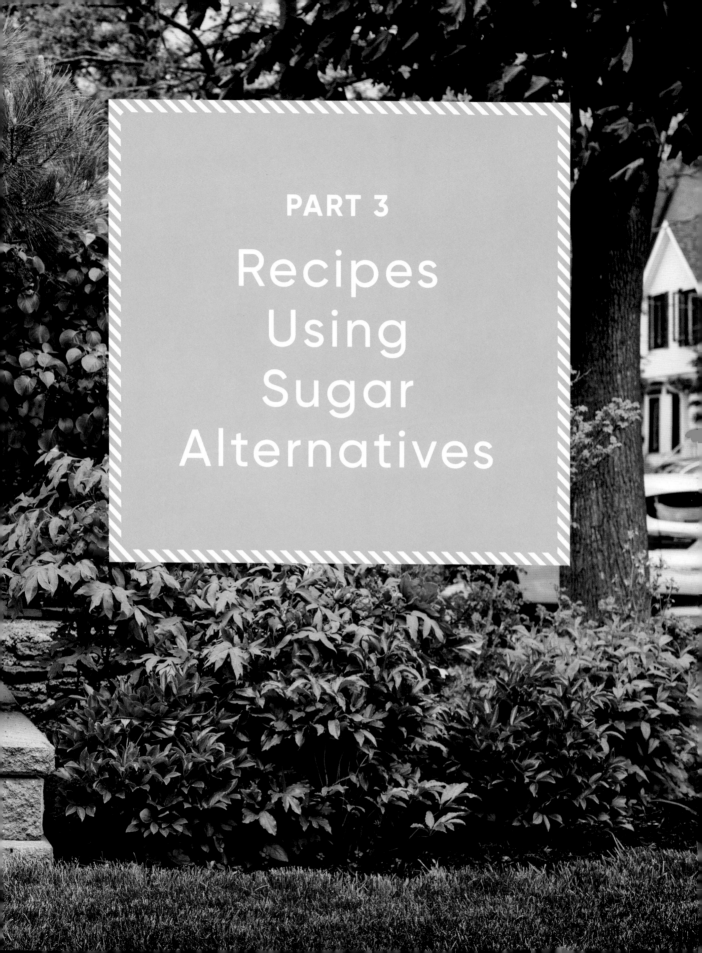

PART 3

Recipes Using Sugar Alternatives

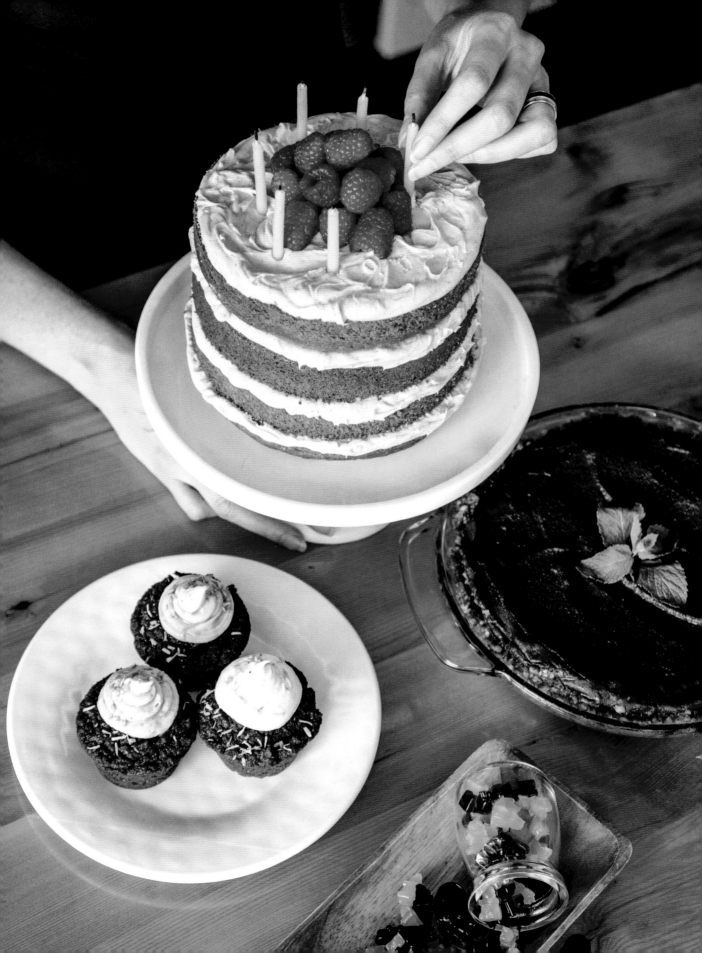

As you're about to embark on this journey, let's set a positive intention for your healing. It feels awesome to anticipate the results you will get from going sugar-free with enthusiasm, strength and a little sparkle of mystery. I can't wait for you to try these delicious recipes that use a bounty of alternative sweeteners that range from zero to moderate levels of carbohydrate. I start with delicious beverages that have low carb options. As we do not perceive sugar calories when they are delivered in beverage form, I recommend that you choose the "no sugar added" option to improve your health whenever possible. The breads and crackers will help you stay away from white flour, which rapidly breaks down into sugar, and the cookies and squares will provide daily treats so that you can treat yourself instead of cheat yourself. I would like you to focus on the crave-busting mains and sides, because real food provides all of the nutrients you need to heal. I made sure to create some tasty special occasion treats so you can splash out when you need something fancy. These recipes are straight from my kitchen to yours and will allow you to have the flavours you crave while getting the health you deserve.

At the beginning of each recipe, the following symbols will offer clarity on dietary designations, restrictions and options:

 Free of grain and its derivatives

 Free of eggs and egg products

 Free of soy and its derivatives

 Free of peanuts and tree nuts

 Free of dairy and its derivatives

 Vegan (free of animal products and their derivatives)

 No sugar added

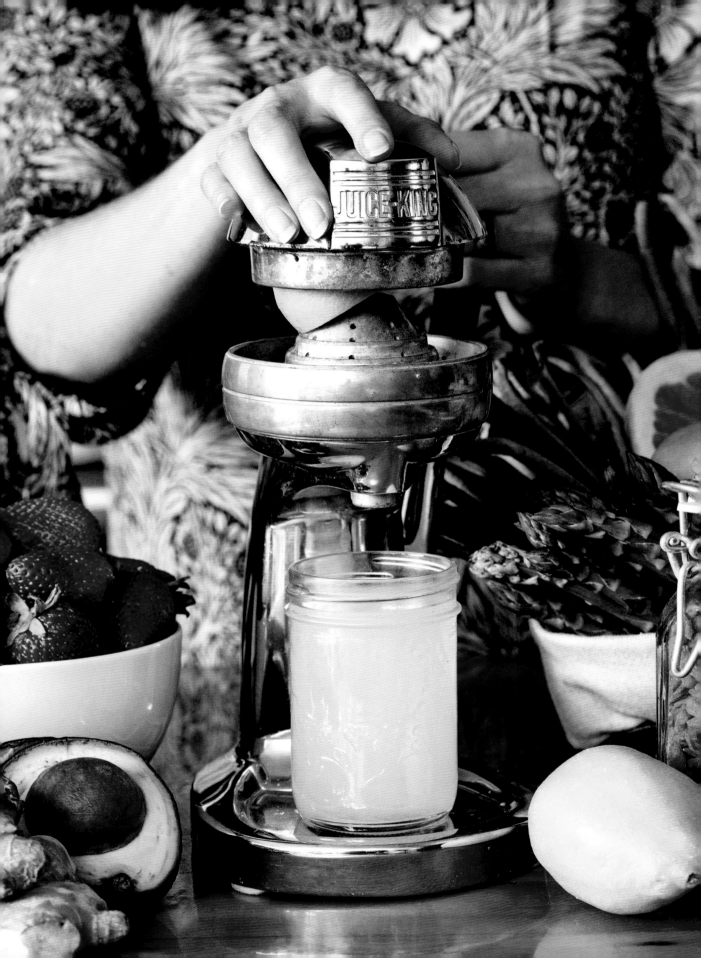

Liquid Healing

Liquid Happiness

     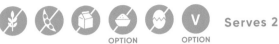   Serves 2

Chocolate has an almost magical power to shift your mood. It not only tastes great but also contains phenylethylamine (PEA), which boosts the release of the feel-good neurotransmitters serotonin and dopamine. Perhaps this is why so many people are addicted to chocolate. But beware of the white sugar and poor-quality oils in conventional chocolate. If you find yourself reaching for chocolate for the good feelings, this shake brings all the fun without the sugar-related crash.

2 cups unsweetened non-dairy milk, warm or cold

⅔ cup fresh or thawed frozen pitted dark cherries

1 tablespoon + 1½ teaspoons raw cacao powder

¼ teaspoon pure monk fruit extract (or 2 teaspoons yacón, raw honey or coconut nectar)

2 tablespoons unsweetened nut or seed butter

1 teaspoon pure vanilla extract

1 teaspoon cinnamon

2 tablespoons collagen or vegan protein powder

Optional Boosters (use 1 to 4)

1 tablespoon ground flaxseed or chia seeds (thickens it nicely)

1 teaspoon maca powder

½ teaspoon ground ginger

1 cup packed baby spinach

1. Place all ingredients, and any boosters, in a high-speed blender and blend until smooth. Pour into 2 glasses. Serve warm or cold.

No Sugar Added Option: Use pure monk fruit extract.

Vegan Option: Use vegan protein powder and omit the honey.

Jolly Roger Juice

 Serves 2

Vegetable juices help to cut down on our sugar cravings, and whichever veggies you choose, you will be ready for your next adventure with more energy. Celery and ginger are both shown to reduce stomach upset, so reach for this drink when your tummy is unhappy. If you have an active stomach ulcer, omit the lemon but don't worry—as your stomach lining heals, sour foods can be reintroduced. You can swap the apple for a few drops of monk fruit to reduce the carbs.

3 stalks kale or romaine lettuce (or 3 cups chopped green cabbage)
3 stalks celery
1 medium English cucumber
½ lemon, peeled
1 large apple, cored (or 4 drops pure monk fruit extract)

Optional (use 1 to 4)
1-inch piece fresh ginger
Pinch of ground nutmeg
½ cup fresh flat-leaf or curly parsley
1 cup chopped fennel, bulb and/or fronds

1. Chop all of the vegetables and fruits to fit the opening of your juicer.

2. Starting with the kale, run the ingredients and, if desired, the optional ingredients through the juicer a handful at a time. If desired, run the pulp through the juicer a second time to extract the maximum amount of juice. Pour into 2 glasses and serve.

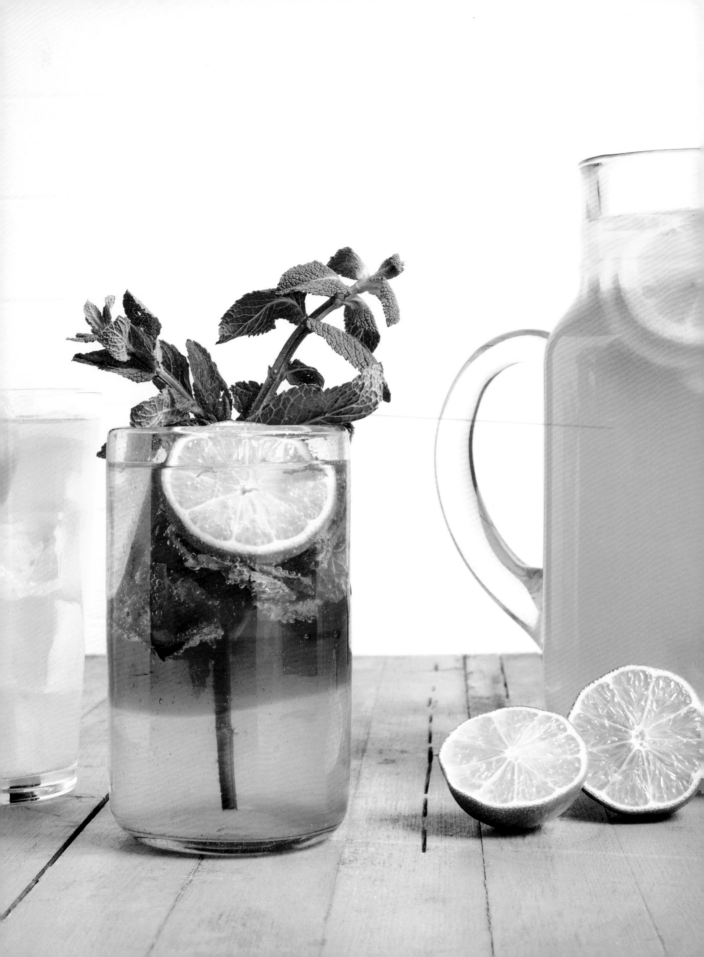

Keto Mock Mojito

   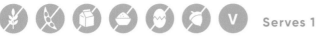   **Serves 1**

I love that this drink is a great alternative when you don't want to consume alcohol or sugar at social events. It has become my favourite drink to order, as most bars have sparkling mineral water, mint leaves and fresh lime juice. I add monk fruit sweetener, which I carry in my purse. Rum is made from fermented cane sugar, so it is important to avoid it when embracing a sugar-free lifestyle. You can double this recipe and use a standard bottle of sparkling mineral water for a great party share.

½ cup fresh mint leaves

2 to 3 tablespoons lime juice (1 to 2 limes)

8 to 10 drops pure monk fruit extract (or 4 to 5 drops liquid stevia)

1 teaspoon inositol powder (optional)

½ cup ice cubes

1½ cups sparkling mineral water

1. Place the mint in a sturdy 16-ounce glass and bruise it with a wooden muddle or spoon. Place half of a squeezed lime in the bottom of the glass.

2. Add the lime juice, monk fruit and inositol powder (if using). Muddle, add the ice cubes and top with sparkling mineral water. Adjust sweetness to taste and serve cold.

Nutmeg Vegan Nog

      Serves 2

OPTION   OPTION

This low-carb, vegan twist on a holiday classic is a favourite at my holiday gatherings. The monk fruit version is thirty calories per cup, making it the gift that keeps on giving. In the spirit of giving, pass this tasty anti-inflammatory recipe along to a friend for their next party. But don't just leave this drink for festive gatherings. It tastes so good warmed in the winter and over ice in the summer.

3 cups unsweetened cashew or coconut beverage, warm or cold

¼ to ½ teaspoon pure monk fruit extract (or 3 tablespoons pure maple syrup or coconut nectar)

1 teaspoon pure vanilla extract

½ to 1 teaspoon cinnamon

¼ teaspoon ground nutmeg

⅛ teaspoon ground turmeric

Optional (use 1 to 3)

Swirl of Coconut Whipping Cream (page 227)

¼ teaspoon ground cardamom

Pinch of cinnamon or ground nutmeg

1. Place all ingredients in a high-speed blender and blend until well mixed and frothy.

2. Pour into 2 glasses and, if desired, top with Coconut Whipping Cream and sprinkle with cardamom, cinnamon or nutmeg. Serve warm or cold.

No Sugar Added Option: Use pure monk fruit extract.

Shamrock Shake

      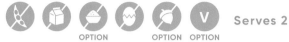 Serves 2

OPTION   OPTION OPTION

My fellow nutritionist Katie Stewart created this super-healthy and sweet mint shake for St. Patrick's Day. I decided to adapt it to provide a low-carb option by using chia seeds as a banana replacement and monk fruit to reduce the carbs while keeping all of the creamy flavour. I drink the higher carb version on days when I need extra energy—great for gym days—and the lower carb version the rest of the time. By keeping my morning drinks sugar-free, I have greater mental focus and improved moods throughout my workday.

1½ cups unsweetened coconut or cashew milk

2 tablespoons ground chia seeds (or 1 large banana)

½ avocado, peeled and pitted (or ½ cup frozen avocado chunks)

½ cup packed baby spinach

1 tablespoon collagen or vegan protein powder

¼ teaspoon pure monk fruit extract (or 1 tablespoon raw honey)

1 teaspoon Hawaiian spirulina or chlorella powder

½ to 1 teaspoon pure mint extract

Pinch of unrefined pink salt

1 tablespoon pumpkin seeds or hemp hearts, for serving (optional)

1. Place all ingredients, except the pumpkin seeds, in a high-speed blender, and blend until smooth.

2. Adjust sweetener and thickness, if desired. Pour into 2 glasses. Top with the pumpkin seeds, if using.

No Sugar Added Option: Use pure monk fruit extract.

Vegan Option: Use vegan protein powder and omit the honey.

Meal Augmentation Shake

     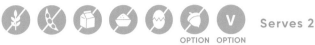 Serves 2

OPTION OPTION

The green colour of this shake comes from the spirulina or chlorella, types of algae that are very nutritious. They are high in antioxidants that help reduce the amount of oxidative damage to cells in the body. With today's increasingly stressful and toxic environment, antioxidants play a key role in helping to repair the body from these effects. Spirulina is also high in protein and is a complete source of all essential amino acids, making it especially beneficial to those who follow a vegan diet.

½ avocado, peeled and pitted

1½ cups unsweetened non-dairy beverage (coconut beverage or almond or cashew milk)

1 tablespoon coconut oil or butter

1 tablespoon + 1½ teaspoons unsweetened nut or seed butter

1 tablespoon + 1½ teaspoons collagen or vegan protein powder

1 tablespoon + 1½ teaspoons lemon juice

1 teaspoon sunflower lecithin powder

1 teaspoon Hawaiian spirulina or chlorella

1 teaspoon pure vanilla or peppermint extract

¼ teaspoon pure monk fruit extract (or ⅛ teaspoon liquid stevia)

⅛ teaspoon ground ginger

Pinch of ground turmeric

Pinch of unrefined pink salt

Optional Boosters (use 1 to 3)

1 to 2 tablespoons pumpkin seed protein powder

1 teaspoon inositol powder

½ banana

1. Place all ingredients, and any boosters, in a high-speed blender and blend until smooth. Pour into 2 glasses.

Vegan Option: Use vegan protein powder.

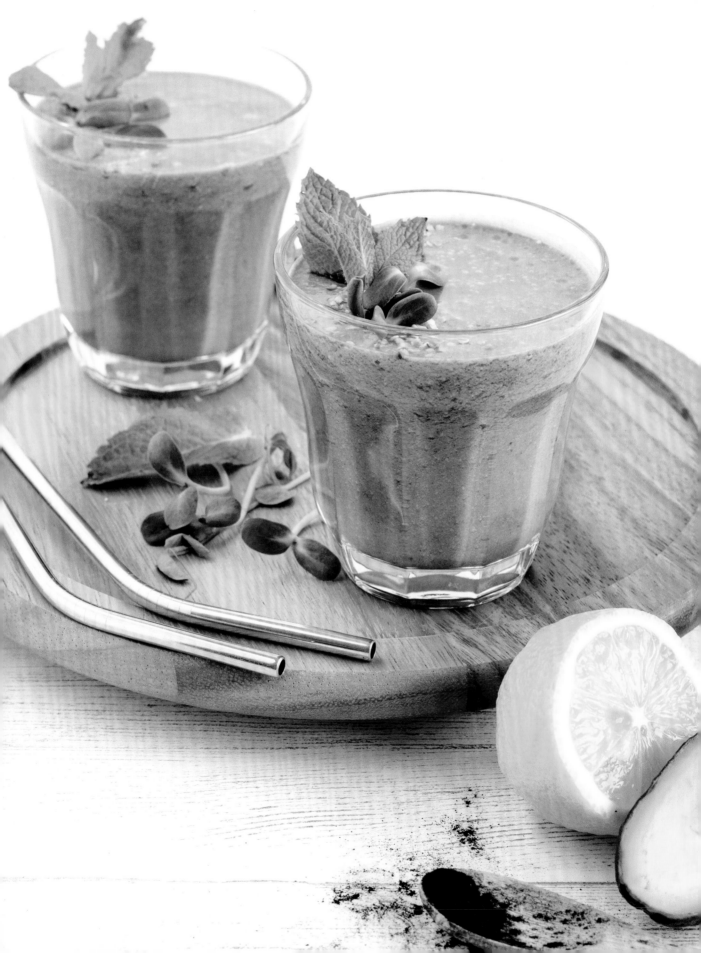

Mocha Elixir

   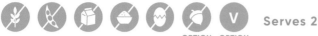

Serves 2

OPTION OPTION

Coconut and cocoa make this creamy chocolatey treat especially beneficial before or after a workout. This is my husband's creation, and he just loves that it is healthier than standard coffee. Cocoa powder contains caffeine, which has been shown to delay the onset of muscle fatigue. Coconut is high in medium-chain triglycerides (MCTs), which are rapidly absorbed by the body and immediately converted into fuel for the body. I love to add avocado and make it into a dreamy avocado coffee! Don't hesitate to use the optional mushroom powder, as it has tremendous health benefits. For example, lion's mane is great for cognition, reishi helps with immunity and cordyceps boosts energy.

1 cup organic brewed coffee, hot

1 cup unsweetened coconut milk, warm (see Tip)

1 tablespoon unsweetened cashew or pumpkin seed butter

2 teaspoons cocoa powder

¼ teaspoon cinnamon

1 teaspoon pure vanilla extract

Pinch of unrefined pink salt

Optional Sweetener

15 to 35 drops pure monk fruit extract (or 10 to 20 drops chocolate- or vanilla-flavoured stevia)

Optional Boosters (use 1 to 5)

½ avocado, peeled and pitted, or ½ cup frozen avocado chunks

½ teaspoon dried mushroom powder of choice

¼ teaspoon ground ginger

½ teaspoon gelatinized maca powder

2 tablespoons collagen powder

1 tablespoon mesquite powder (if using, you can reduce the amount of sweetener)

1. Place all ingredients, and any sweetener or boosters, in a high-speed blender and blend until smooth. Pour into 2 glasses.

Tips:

1. Instead of using brewed coffee, you can use 1 to 2 teaspoons (depending on desired strength) organic instant coffee powder mixed with 1 cup of hot water.

2. If you prefer to use coconut beverage, skip the water and use 2 cups of warm coconut beverage.

Vegan Option: Omit the collagen powder option.

No Monkey Business

      Serves 2

OPTION OPTION

How many smoothie recipes rely on banana to make things taste good? I made a point of making this recipe without banana to prove that the texture and satisfaction of a smoothie can be created in other ways. The added benefit is that no-banana smoothies are perfect for those following a low-carb or keto diet. The flaxseed and nut butter provide the texture of a banana-thickened smoothie, and the optional spices create a beautiful chai flavour that will keep you coming back for more.

1½ cups unsweetened non-dairy beverage (coconut beverage or almond or cashew milk)

½ cup canned full-fat coconut milk

1 to 2 tablespoons collagen or vegan protein powder

2 tablespoons unsweetened nut or seed butter

1 tablespoon + 1½ teaspoons ground flaxseed or chia seeds

½ teaspoon cinnamon

¼ teaspoon liquid stevia (or ½ teaspoon pure monk fruit extract)

1 teaspoon pure vanilla extract

⅛ teaspoon unrefined pink salt

Optional Boosters (use 1 to 5)

¼ teaspoon ground nutmeg

¼ teaspoon ground ginger

¼ teaspoon ground cardamom

Pinch of ground turmeric

1 teaspoon sunflower lecithin powder

1. Place all ingredients, and any boosters, in a high-speed blender and blend until smooth. Pour into 2 glasses.

Vegan Option: Use vegan protein powder.

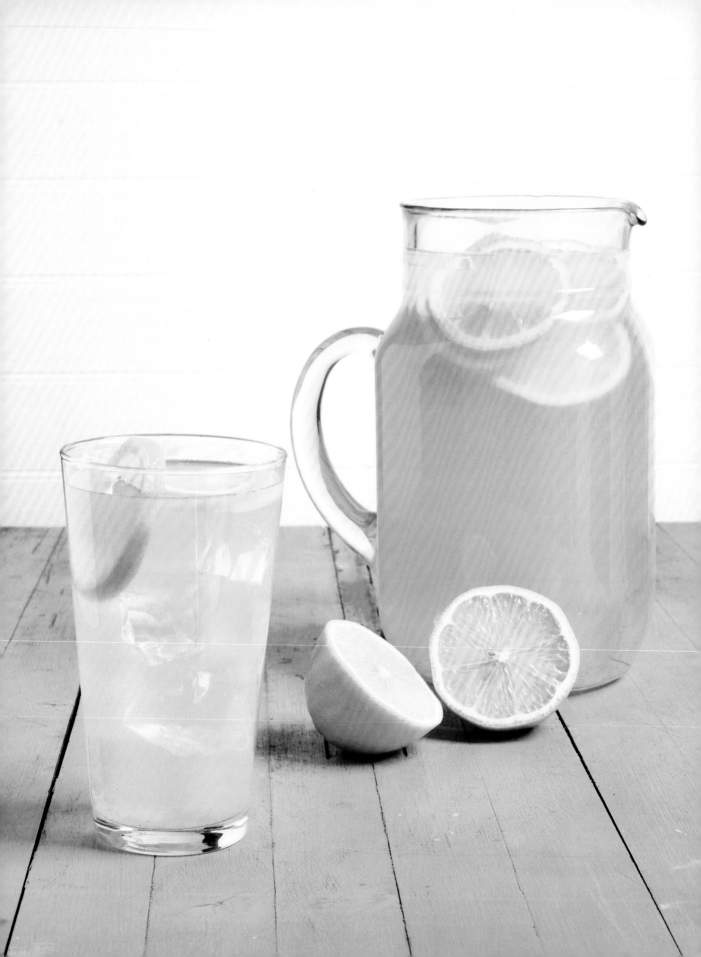

Jules's Soft Lemonade

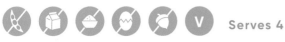 Serves 4

Have you ever tried fresh-pressed lemonade at farmers' markets or festivals? My husband has been selling this recipe at our local farmers' market for a decade, and now I'm sharing our recipe with you. I recommend fresh juice over bottled because the antioxidants are higher, but it will still taste good if that is all you can muster. Lemons reduce inflammation, balance your blood sugar and taste great with stevia. Avoid using lemon juice packed in plastic, as the acidity can pull toxins, such as bisphenol A, from the plastic into the juice.

1 lemon, sliced
4 cups water
Juice of 3 lemons (about ⅔ cup)
½ teaspoon liquid stevia
Pinch of ground turmeric
  (optional)
A pinch or ⅛ teaspoon
  unrefined pink salt
1 teaspoon electrolyte powder
  (a mix of magnesium, calcium
  and potassium is ideal)
  (optional)
1 cup ice cubes or 1 cup frozen
  blueberries

1. Add the lemon slices to a pitcher. Pour in the water, then add the lemon juice.

2. Add the stevia, turmeric and/or electrolyte (if using) and salt. Stir well, adding the ice just before serving.

3. If using frozen blueberries, place them in a blender, top with the lemonade and blend until smooth. You can also reduce the water by 2 cups and add 1 cup ice and 1 cup blueberries to create a blueberry lemonade slushie.

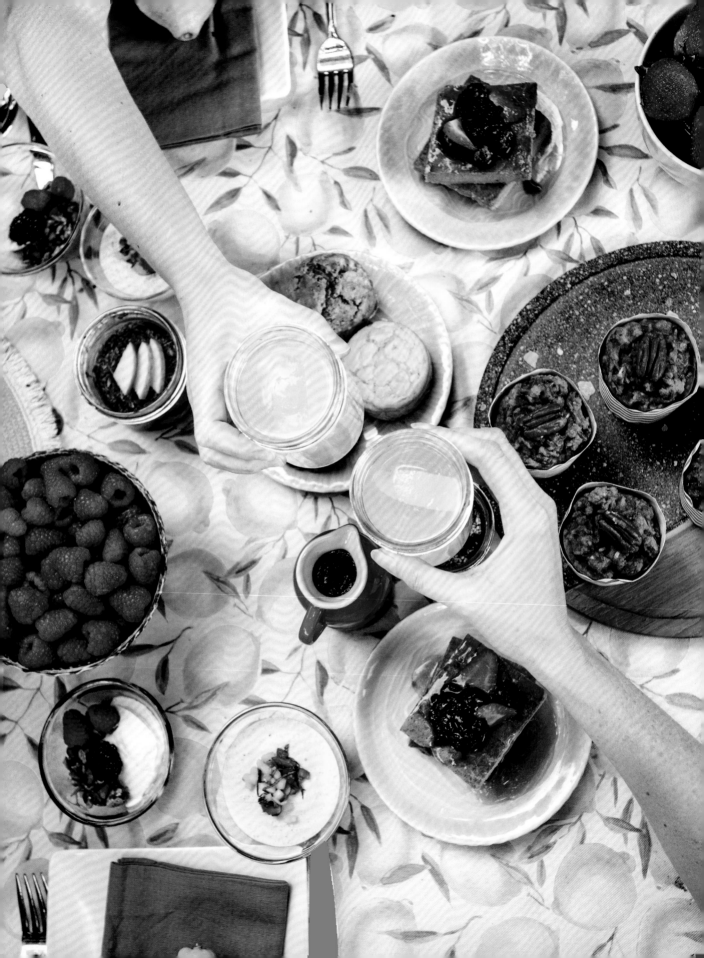

Meals That Start the Day

Five-Minute Faux Yogurt

OPTION OPTION   Makes 3 cups

Let's face it, store-bought non-dairy yogurt is expensive and a bit of a science experiment to make at home. In this recipe, I use gelatin or agar agar as the gelling agent, creating consistent and delicious results every time. This allows you to add the beneficial probiotic bacteria as you serve it, which takes away the guesswork of "is it done yet?" when making non-dairy yogurt.

1 cup raw cashews or coconut cream (about 1 cup coconut cream from a chilled 14-ounce can of full-fat coconut milk)

2 cups hot water

1½ teaspoons gelatin powder (or 3 tablespoons agar agar if using cashews or 1 tablespoon agar agar if using coconut cream)

1 teaspoon pure vanilla extract

Pinch of unrefined pink salt

⅛ teaspoon pure monk fruit extract

Optional Boosters (use 1 to 2)

⅛ teaspoon beet powder (for a pink colour)

⅛ teaspoon Blue Majik algae powder (for a blue colour)

1 capsule probiotic bacteria

Optional Toppings

Chocolate Crunch Low-Carb Granola (page 176)

½ to 1 cup fresh berries (raspberries, strawberries, blueberries, blackberries)

1. If using coconut cream, chill the can of coconut milk in the fridge for at least 4 hours. When ready to use, open the can and scoop out the solid coconut cream. (Reserve the coconut water for smoothies or other recipes.) If using cashews, you can soak them for 4 hours for improved digestibility, but it is not necessary for this recipe. If you use soaked cashews, reduce the hot water by ½ cup.

2. Combine all ingredients and any boosters, except the probiotic (if using), in a high-speed blender and blend on high for 2 minutes until smooth.

3. Pour into wide-mouth mason jars, cover and chill in the refrigerator until it reaches your preferred consistency. If desired, open a probiotic capsule and stir its contents into your serving of yogurt. Add desired toppings.

Vegan Option: Use agar agar.

Baked Porridge-in-a-Jar

    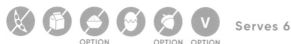 **Serves 6**

OPTION   OPTION   OPTION

What I love about this healthy breakfast is how it makes eating well on the run possible. If you are a person who does not eat breakfast until you arrive at work or school, this portable aromatic jar of goodness is a real time saver, as you can make it on the weekend and enjoy it during the week. I adore the flavour options, which keep your mornings exciting so that you are likely to stick with this healthy breakfast choice.

1 cup unsweetened shredded coconut (see Tip)

3 tablespoons ground chia seeds or flaxseed

½ teaspoon baking powder

¼ teaspoon unrefined pink salt

1 cup unsweetened coconut beverage

1 tablespoon pure vanilla extract

½ teaspoon pure monk fruit extract (or ¼ teaspoon chocolate-flavoured stevia or 1 tablespoon raw honey, yacón syrup or coconut nectar)

1. Preheat the oven to 350°F. Set out six ½-cup mason jars or three 1-cup mason jars.

2. In a large bowl, mix together the coconut, chia seeds, baking powder and salt.

3. Add the coconut beverage, vanilla and monk fruit. Stir until well combined.

4. Add the ingredients for your preferred flavour option (see the next page), stirring to combine. Set aside for 5 minutes to allow the mixture to meld together. Evenly divide the mixture among the mason jars, leaving about 1 inch at the top. If any milk remains at the bottom of the mixing bowl, divide it equally among the jars.

5. Place the jars on a small baking sheet and bake for 22 to 24 minutes, or until slightly firm and golden on top.

6. Enjoy immediately or let cool completely. Seal with a lid and store in the fridge for up to 5 days or in the freezer for up to 3 months.

Tip: If you prefer a higher carb option and enjoy gluten-free grains, you can swap the coconut for rolled quinoa, millet or buckwheat flakes.

No Sugar Added Option: Use pure monk fruit extract or stevia.

Vegan Option: Omit the honey.

Recipe continues

FLAVOUR OPTIONS

Apple Cinnamon: 1 cup cored and chopped apple, ⅓ cup raw pumpkin seeds or chopped raw almonds, 1 teaspoon cinnamon and ¼ teaspoon ground nutmeg. (Omit the apple to make it keto-friendly.)

Blueberry Nutmeg: 1 cup wild blueberries (fresh or thawed), ⅓ cup hemp hearts, ½ teaspoon cinnamon and ¼ teaspoon ground nutmeg.

Ginger Peach: 1 cup pitted and chopped peaches (fresh or thawed), ⅓ cup chopped raw pecans, ¼ to ½ teaspoon ground ginger and ½ teaspoon cinnamon.

Cherry Chocolate: 1 cup pitted cherries cut in half, 2 teaspoons cocoa powder and ¼ cup sugar-free chocolate chips.

Banana Walnut: 1 cup sliced banana, ⅓ cup raw walnuts, ½ teaspoon cinnamon and ¼ teaspoon ground nutmeg.

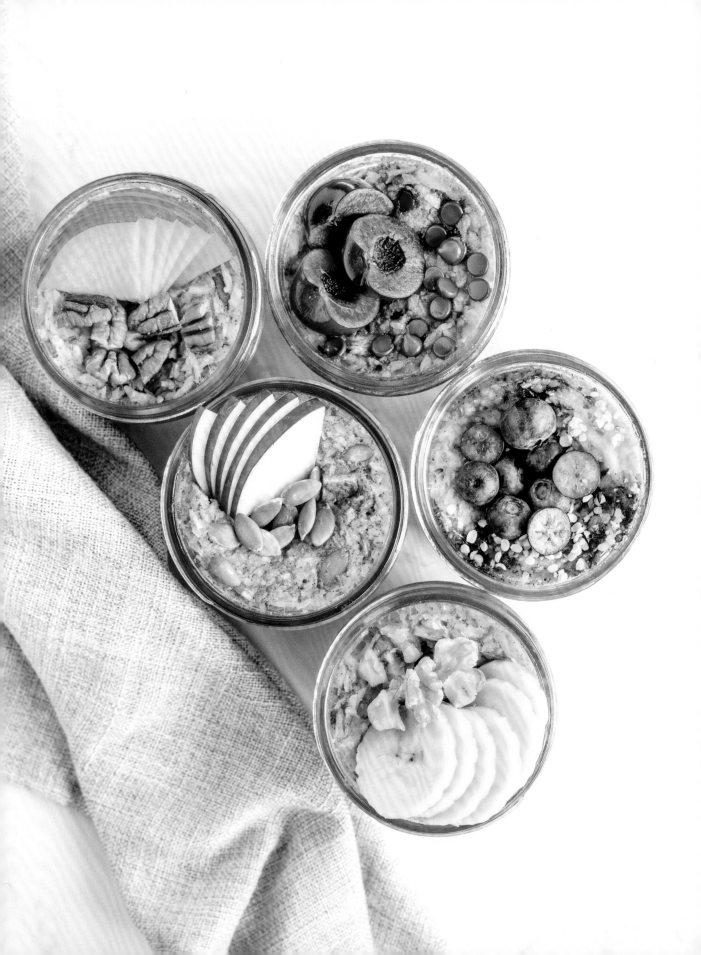

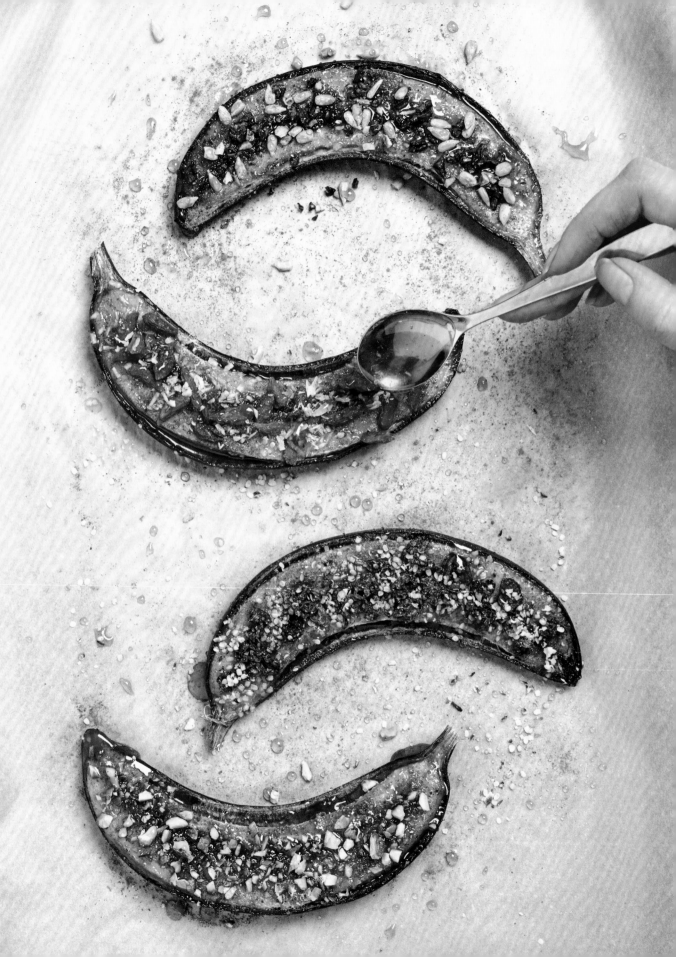

Baked Bananas

V OPTION   Serves 4

This is a healthy variation of Bananas Foster that I made on my TV show, *Healthy Gourmet*. One banana contains a large amount of your daily needs of vitamin B6, a critical vitamin for the metabolism of estrogen, so enjoy this recipe when PMS strikes and has you craving sweets. The spices and optional toppings are anti-inflammatory and bring the flavour over the top! (Shown in the photo served with Faux Maple Syrup, page 225.)

2 large skin-on ripe bananas
3 to 5 drops chocolate-flavoured liquid stevia or pure monk fruit extract (or 1 teaspoon lúcuma or mesquite powder)
1 teaspoon coconut oil
¼ teaspoon cinnamon
¼ teaspoon ground ginger or nutmeg
Pinch of unrefined pink salt

Optional Toppings (use 1 to 6)
Cocoa nibs
Unsweetened shredded coconut
Freeze-dried, sugar-free cranberries or dried goji berries
Seeds (sesame and/or sunflower)
Hemp hearts
Raw chopped nuts (hazelnuts, almonds, walnuts, pecans, pistachios)

1. Preheat the oven to 350°F. Line a baking sheet with unbleached parchment paper.

2. Slice the bananas in half lengthwise, leaving the skin on. Place the banana halves skin side down on the prepared baking sheet.

3. In a small bowl, mix together the stevia and coconut oil. Using the back of a spoon, rub equal amounts of the mixture over the banana halves. Evenly sprinkle the cinnamon, ginger and salt over the banana halves. If using an alternative sweetener powder, evenly sprinkle a ¼ teaspoon of your choice overtop each banana half. Bake for 18 minutes until the bananas are soft. Sprinkle with the desired toppings and serve immediately.

Baked Gingerbread Pancakes

OPTION   **Makes 6 to 8 square pancakes**

Do you adore brunch as much as I do? It is so fun to entertain on a Sunday, but making pancakes for a crowd can be challenging. This recipe comes together as fast as a smoothie and comes out of the oven all at once so that everyone can eat at the same time. Full of delightful spices that also improve digestion, these pancakes provide a nice nutritional balance of slow-burning carbs, healthy fats and protein.

1 tablespoon avocado oil, for greasing the dish

5 large eggs

¼ cup unsweetened non-dairy milk

½ cup unsweetened nut or seed butter

1 cup unsweetened applesauce

¼ teaspoon pure monk fruit extract

2 teaspoons baking powder

1 teaspoon cinnamon

½ to 1 teaspoon ground ginger

½ teaspoon ground nutmeg or allspice

¼ teaspoon ground turmeric (optional for colour)

Pinch of unrefined pink salt

½ cup raw almond, hazelnut or sunflower seed flour

For serving

Fruit Compote (page 170)

Coconut Whipping Cream (page 227; optional)

Faux Maple Syrup (page 225)

1. Preheat the oven to 400°F. Line a 13- × 9-inch glass baking dish with unbleached parchment paper. Spread the avocado oil evenly across the paper.

2. Combine the eggs, milk, nut butter, applesauce, monk fruit, baking powder, cinnamon, ginger, nutmeg, turmeric (if using) and salt in a blender. Blend until well mixed. Add the nut or seed flour and blend again to combine.

3. Pour the batter into the prepared baking dish. Shake to evenly disperse the batter around the dish.

4. Bake for 26 minutes until the top is dry and slightly golden on the edges. Let cool, then cut into 6 to 8 pieces.

5. To serve, top each slice of pancake with the Fruit Compote and/or Coconut Whipping Cream, if using. Store the pancakes in an airtight container in the refrigerator for up to 4 days. They freeze well for up to 1 month and refresh nicely when toasted.

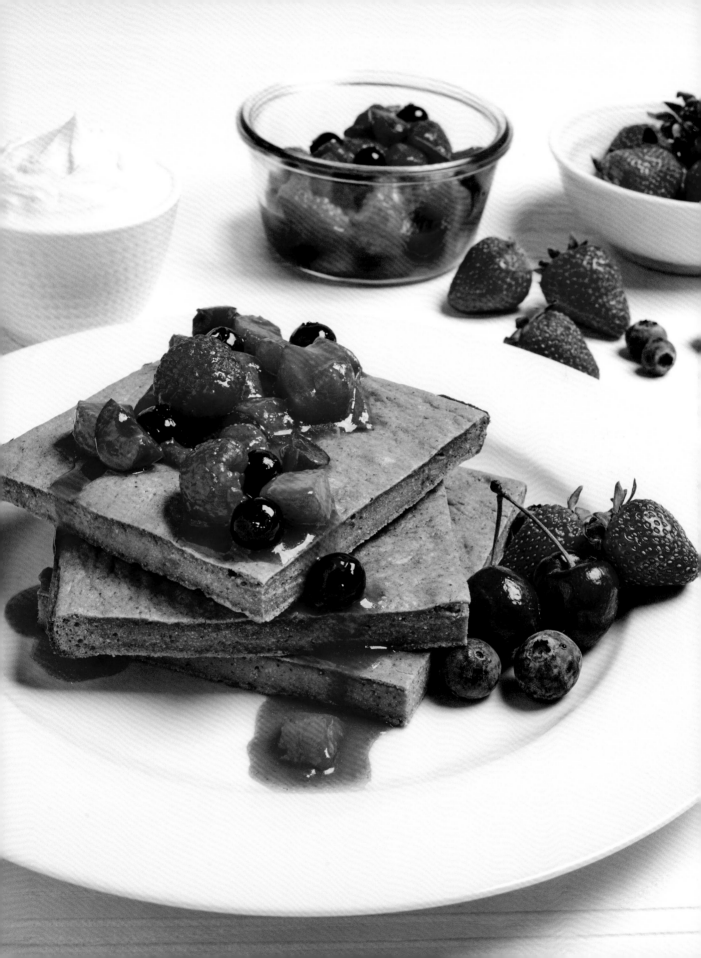

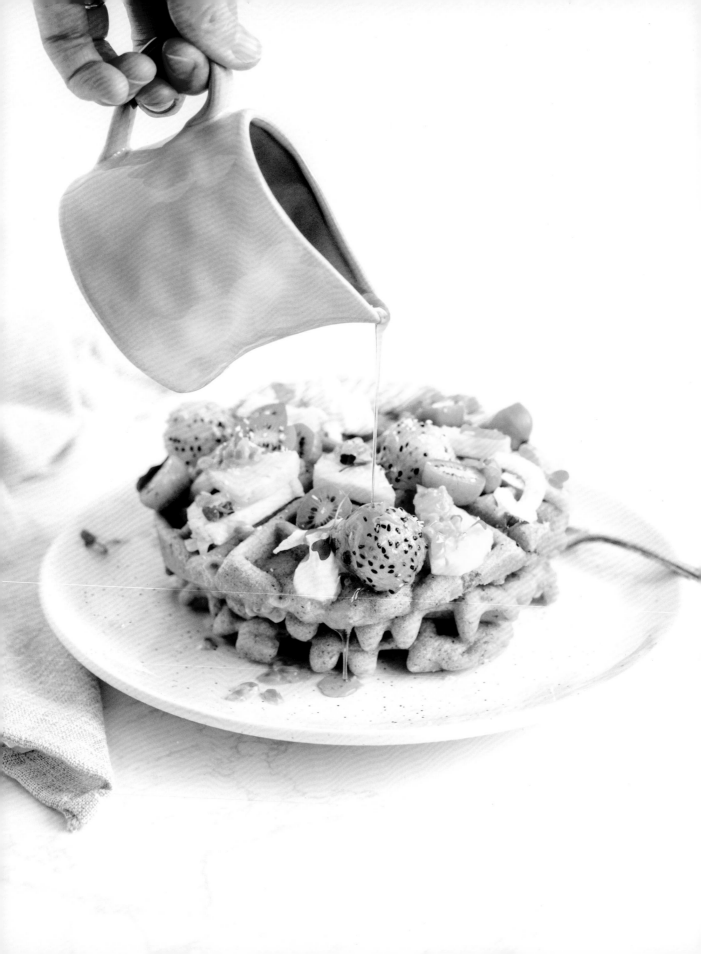

Wonderful Grain-Free Waffles

   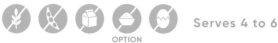
OPTION
Serves 4 to 6

I wanted to make classic waffles for my sister-in-law Coreene, who has celiac disease, a serious auto-immune disease where the ingestion of gluten causes damage in the small intestine. It is now estimated to affect 1 in 100 people worldwide, yet many people go undiagnosed. If you have consistent digestive problems, chronic pain or exhaustion, it is a good idea to check if avoiding gluten will make a difference for you. Family members and clients have benefited enormously from a grain-free menu.

These waffles are tasty enough to convert picky eaters to a sugar-free lifestyle, especially when served with Faux Maple Syrup (page 225). This recipe makes about four to six waffles but may vary depending on the size of your waffle iron. You can freeze the cooked waffles, then reheat them in a toaster, toaster oven or regular oven when ready to serve.

1 cup almond or hazelnut flour
½ cup cassava flour
1½ teaspoons baking powder or soda
1 teaspoon cinnamon
½ teaspoon unrefined pink salt
3 large eggs
½ cup coconut beverage or water
6 tablespoons avocado oil, more for the waffle iron
2 tablespoons coconut syrup (or ½ teaspoon pure monk fruit extract or ¼ teaspoon liquid stevia)

Optional Boosters (use 1 or 2)
1 teaspoon pure vanilla extract
1 to 2 teaspoons cocoa powder

Optional Toppings (use 1 to 5)
Fresh berries (raspberries, blueberries, blackberries)
Unsweetened nut butter
Chopped raw nuts and/or seeds
Faux Maple Syrup (page 225)
Coconut Whipping Cream (page 227)

1. Preheat the waffle iron on high heat. Preheat the oven to 200°F. Line a baking sheet with unbleached parchment paper.

2. In a medium bowl, combine the almond flour, cassava flour, baking powder, cinnamon and salt.

3. In a large bowl, whisk together the eggs, coconut beverage, coconut oil, coconut syrup and any boosters (if using), then pour the mixture into the dry ingredients and mix until well combined.

4. Brush both sides of the waffle iron with a thin coating of avocado oil. Pour about ½ cup of batter per waffle into the centre of the waffle iron, gently spreading evenly before closing. Cook until the waffles are lightly brown (see Tip). Transfer to the prepared baking sheet and keep warm in the oven. Repeat with the remaining batter.

5. Serve the waffles with the desired toppings. Alternatively, store cooked waffles in an airtight container in the fridge for up to 4 days or in the freezer for up to 1 month.

Tip: Follow the manufacturer's instructions to learn the doneness indicator. If your waffle iron doesn't have one, a good tip is that the waffle will be done when the steam stops.

No Sugar Added Option: Use pure monk fruit extract or stevia.

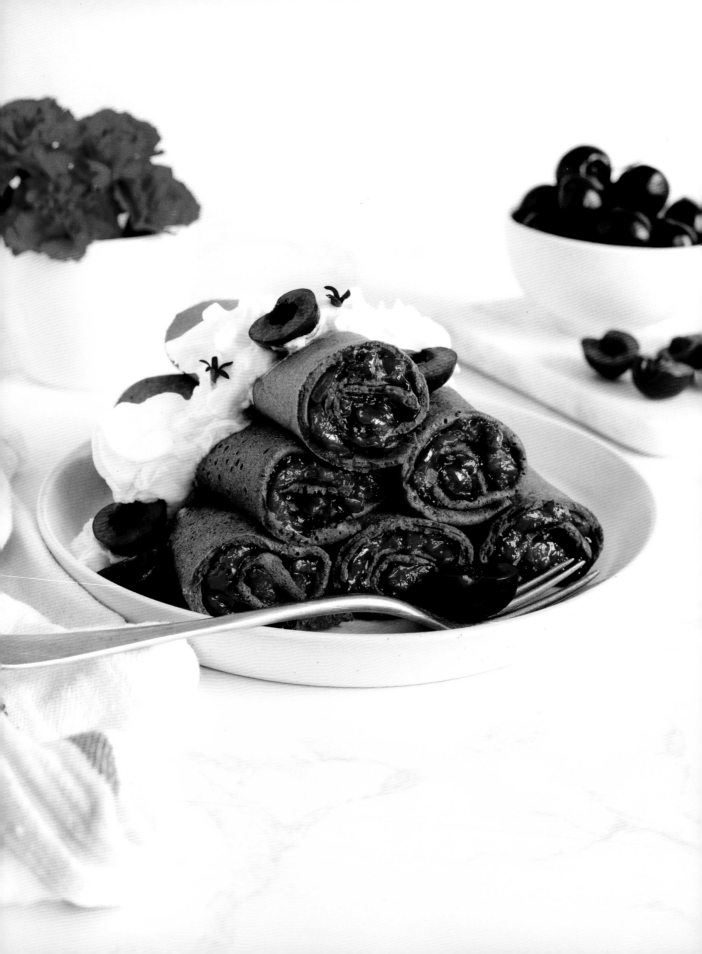

Black Forest Crepes

    Makes 4 crepes

OPTION

These dark-coloured crepes look dramatic at the breakfast table, but they are much healthier than regular crepes because they are both grain-free and low on the glycemic index. By avoiding a sugar rush in the morning, you are better able to stay away from sugar all day long. In addition, the combination of cherries and chocolate will have you craving these crepes on a Sunday morning.

4 large eggs

1 cup unsweetened coconut beverage

¾ cup almond or hazelnut flour

¼ cup cassava flour

½ teaspoon baking powder

½ teaspoon cinnamon

Pinch of unrefined pink salt

2 tablespoons cocoa powder

2 tablespoons coconut or yacón syrup (or ⅛ teaspoon pure monk fruit extract)

1 tablespoon avocado oil, for greasing the pan

Toppings

Cherry Filling (page 170)

Coconut Whipping Cream (page 227)

1. Preheat the oven to 200°F. Line a baking sheet with unbleached parchment paper.

2. Starting with the eggs, combine all ingredients except the avocado oil in a blender and blend until well combined.

3. Heat a small amount of the avocado oil in a 10-inch skillet or crepe pan over medium-high heat.

4. Add ¼ cup of the batter to the pan, tilting the pan gently to spread the batter evenly across the hot pan. It's like making a thin, large pancake.

5. Cook the crepe until the edges start to set, about 5 minutes. Then gently flip the crepe and cook for another 2 minutes until it easily releases from the pan. Transfer the crepe to the prepared baking sheet and keep warm in the oven while you cook the remaining crepes.

6. Serve the crepes with Cherry Filling and/or Coconut Whipping Cream. Store leftovers in an airtight container in the refrigerator for up to 3 days.

Tip: A large crepe pan makes about 5 crepes. Depending on the size of your pan, you can make smaller ones and more of them.

No-Sugar Added Option: Use pure monk fruit extract.

Cherry Filling   Makes 2 cups

Cherries have been shown to decrease levels of hemoglobin A1C, the marker that shows damage from long-term sugar exposure. The red pigment in cherries is created by anthocyanins, which have been shown to reduce the inflammatory markers in the blood. This could create a reduction in the inflammation of your joints and, ultimately, a reduction in pain. Enjoy this filling as a wonderful alternative to sugary jam.

2 cups fresh or frozen pitted whole sweet cherries

⅛ teaspoon pure monk fruit extract (or 2 tablespoons coconut nectar, yacón syrup or raw honey)

2 teaspoons ground flaxseed or chia seeds

1 tablespoon lemon juice

½ teaspoon pure vanilla extract

1. Place all ingredients in a large saucepan over medium heat. Cook, stirring often, until glossy and thickened, 5 to 10 minutes.

2. Taste to adjust sweetener if desired, then remove the pan from the heat and serve. Store in a mason jar in the fridge for up to 2 weeks.

No Sugar Added Option: Use pure monk fruit extract.

Vegan Option: Omit the honey.

Fruit Compote   Makes 1 cup

It is so fast and easy to make your own fruit compote to replace sugar-filled jam. When you use frozen fruit, you save money and enjoy a taste of summer all year long. Berries are very anti-inflammatory because they contain polyphenols that can improve digestion issues, diabetes, memory and the heart. This recipe pairs nicely with Baked Gingerbread Pancakes (page 164) or is a nice jam replacement for muffins.

1 tablespoon + 1½ teaspoons coconut oil

3 cups fresh or frozen fruit (any combination of oranges, pears, apples, raspberries, blueberries, blackberries or cherries)

1 teaspoon cinnamon

½ teaspoon ground ginger

½ teaspoon pure monk fruit extract (or ¼ teaspoon liquid stevia)

1. In a medium pot, melt the coconut oil over medium heat.

2. Prepare your fruit choices by peeling, coring and roughly chopping larger fruit into ½-inch cubes. Add the fruit, cinnamon, ginger, and monk fruit to the pot and cook for 5 to 10 minutes, stirring often, until the fruit is soft but still holding its shape. Store in an airtight container in the fridge for up to 1 week or in the freezer for up to 1 month.

Chocolate Banana Breakfast Cookies

       Makes 10 cookies

OPTION OPTION

If a breakfast smoothie married a cookie, this would be their love child. Bananas are high in potassium, making these cookies a great snack for energetic activities and sports. If you make them with sunflower seed flour, they become an allergen-free snack that can feed the whole team. These cookies provide a nice balance of protein, carbohydrates and fats and keep well in the freezer, ready to go when your hungry crew needs them most.

3 ripe bananas, divided

1¼ cups almond or sunflower seed flour (see Tip)

3 tablespoons cocoa powder

½ teaspoon baking soda

½ teaspoon pure monk fruit extract or chocolate-flavoured liquid stevia

¼ teaspoon unrefined pink salt

2 tablespoons collagen powder (or ⅓ cup pumpkin or hemp protein powder)

½ cup sugar-free chocolate chips

1½ teaspoons lúcuma or mesquite powder (optional)

1. Preheat the oven to 350°F. Line a baking sheet with unbleached parchment paper.

2. Mash 2 of the bananas in the bowl of a stand mixer. Add the almond flour, cocoa powder, baking soda, monk fruit, salt and collagen powder and lucuma powder (if using) and mix until well combined.

3. Mix in the chocolate chips. Using a large spoon or ice cream scoop, measure about 2 tablespoons of the mixture onto the prepared baking sheet. Flatten the dough into a round cookie shape. Repeat with the remaining dough.

4. Slice the remaining banana crosswise into 10 rounds. Place a round of banana on top of each cookie.

5. Bake for 18 to 20 minutes, then transfer to a wire rack to cool. Store in an airtight container on the countertop for 4 days or in the freezer for up to 3 months.

Tip: One cup of sunflower seeds makes 1½ cups sunflower seed flour.

Vegan Option: Use pumpkin or hemp protein powder.

Fast English Muffins

OPTION   Makes 1 English Muffin

This recipe is so simple to make, it is great for a quick morning breakfast. Eggs are proven to keep you satiated, and it is fun that each guest can decide what flavour to try. You can serve both sweet and savoury English muffins in the same sitting and see which is considered the most impressive. They are great for brunches or group breakfasts, as you can simply multiply the ingredients below by the number of people. It is easier to make them in ramekins rather than mix them in one big bowl and then divide it. Feel free to serve with your favourite nut or seed butter or with a fried egg and sliced avocado.

Coconut oil, for greasing the
    pan
1 large egg
1 tablespoon + 1½ teaspoons
    coconut flour (or
    2 tablespoons almond flour)
Pinch of baking soda
Pinch of unrefined pink salt

1. Preheat the oven to 400°F. Grease a small ramekin with the coconut oil.

2. In the ramekin, using a fork, mix together the egg, coconut flour, baking soda, salt and ingredients from your flavour option, ensuring that there are no lumps and scraping down the sides to ensure a clean edge.

3. Bake for 19 minutes, or until a toothpick inserted in the middle comes out clean. Store it in an airtight container in the fridge for up to 1 week or in the freezer for up to 1 month.

FLAVOUR OPTIONS

Sweet: Add 2 to 3 drops pure monk fruit extract.

Nutty: Add 2 teaspoons unsweetened nut butter + 2 drops pure monk fruit extract.

Sweet Cinnamon: Add 1 teaspoon cinnamon + 2 drops pure monk fruit extract.

Italian Seasoning: Add ½ teaspoon Italian seasoning + 1 tablespoon minced softened sun-dried tomatoes.

French Seasoning: Add ½ teaspoon herbs de Provence + ¼ teaspoon onion powder.

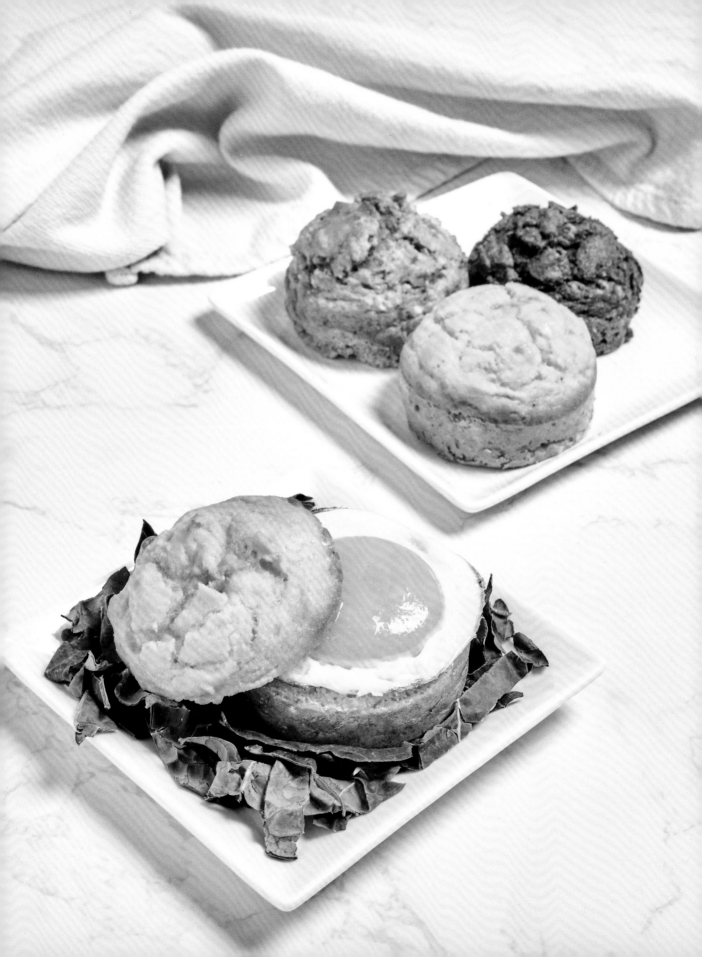

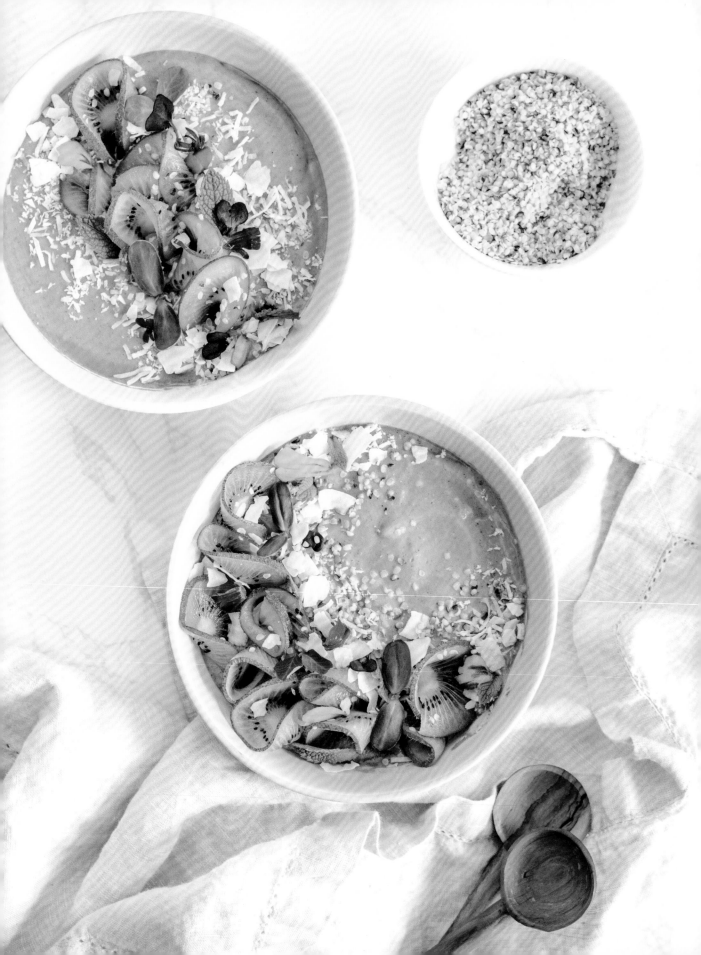

Green Dragon Smoothie Bowl

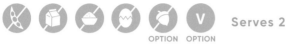

OPTION   OPTION   **Serves 2**

Smoothie bowls are great when you prefer to eat rather than drink your blended breakfast, and this one packs in a lot of nutrients that will keep you satisfied and fuelled for hours. The avocado makes it super creamy and the tropical fruit will make you feel like you are waking up on a balmy beach. Protein is a great way to feel full for a longer period, so enjoy the collagen or vegan protein powder to sustain your energy and bust any mid-morning cravings.

1 ripe avocado, peeled and pitted

1 frozen banana

1 cup frozen mango chunks

1 cup canned full-fat coconut milk

1½ cups packed baby spinach

1 tablespoon ground flaxseed or chia seeds

4 tablespoons vegan protein or collagen powder

2 tablespoons unsweetened nut or seed butter

½ teaspoon pure vanilla extract

⅛ teaspoon pure monk fruit extract (or 1 to 2 teaspoons lúcuma powder) (optional)

2 tablespoons lemon juice

Pinch of unrefined pink salt

Optional Toppings

Unsweetened shredded coconut

Kiwi slices

Hemp hearts

Edible flowers and/or fresh mint leaves

1. Combine all smoothie ingredients in a high-speed blender and blend until smooth.

2. Divide between 2 bowls and top with desired toppings.

Vegan Option: Use vegan protein powder.

Chocolate Crunch Low-Carb Granola

        Makes 8 cups

My dad loves granola so much that he would enjoy two servings in a sitting, only to learn that he had eaten 60 grams of carbs (25 grams of refined sugar) that left him tired and craving a lift from caffeine or sugar in the afternoon. When he went sugar-free, one of his biggest requests was a replacement for granola, and I managed to create one that is tasty yet slim on carbohydrates. After losing twenty-five pounds, he once again has the energy to work at his demanding job with a smile, which is awesome considering he just celebrated his seventy-eighth birthday. He is such an inspiration to me and a good example of how going sugar-free can produce big benefits at any age.

¾ cup ground chia seeds (about ½ cup whole chia seeds)

1 teaspoon chocolate, vanilla flavoured or plain liquid stevia (or 2 teaspoons pure monk fruit extract)

1½ cups unsweetened coconut beverage

1 cup unsweetened shredded coconut

1½ cups raw sunflower seeds

1 cup raw pumpkin seeds

1 cup raw cashew pieces, chopped hazelnuts or more sunflower or pumpkin seeds

¼ cup cocoa powder

1 teaspoon cinnamon

½ teaspoon ground ginger

½ teaspoon ground cardamom or allspice

¼ to ½ teaspoon ground turmeric

1 tablespoon lúcuma or mesquite powder (optional)

¼ teaspoon unrefined pink salt

½ cup unsweetened cashew butter or other nut or seed butter

1. Preheat the oven to 170°F. Line 2 baking sheets with unbleached parchment paper.

2. In a medium bowl, combine the chia seeds, stevia and coconut beverage. Stir well and let sit until a gel forms, about 5 minutes. You can use the chia seed mixture as is or, if you want a smoother texture for easier mixing, transfer it to a blender, blend on high speed until smooth, then transfer the mixture back to the bowl.

3. Meanwhile, in a large bowl, combine the coconut, sunflower seeds, pumpkin seeds, cashews, cocoa powder, cinnamon, ginger, cardamom, turmeric, lucuma (if using) and salt. Mix until well combined.

4. Add the cashew butter mixture to the chia seed mixture, then fold the mixture into the dry ingredients and stir until you reach a cookie dough consistency.

5. Using your fingers, break the mixture into small clumps and spread it evenly over the prepared baking sheets. Leave as much space between the clumps as you can.

6. Bake for 6 hours, then turn off the oven and leave the granola in the oven overnight or until completely dry. Store in an airtight container on the countertop for up to 1 month.

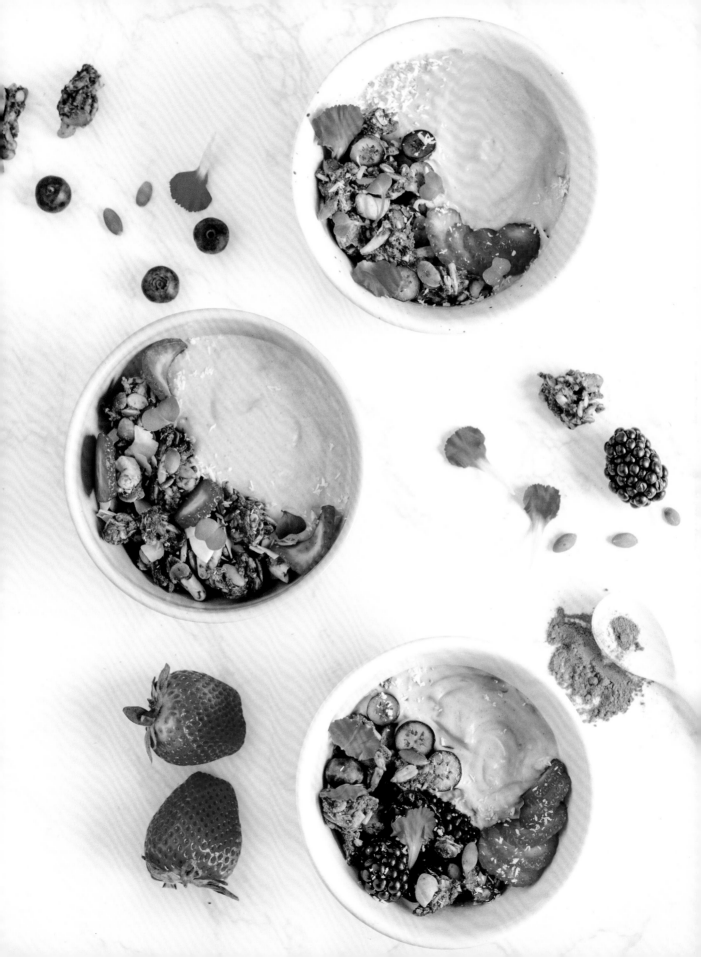

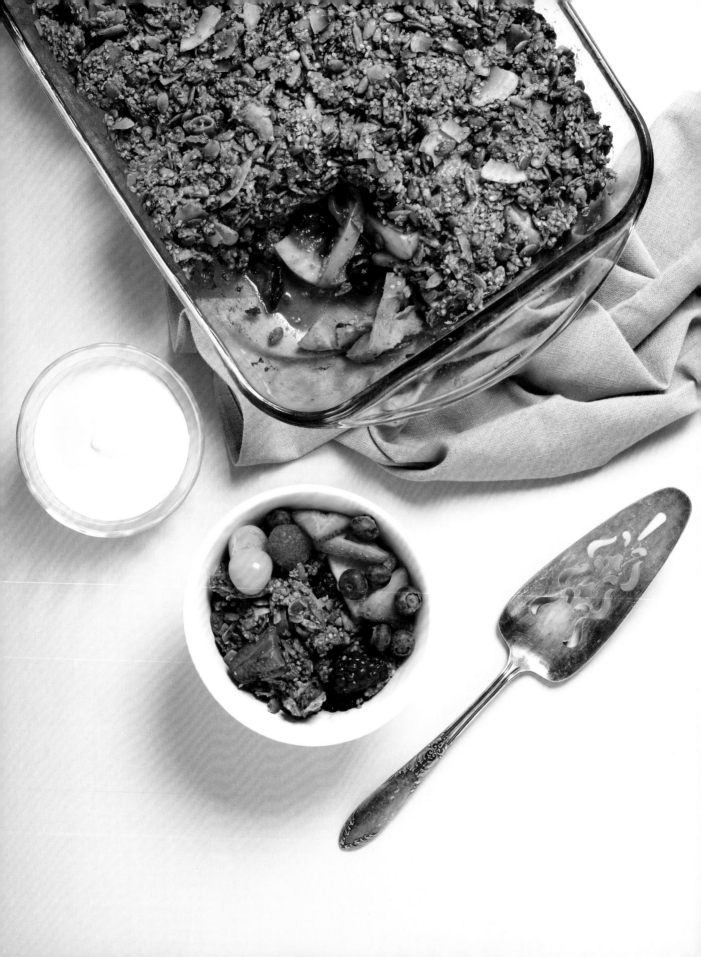

Fabulous Fruit Crisp

      OPTION OPTION **Serves 10**

I created this fruit crisp with a granola-like topping so that my dad could have a quick breakfast when on the run. This dish is not keto-friendly, but if you use the monk fruit in the topping you reduce an incredible amount of carbs in your first meal of the day. Berries are lower in carbs than other fruits, and apples help us balance our hormones because they are rich in fibre and calcium D-glucarate, which helps the body get rid of excess hormones, such as estrogen, before they are reabsorbed.

4 cups apples and/or pears, sliced into bite-size pieces

3 to 4 cups frozen fruit (blueberries, raspberries, blackberries, peaches, cherries)

¼ cup unsweetened nut or seed butter

1 teaspoon cinnamon

¼ teaspoon liquid stevia (or ½ teaspoon pure monk fruit extract or ¼ cup liquid honey)

½ cup unsweetened coconut beverage

Toppings

1½ cups unsweetened coconut flakes

1 cup unsweetened nut or seed butter

1 cup hemp hearts

1 cup raw sunflower seeds

1 cup raw pecans or pumpkin seeds

1 tablespoon cinnamon

½ teaspoon unrefined pink salt

1 teaspoon pure monk fruit extract (or ½ cup raw honey)

1. Preheat the oven to 325°F.

2. In a 13- × 9-inch baking dish, mix together all of the fruit, the nut butter, cinnamon and stevia. Top with the coconut beverage.

3. In a large bowl, mix together all of the topping ingredients until well combined. Evenly spread the topping mixture over the fruit base.

4. Bake for 50 minutes, or until the topping begins to turn golden brown.

5. Serve immediately or cool completely. Store, covered, in the fridge for up to 5 days or in the freezer for up to 1 month.

No Sugar Added Option: Use pure monk extract or liquid stevia.

Vegan Option: Omit the honey.

Mango Gello Pudding Cups

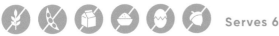 Serves 6

You know a recipe is good when you think about it often and carve out time to make it. This one is simple to make and absolutely delicious. It comes together as quickly as a smoothie and has become a family favourite in our home. Mango is a good source of vitamin A, which benefits our eyes, skin and respiratory system, so enjoy this recipe knowing that it is healthy and delightful.

⅓ cup cold water

2 tablespoons gelatin powder

1 can (14 ounces) full-fat coconut milk

2 cups fresh or thawed frozen mango chunks (about ⅔ pound)

Pinch of unrefined pink salt

⅛ teaspoon pure monk fruit extract

Optional Booster

1 teaspoon pure vanilla extract

Optional Toppings (use as many as you like)

Raspberries

Fresh mango, thinly sliced

Unsweetened flaked or shredded coconut

Edible flowers

1. Combine the water, gelatin and coconut milk in a blender or high-speed blender and blend well.

2. Add the mango and blend until very smooth. If you are using a high-speed blender, you do not need to thaw the mango completely. Add the salt, monk fruit and vanilla, if using.

3. Divide the mixture evenly among six ½-cup mason jars. Top with the desired toppings, cover and chill until set, about 1 hour. Store in an airtight container in the fridge for up to 10 days.

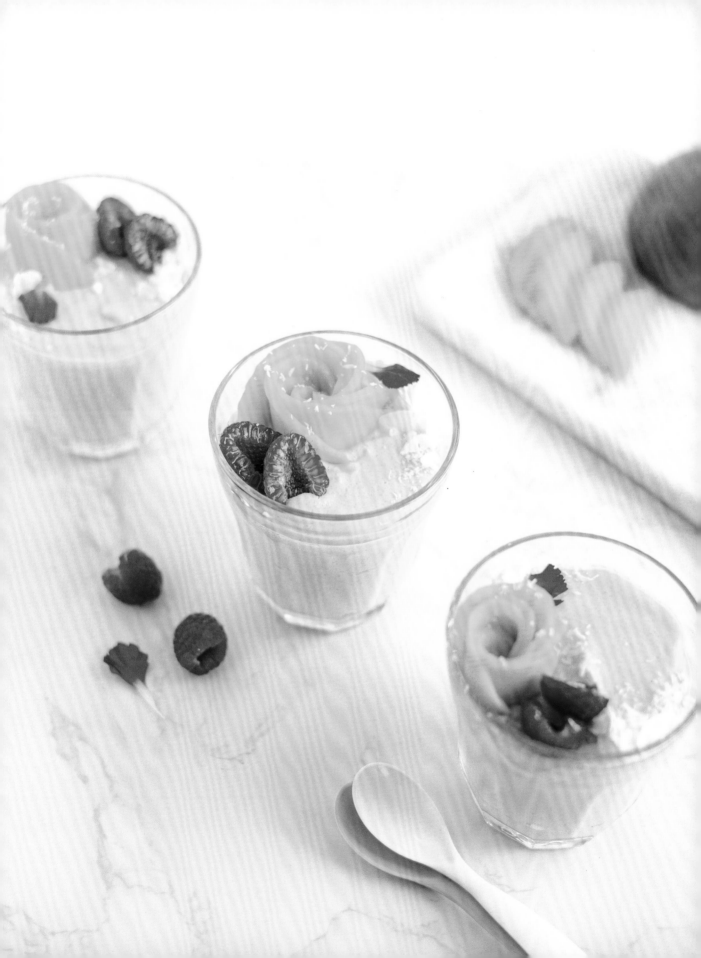

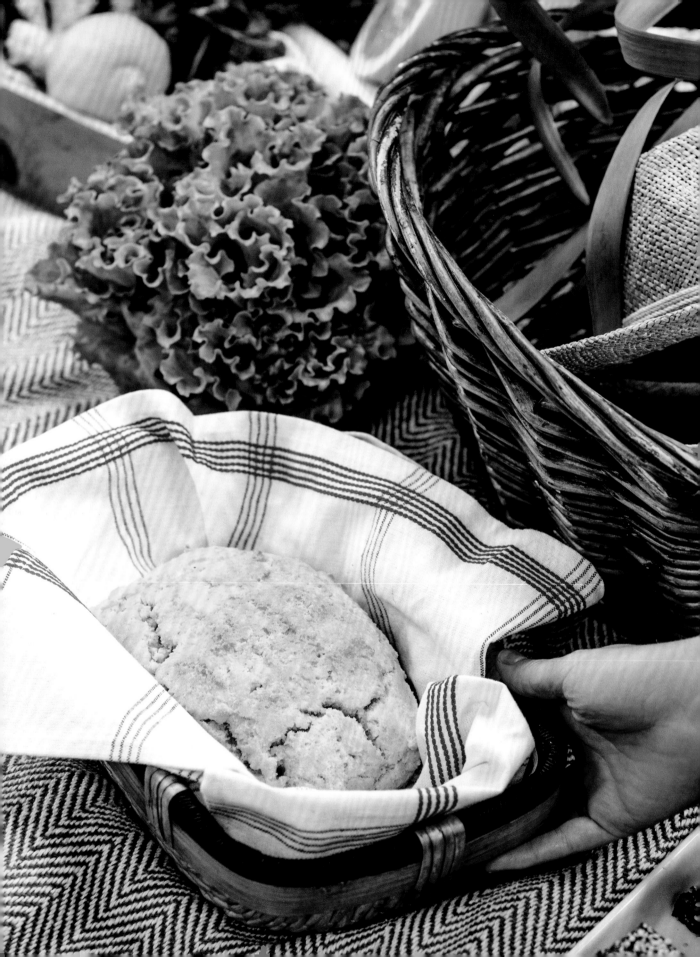

Breads, Chips and Crackers

Cassava Tortillas

       Makes 10 tortillas

This is the perfect recipe to keep on hand when you are short on time but want to have something fresh and delicious for the whole family. Cassava is a hypoallergenic root that works well as a flour for people with allergies or autoimmune disorders. It has a low glycemic index of 46, which means that it is less likely than other foods to cause a rapid rise in blood sugar levels. When you keep your blood sugar balanced, you are less likely to crave sugar. Try using these tortillas as a pizza crust or as a dipper for my Pizza Dip (page 269).

2 cups cassava flour (see Tip)

1 cup canned full-fat coconut milk

⅓ cup avocado oil, more for cooking

½ cup water

1 teaspoon unrefined pink salt, or to taste

2 teaspoons garlic, curry or paprika powder (optional)

1. In a medium bowl, mix together all ingredients until well combined, creating a dough that is smooth and sticks together. If the dough is too stiff, add 1 teaspoon of water at a time until the desired consistency is reached.

2. Divide the dough into 10 equal portions and shape into balls. Cut out 2 squares of unbleached parchment paper and place a dough ball between them. Using the side of a tall glass or a rolling pin, roll the dough into a flat, round tortilla. If the dough is too sticky, sprinkle lightly with cassava flour. Repeat with the remaining dough balls.

3. Heat a 10-inch frying pan over medium-low heat. Drizzle lightly with avocado oil, then transfer the tortillas to the hot pan. You will need to cook the tortillas in batches.

4. Cook the tortillas to your personal preference: about 4 minutes per side for soft tortillas or 5 or more minutes per side for crispier tortillas. Store in an airtight container in the fridge for up to 1 week or in the freezer for up to 1 month.

Tip: Cassava flour cannot be substituted with tapioca flour in this recipe.

Banana Bread Cookie Crackers

       Makes 70 crackers

Do you love banana bread? I adore the spices and the sweet taste, but it is time to ditch the sugar and flour. I call these cookie crackers because they are sweet like a cookie yet sturdy and shaped like a cracker. Healthy treats are often in short supply when you are travelling, so I suggest you make a double batch of these before a trip. The crackers can be eaten on their own or used as a base for dips and spreads. The dates provide electrolytes and stabilize blood sugar.

½ cup water
1 cup mashed ripe banana
¾ cup ground golden flaxseed
   or ground white chia seeds
¾ cup pitted Medjool dates,
   chopped
½ teaspoon unrefined pink salt
½ teaspoon cinnamon
¼ teaspoon ground ginger
¼ teaspoon ground nutmeg
1 cup sesame seeds (see Tip)
½ cup unsweetened shredded
   coconut

1. Preheat the oven to 250°F. Line a baking sheet with unbleached parchment paper.

2. Combine the water, banana, flaxseed, dates, salt, cinnamon, ginger and nutmeg in a food processor and purée.

3. Add the sesame seeds and coconut and pulse until well combined.

4. Spread the stiff batter evenly onto the prepared baking sheet.

5. Using a butter knife, score the crackers into the desired size and shape.

6. Bake for 2 hours, then flip, peeling the crackers off the parchment paper. Bake for another 1½ to 2 hours, then turn off the oven, keeping the door closed. Leave the crackers in the oven overnight or until completely dry.

7. Allow the crackers to cool completely before storing them in an airtight container on the countertop for up to 2 months.

Tip: Hemp hearts can be substituted for sesame seeds for extra nutrition.

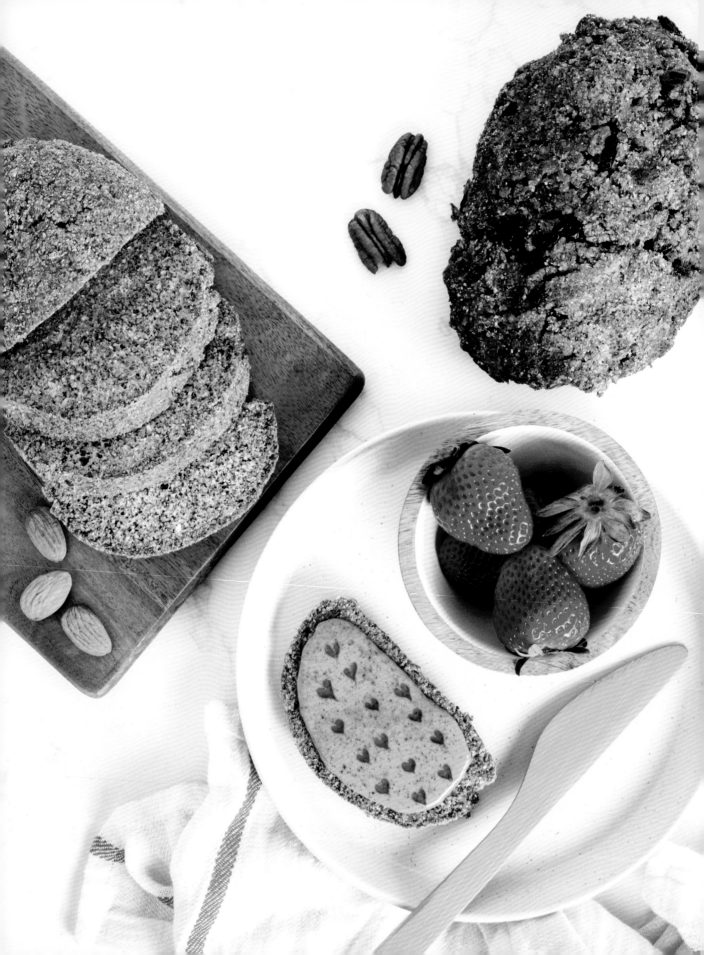

Baba's Bread

        Makes 2 small loaves

My mom is Ukrainian and is known affectionately as Baba, so when she came up with this great recipe, we had to honour her by calling it Baba's Bread. I don't suggest using pre-made almond flour or the bread will turn out very dense and wet. Making your own almond flour is less expensive and results in a lighter bread that is perfect for toasting. Be sure to use frozen nuts, which prevents them from turning into a paste. Simply toss them in the freezer the night before making this bread. The best part about this bread is that it is super low carb yet deeply satisfies cravings. Baba makes it every week because the family can't get enough.

2½ cups raw almonds, hazelnuts or pecans, frozen overnight
⅓ cup flax seeds (see Tip)
½ cup coconut flour
½ cup psyllium husks
1 tablespoon baking powder
1 teaspoon unrefined pink salt
2 cups water
1 tablespoon extra-virgin olive oil
2 teaspoons apple cider vinegar

Optional Savoury Flavour
1 cup green or black olives, well drained, pitted and sliced
2 tablespoons chopped fresh rosemary

Optional Sweet Flavour
1 tablespoon cinnamon
1 cup raisins, chopped

Tip: I suggest you freshly grind your flax seeds for best results. If you don't have a grinder, use ½ cup ground flaxseed. Store ground flaxseed in an airtight container in the freezer to preserve freshness.

1. Position a rack in the middle of the oven. Preheat the oven to 400°F. Line a baking sheet with unbleached parchment paper.

2. Place the frozen nuts in a food processor and grind them into a rough meal, about 2 minutes. Make sure to pulse the processor and keep checking to make sure you have not turned the nuts into a paste or butter. They should have a cornmeal-like texture.

3. Place the nut meal in a large bowl.

4. Grind the flax seeds in a clean coffee grinder and add them to the bowl. Mix in the coconut flour, psyllium, baking powder and salt.

5. In another large bowl, whisk together the water, olive oil, and apple cider vinegar. Add the dry mixture to the wet mixture and combine thoroughly but do not overmix. Add savoury or sweet ingredients (if using) and mix again.

6. Divide the dough into 2 portions and form into loaves on the prepared baking sheet. You can smooth the tops, but make sure not to press too firmly on the dough. This bread does not rise very much, if at all, so form the loaves as you want them to look once baked.

7. Set aside for 10 minutes so that the fibre completely absorbs any liquid, then bake for 60 minutes.

8. Using the parchment paper, transfer the loaves to a cooling rack and let cool completely before slicing. Store covered on the countertop for up to 2 days or slice and freeze for up to 3 months.

Chewy Baguette or Buns

      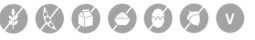 Makes 1 to 2 baguettes or 8 buns

I last ate conventional bread in France nearly a decade ago, and I'll never forget it. This baguette has the familiar chew and smooth gluey texture that many bread eaters crave. I used Baba's Bread (page 187) as inspiration to create this nut-free version, and the great news is that it is easier to make than muffins. This bread is very low carb and free of all common allergens, so it makes it great to share with people who are following an anti-inflammatory diet.

2½ cups raw sunflower seeds
⅓ cup flax seeds (see Tip)
¾ cup coconut flour
¼ cup psyllium seed powder
1 tablespoon baking powder
1 teaspoon unrefined pink salt
2 cups water or unsweetened non-dairy milk
1 tablespoon avocado oil
2 teaspoons apple cider vinegar

Tip: I suggest you freshly grind your flax seeds for best results. If you don't have a grinder, use ½ cup ground flaxseed. Store ground flaxseed in an airtight container in the freezer to preserve freshness.

1. Position a rack in the middle of the oven. Preheat the oven to 400°F. Line a baking sheet with unbleached parchment paper.

2. Grind the sunflower seeds in a clean coffee grinder or high-speed blender and transfer to a large mixing bowl.

3. Grind the flax seeds in a clean coffee grinder and add to the bowl with the sunflower seed flour. Add the coconut flour, psyllium, baking powder and salt and mix well.

4. In a medium bowl, whisk together the water, avocado oil and apple cider vinegar. Add the wet mixture to the dry mixture and mix thoroughly.

5. Shape the dough into 1 long loaf, 2 small loaves or 8 buns and place on the prepared baking sheet. Smooth out the tops if making buns, but make sure not to press too firmly on the dough. If you'd like a smoother texture for your baguette, roll the excess parchment paper over the formed loaf. Using your hands, gently squeeze the loaf from the middle to the ends until you reach the desired shape and thickness.

6. Set aside for 10 minutes so that the fibre completely absorbs any liquid, then bake for 60 minutes for the loaf or loaves or 45 to 50 minutes for the buns.

7. Using the parchment paper, transfer the bread to a cutting board and let cool completely before slicing. Store covered on the countertop for up to 2 days or slice and freeze for up to 3 months.

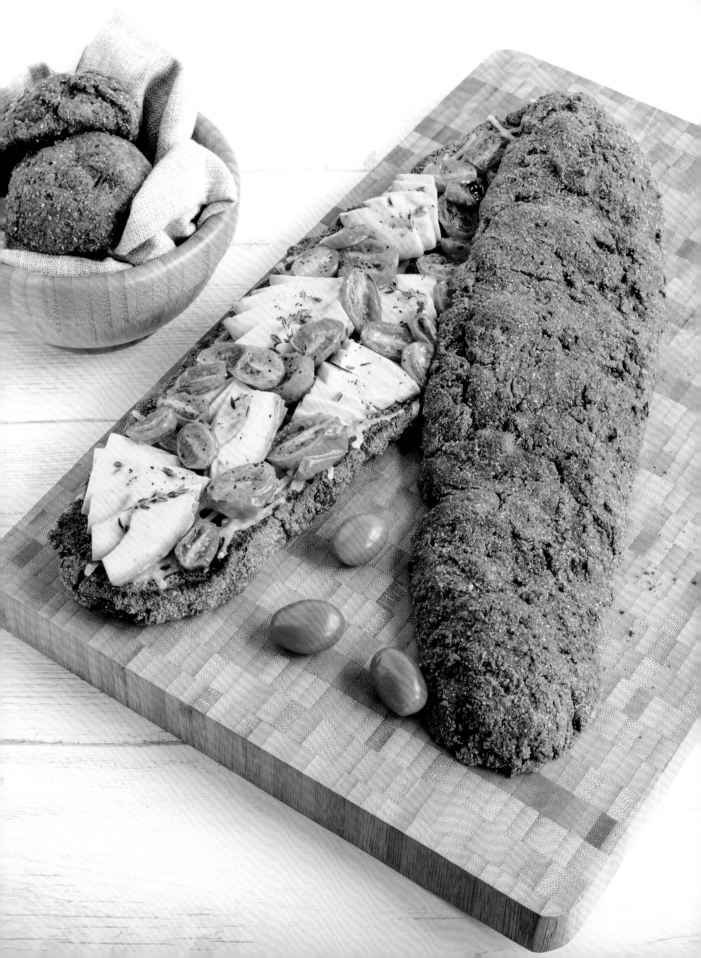

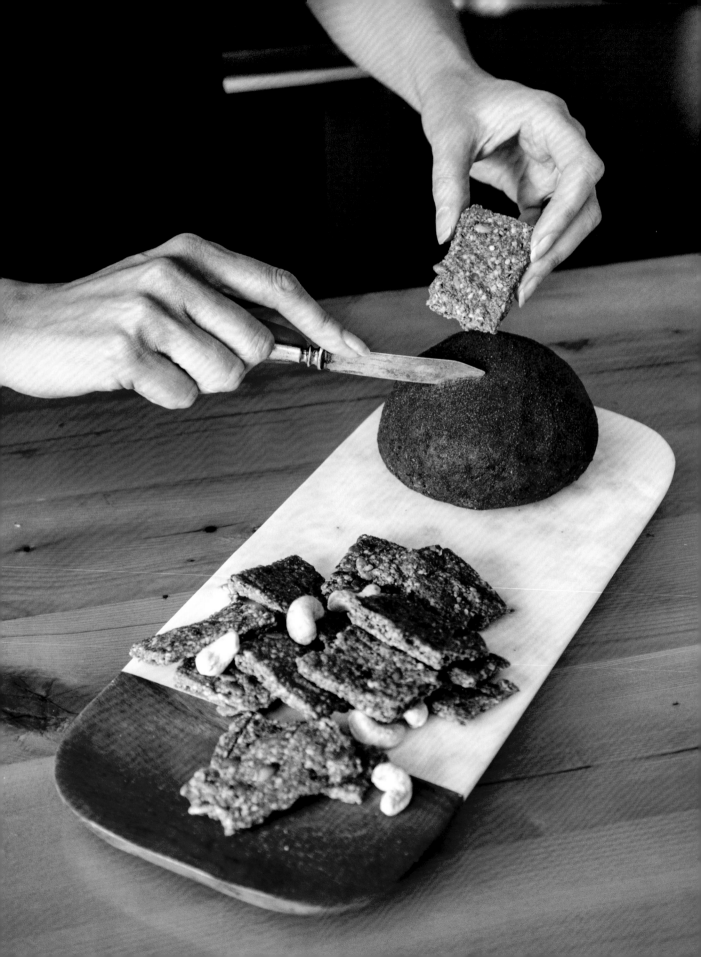

Keto Seed Crackers

       Makes 25 to 30 crackers

This low-carb cracker has an awesome sesame taste and makes a lovely combination when paired with Pizza Cheese (page 266). These crackers have heaps of fibre and are best enjoyed with a healthy beverage to maximize their digestive benefits. They are also safe in schools, as they are nut-free. This is my favourite cracker recipe and is as easy to make as cookies. I love to serve these crackers alongside dips and veggies at parties or as a substitute for chips or popcorn during a movie.

⅔ cup raw sunflower seeds, ground into flour

⅓ cup raw pumpkin seeds

⅓ cup ground golden flaxseed or white chia seeds

⅓ cup sesame or hemp seeds

1 tablespoon psyllium husk powder

1 teaspoon unrefined pink salt

1 tablespoon coconut oil

¾ cup boiling water

1. Position a rack in the lower third of the oven. Preheat the oven to 300°F. Line a baking sheet with unbleached parchment paper.

2. In a large bowl, mix together the ground sunflower seeds, pumpkin seeds, flaxseed, sesame seeds, psyllium and salt. Add the coconut oil and boiling water and mix with a spatula. Alternatively, you can mix everything together in a stand mixer.

3. Using your fingers, spread out the dough thinly, about ¼-inch thick, on the prepared baking sheet. Using a butter knife, score the crackers into 2-inch squares.

4. Bake for 50 to 60 minutes, then turn off the oven, keeping the door closed. Let sit in the oven to dry for another 20 to 30 minutes until golden brown, checking occasionally to make sure that they don't brown too much. Remove from the oven and let cool completely before breaking into pieces. Store in an airtight container on the countertop for up to 3 weeks.

Divine Grain-Free Crackers or Flatbread

OPTION

Makes 48 crackers or 20 flatbreads

I created these crackers to have something nourishing on the road that did not need refrigeration. I recommend making a double or triple batch, as they last for weeks. They are the perfect blend of salt, sweet and fat that satisfies the bliss point. I love knowing that my nutrition is covered with the omega-3 in the flaxseed and the anti-inflammatory spices. Also, the sweet potato makes these crackers appealing to kids and seniors with picky palettes.

1 cup ground flaxseed

¾ cup water

½ cup unsweetened nut or seed butter

1 teaspoon unrefined pink salt

10 black or green olives, pitted

2 cups roughly chopped fresh herbs (basil, chives, parsley) (or ½ cup mixed dried herbs of choice)

3 tablespoons yellow mustard

3 cups grated sweet potato

1 cup cassava flour or ground unsweetened coconut shreds (making a full-fat coconut flour)

1 cup sesame seeds or hemp hearts

1 cup sunflower seeds

1. Preheat the oven to 350°F. Line a baking sheet with unbleached parchment paper.

2. In a small bowl, soak the ground flaxseed in the water for 15 minutes.

3. Add the soaked flaxseed mixture, nut butter, salt, olives, herbs and mustard to a food processor and pulse to mix well. Add the sweet potato, cassava flour, sesame seeds and sunflower seeds and blend to a paste-like consistency, scraping down the sides as needed.

4. Spread the mixture evenly and smoothly to ¼-inch thickness on the prepared baking sheet. The mixture may be sticky. If it is difficult to spread evenly, do the best you can, then wet the back of a spatula to finish. Once smooth and even, use a fork to poke holes on the surface. Using a butter knife, score into 2- × 3-inch crackers or 4-inch square flatbreads. Bake for 60 minutes. Turn off the oven, flip the crackers and return to the warm oven for another 60 minutes or until very dry. If you used fresh herbs, you may need more time for a crisp cracker. (Alternatively, you can dehydrate the crackers at 120°F for 8 hours.)

5. Remove the crackers from the oven and let cool. When fully cooled, the crackers should be dry and crunchy. If you like a softer cracker, bake for a shorter period or use fresh herbs. Store in an airtight container on the countertop for up to 3 weeks.

Light Me Up Bread

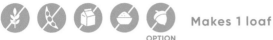 Makes 1 loaf

OPTION

The large number of eggs in this recipe dramatically increases the protein per slice, making this bread a great choice for breakfast. I like to bake two loaves at a time, then freeze the slices for meals on the run, as they toast well. The almond or sunflower seed flour makes this bread very low carb, with 1.5 net carbs per slice.

5 large eggs
¼ teaspoon cream of tartar (or ½ teaspoon lemon juice)
¼ cup coconut oil, melted
1¾ cups almond flour (or 2 cups sunflower seed flour)
⅓ cup coconut flour
2 teaspoons baking powder
Pinch of unrefined pink salt

1. Preheat the oven to 375°F. Line a 9- × 4-inch loaf pan with unbleached parchment paper, leaving an overhang on 2 sides.

2. In a large bowl or stand mixer fitted with the whisk attachment, separate the egg whites from the yolks. Reserve the yolks in a small bowl. Don't worry about precisely separating the eggs, since you will be folding everything back together soon enough (the egg whites give this loaf height).

3. Add the cream of tartar to the egg whites and whisk until soft peaks form. This step ensures that the egg whites stabilize. Set aside two-thirds of the whisked egg whites in a small bowl.

4. To the large bowl containing one-third of the whisked egg whites, add the reserved egg yolks, coconut oil, almond flour, coconut flour, baking powder and salt and stir until combined.

5. Gently fold in the remaining two-thirds of the whisked egg whites until fully incorporated. Be careful not to overmix, or the air bubbles in the whipped egg whites will collapse.

6. Pour the mixture into the prepared loaf pan. Bake for 35 to 38 minutes until golden on top, or until a toothpick or knife inserted in the middle comes out clean. Using the parchment paper, remove from the pan and let cool completely before slicing. Store in an airtight container in the fridge for up to 1 week or slice and keep in the freezer for up to 3 months.

Poppy Seed Lemon Loaf

    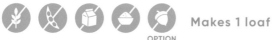

OPTION   Makes 1 loaf

This is a sweet variation of Light Me Up Bread (page 193). It tastes like a lovely pound cake and is great to serve with tea at a gathering. Poppy seeds are a rich source of vitamins B1 and B9 and essential minerals, including calcium, iron, magnesium, manganese, phosphorus and zinc.

Poppy Seed Lemon Loaf

5 large eggs

¼ teaspoon cream of tartar (or ½ teaspoon lemon juice)

¼ cup melted coconut oil

2¼ cups almond, hazelnut or sunflower seed flour

2 teaspoons baking powder

Pinch of unrefined pink salt

1 teaspoon lemon zest

¼ cup lemon juice

1 teaspoon pure monk fruit or stevia extract

1 tablespoon poppy seeds

Lemon Glaze

½ cup powdered monk fruit or erythritol sweetener

2 tablespoons lemon juice

1 teaspoon arrowroot flour, to thicken (optional)

1. To make the poppy seed lemon loaf, preheat the oven to 375°F. Line a 9- × 4-inch loaf pan with unbleached parchment paper, leaving an overhang on 2 sides.

2. In a large bowl or stand mixer fitted with the whisk attachment, separate the egg whites from the yolks. Reserve the yolks in a small bowl. Don't worry about precisely separating the eggs, since you will be folding everything back together soon enough (the egg whites give this loaf height).

3. Add the cream of tartar to the egg whites and whisk until soft peaks form. This step ensures that the egg whites stabilize. Set aside two-thirds of the whisked egg whites in a small bowl.

4. To the large bowl containing one-third of the whisked egg whites, add the reserved egg yolks, coconut oil, almond flour, baking powder and salt and stir until combined. Add the lemon zest and juice, monk fruit and poppy seeds and stir until combined.

5. Gently fold in the remaining two-thirds of the whisked egg whites until fully incorporated. Be careful not to overmix, or the air bubbles in the whipped egg whites will collapse.

6. Pour the mixture into the prepared loaf pan. Bake for 30 to 35 minutes until golden on top, or until a toothpick or knife inserted in the middle comes out clean. Using the parchment paper, remove from the pan and let cool completely before glazing.

7. Meanwhile, make the lemon glaze. In a small bowl, whisk together the monk fruit, lemon juice and arrowroot flour (if using) until well combined.

8. When the loaf is cool, drizzle the glaze overtop and serve. Store in an airtight container in the fridge for up to 1 week or slice and keep in the freezer for up to 3 months.

Corn-Free Tortilla Chips

    Makes 25 chips

When I gave up all grains, it was hard to stare down guacamole with just chopped veggies as a dipper. You are going to love how flexible this recipe is, because you can season it any way you like. Make sure to check the chips frequently when baking, especially the first couple of times you make them, until you get to know the timing in your oven. They go from lightly toasted to overdone in less than a minute. Roll out the dough thinly if you want tortilla chips or a bit thicker if you want them to be more like a pita chip.

2 large eggs (or 4 egg whites)
2 cups almond or hazelnut flour (see Tip)
1 teaspoon unrefined pink salt

Nacho Seasoning
2 tablespoons nutritional yeast
½ teaspoon garlic powder
½ teaspoon smoked paprika
Pinch of freshly cracked pepper

Curry Seasoning
½ teaspoon smoked paprika
½ teaspoon ground turmeric
½ teaspoon ground cumin
Pinch of cayenne pepper

1. Preheat the oven to 350°F. Line a baking sheet with unbleached parchment paper.

2. In a large bowl, combine the eggs, almond flour, salt and any desired seasoning. Mix until smoothly combined.

3. Transfer the dough to the prepared baking sheet. Lay a sheet of parchment paper over the dough and, using a rolling pin or the side of a tall glass, roll the dough to the desired thickness. The thinner the dough, the crispier the chip.

4. Once you have rolled the dough into an even sheet, use a butter knife to score it into triangles, cleaning up the edges to make an even and uniform chip shape.

5. Bake for 10 minutes for tortilla chips or 15 to 20 minutes for pita-style chips, until golden. Watch them carefully, as they can go from perfect to overdone very quickly.

Tip: Two cups of unsweetened shredded coconut ground into flour using a clean coffee grinder or small food processor works as a substitute for 1 cup almond or hazelnut flour, but you need to add 1 tablespoon of white chia seeds or golden flaxseed to the mix to help bind it together. Do not use store-bought coconut flour or the chips will be too dry.

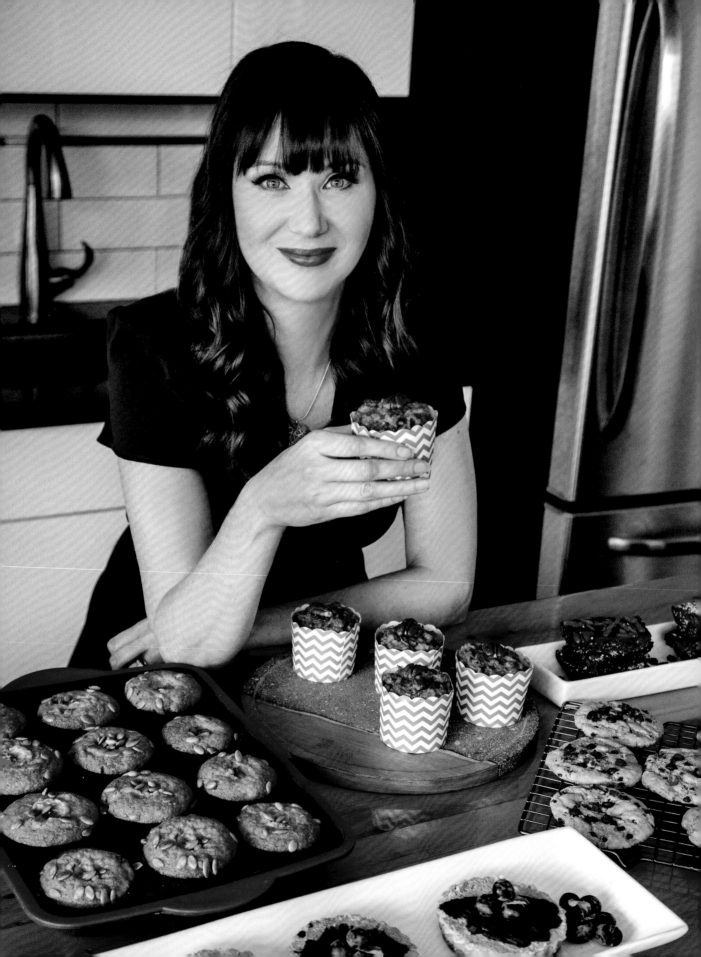

Cookies, Cakes, Squares and Muffins

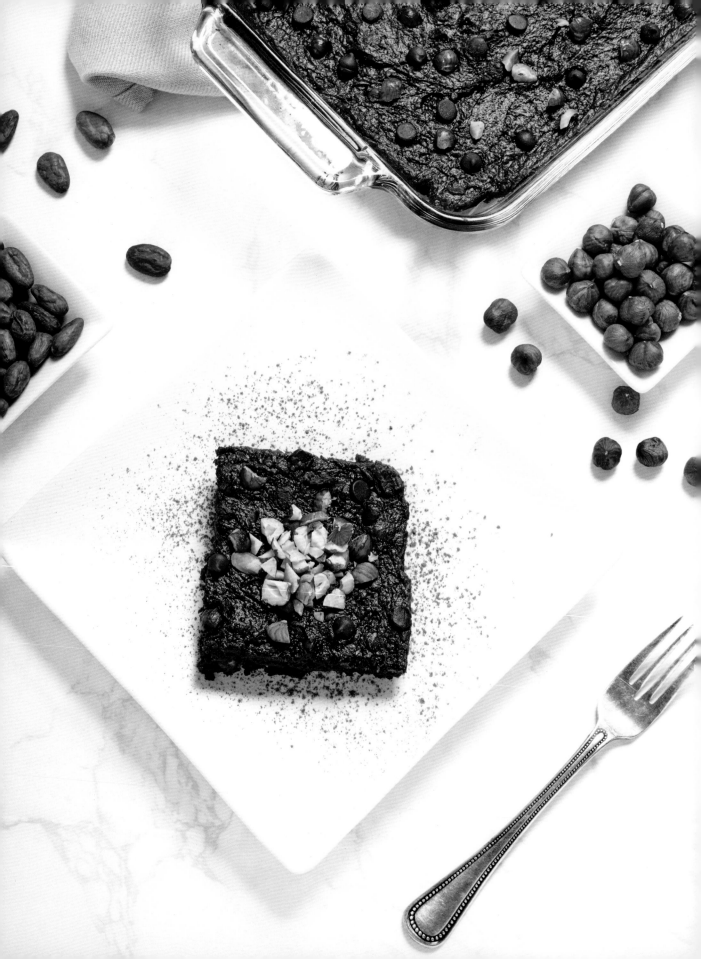

Avocado Keto Brownies

      Makes 9 brownies

Avocados truly are nutrition powerhouses. They are a great source of many vitamins, such as vitamins B-complex, E and K. They are also high in healthy fats, known as monounsaturated fats, which are great for the heart and help with the absorption of other nutrients. In these brownies, avocados provide a creamy and fudgy texture that will please even the most skeptical brownie lover. Serious sugar lovers taste-tested these brownies and they gobbled them up.

1 cup Coconut Whipping Cream (page 227; see Tip)

1 cup unsweetened creamy nut or seed butter

1 cup mashed ripe avocado

¼ cup ground flaxseed or chia seeds

½ cup almond, hazelnut or sunflower seed flour (see Tip)

⅓ cup cacao powder

1 teaspoon cinnamon

1 teaspoon pure vanilla extract

½ teaspoon unrefined pink salt

2 teaspoons pure monk fruit extract or chocolate stevia

Optional Add-Ins

½ cup sugar-free chocolate chips

½ cup chopped raw nuts (pecans, hazelnuts, almonds)

1. Preheat the oven to 325°F. Line an 8-inch square baking dish with unbleached parchment paper.

2. Combine the coconut cream, nut butter, avocado, flaxseed, almond flour, cacao powder, cinnamon, vanilla, salt and monk fruit in a food processor or high-speed blender and blend on high until smooth. Transfer to a medium bowl and stir in the chocolate chips and nuts, if using.

3. Scrape the batter into the prepared baking dish. Using the back of a spoon or a sheet of unbleached parchment paper, level out the batter across the dish.

4. Bake for 25 to 28 minutes, or until a toothpick inserted in the middle comes out clean. Remove from the oven and let cool.

5. Cut into 9 squares and serve or store the brownies in an airtight container on the countertop for up to 1 week or in the freezer for up to 3 months.

Tips:

1. If you only have canned coconut milk, place a 14-ounce can of full-fat coconut milk in the fridge overnight. When ready to make the brownies, scoop out the solid coconut cream and add enough coconut water to equal 1 cup. Use the leftover coconut water in smoothies and other recipes.

2. You can make ½ cup sunflower seed flour by placing ⅓ cup sunflower seeds in a clean coffee grinder or high-speed blender, then grinding them for about 30 seconds or until a fine nut flour–like texture is reached.

Banana Muffins

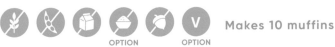

OPTION   OPTION   **Makes 10 muffins**

This muffin recipe is a real crowd-pleaser because it is so balanced and delicious. No one will ever know that it is free of refined flour and sugar. This muffin is wonderful to share with friends who have allergies because the cassava flour is so well tolerated. If you want to reduce the carbohydrates even further, you can substitute almond or hazelnut flour for the cassava flour.

1 cup cassava flour

¼ cup coconut flour

2 teaspoons baking powder

1 teaspoon cinnamon

½ teaspoon unrefined pink salt

1½ cups mashed ripe banana (about 3 large)

¼ cup yacón syrup (see Tip; or ½ teaspoon pure monk fruit extract)

½ cup melted coconut oil

2 large eggs, room temperature (or flax or chia egg; see Tip)

¼ cup full-fat coconut milk

1 teaspoon pure vanilla extract

½ cup sugar-free chocolate chips or raw pumpkin seeds (optional)

1. Preheat the oven to 375°F. Line a muffin tin with paper liners.

2. In a medium bowl, mix together the cassava flour, coconut flour, baking powder, cinnamon and salt.

3. In a large bowl, combine the banana, yacón syrup, coconut oil, eggs, coconut milk and vanilla.

4. Fold the dry mixture into the wet mixture, stirring until fully incorporated. Mix in the chocolate chips or pumpkin seeds, if using.

5. Fill the muffin cups about three-quarters full. Bake for about 28 to 30 minutes, until the edges are golden brown and firm. Let cool for at least 10 minutes before serving. Store, covered, on the countertop for up to 3 days or in the freezer for up to 3 months.

Tips:

1. Coconut nectar can be substituted for the yacón syrup if you are on the slow breakup plan and can tolerate some sucrose.

2. To make the flax or chia egg, in a small bowl, whisk together 2 tablespoons ground flaxseed or chia seeds and 5 tablespoons hot water until well combined. Set aside to soak for 10 minutes so that the flaxseed can swell and absorb the liquid.

No Sugar Added Option: Use pure monk fruit extract.

Vegan Option: Use flax or chia egg substitute.

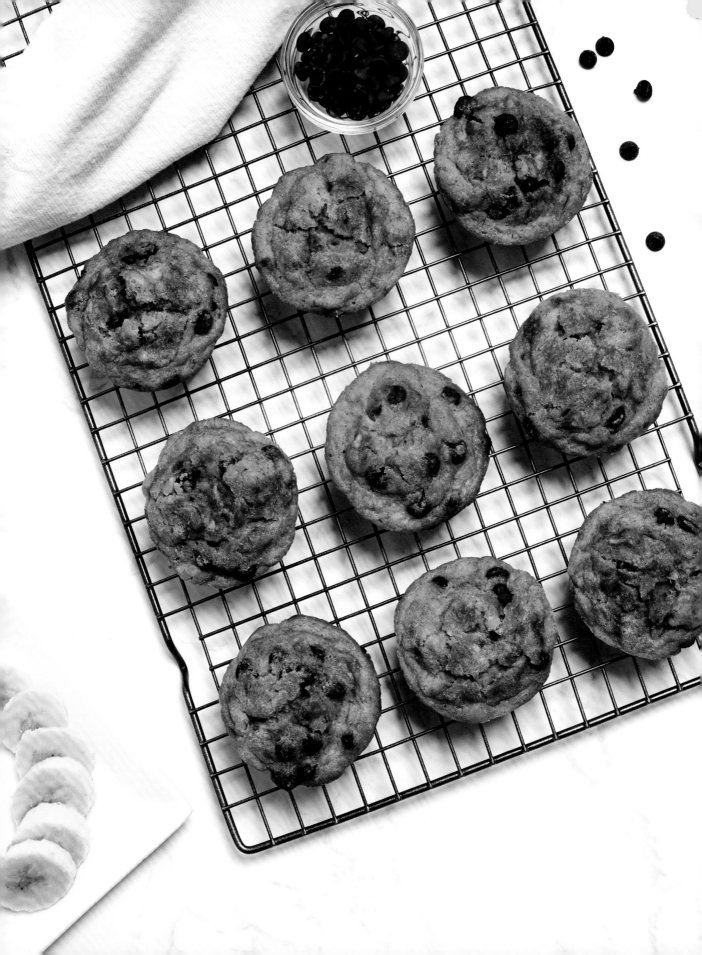

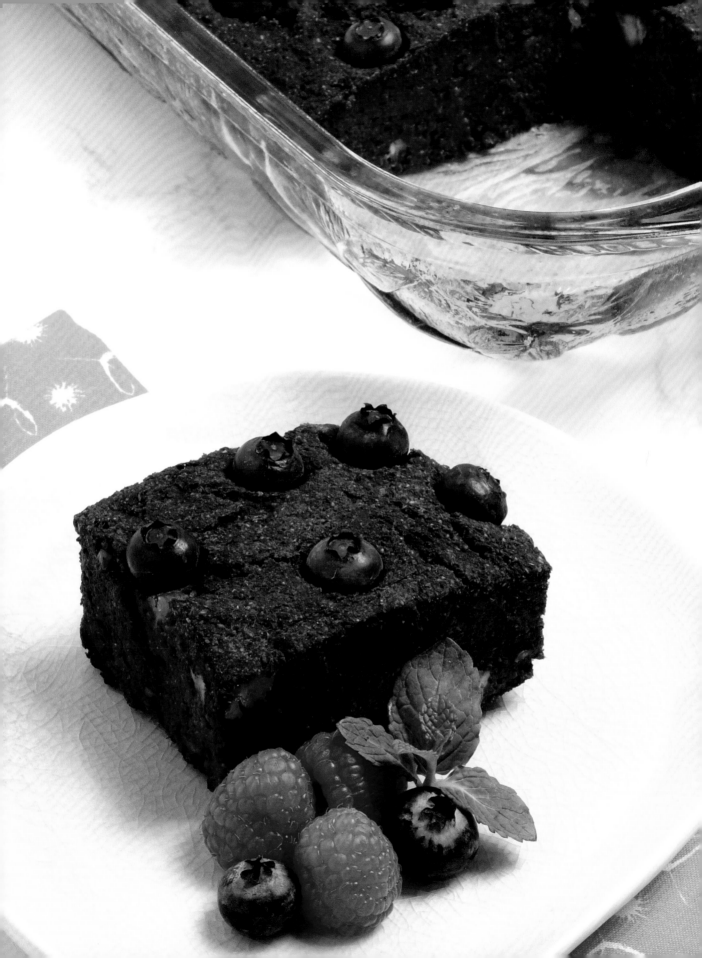

Berry Brownie Cake

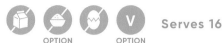 **Serves 16**

My sister, Lynn, is a master grain-free baker who has the knack of figuring out the exact ratios to make cakes, cookies and pies taste heavenly. When she dreamt up this perfectly balanced chocolate birthday cake for her son Kaydn, we knew she had struck gold. It has the perfect balance of fudge to cake texture that will have you dreaming of seconds. I love the monk fruit extract for a no-added-sugar version, but Lynn enjoys using honey to satisfy her kids.

½ cup whole chia seeds

1⅓ cups water or coconut beverage

6 ripe bananas (see Tip)

½ cup coconut oil, melted plus more to grease the pan

½ teaspoon pure monk fruit extract (or ½ cup raw honey)

1 cup raw pecans, chopped

1 cup coconut flour, if using monk fruit (or 1½ cups coconut flour, if using honey)

1 cup cocoa powder

1 teaspoon unrefined pink salt

1 teaspoon baking soda

1 cup fresh or frozen raspberries or blueberries

Tip: I suggest that you freeze the ripe bananas and then thaw them before using them. This cuts down on the guesswork as to the moisture level of the cake.

No Sugar Added Option: Use pure monk fruit extract.

Vegan Option: Omit the honey.

1. Preheat the oven to 350°F. Grease one 13- × 9-inch baking dish or two 10-inch pie plates with coconut oil or line them with unbleached parchment paper, leaving enough overhang for easy removal.

2. Grind the chia seeds in a clean coffee or spice grinder. This will give you about ⅔ cup ground chia seeds, but do not worry about an exact measurement.

3. Place the ground chia seeds in the bowl of a stand mixer. (Alternatively, you can use a hand mixer.) Add the water and blend for 2 minutes to allow the chia to thicken.

4. Mix in the bananas, then add the melted coconut oil, monk fruit and pecans.

5. In a medium bowl, sift together the coconut flour, cocoa powder, salt and baking soda.

6. Slowly add the dry ingredients to the wet ingredients and mix for 1 minute.

7. If using frozen berries, stir them into the batter for 1 minute until lightly combined. Do not overmix, as the chunks of frozen berries, if using, add lovely pops of flavour to the cake. If using fresh berries, press them directly into the top of the cake batter to create a lovely effect.

8. Spread the batter evenly between the dishes. Bake for 30 to 40 minutes, until the cake is firm and springs back when gently pressed. Let cool in the pan before serving. Store in an airtight container on the countertop for 1 week or in the freezer for up to 3 months.

Carrot Cake Muffins

 Makes 12 large or 24 mini muffins

Do you want a decadent muffin that will really wow your family? This cake muffin has all the bells and whistles and is so healthy because you sneak veggies into kids without them noticing. If you would prefer to make this as a cake, use an 11- × 7-inch cake pan. What makes this cake different is that I slashed the carbs by getting rid of the added sugar. It is nice topped with Vegan Buttercream Icing (page 293).

2½ cups almond, pecan, hazelnut or sunflower seed flour

2 teaspoons baking powder

1 teaspoon unrefined pink salt

¼ teaspoon ground turmeric

1 tablespoon cinnamon

1 teaspoon pure monk fruit extract (or ½ teaspoon liquid stevia)

1 cup mashed ripe banana

3 large eggs (or flax or chia egg; see Tip)

1 teaspoon apple cider vinegar

2 teaspoons pure vanilla extract

¼ cup coconut oil, melted

2 cups shredded carrots

1 cup shredded zucchini

¾ cup chopped raw walnuts or pecans

½ cup raisins (optional)

Vegan Option: Use flax or chia egg substitute.

1. Preheat the oven to 350°F. Line 12 large or 24 mini muffin cups with unbleached paper liners.

2. In a small bowl, combine the almond flour, baking powder, salt, turmeric and cinnamon.

3. In the bowl of a stand mixer or blender, combine the monk fruit, banana, eggs, apple cider vinegar, vanilla and coconut oil and blend until well combined.

4. Transfer the wet mixture to a large bowl (or leave in the bowl of a stand mixer, if using), add the dry ingredients and mix until thoroughly combined.

5. Fold in the carrots, zucchini, walnuts and raisins, if using.

6. Fill the muffin cups about three-quarters full. (I like to use 2 spoons for this. Scoop with one spoon and push and fill the cup with the other spoon.)

7. Bake for 30 to 35 minutes for mini muffins, 50 to 60 minutes for large muffins or 70 minutes for a cake, until golden brown on the edges and a knife inserted in the middle comes out clean. Let cool in the muffin tins for 1 hour, then remove from the tins to cool completely. Store in an airtight container on the countertop for up to 3 days, in the fridge for up to 10 days or in the freezer for up to 3 months.

Tip: To make the flax or chia egg, in a small bowl, whisk together 1 tablespoon ground flaxseed or chia seeds and 2½ tablespoons hot water until well combined. Set aside to soak for 10 minutes so that the flaxseed or chia seeds can swell and absorb the liquid. This version of the recipe may increase the cooking time for both muffins and cake by 5 minutes.

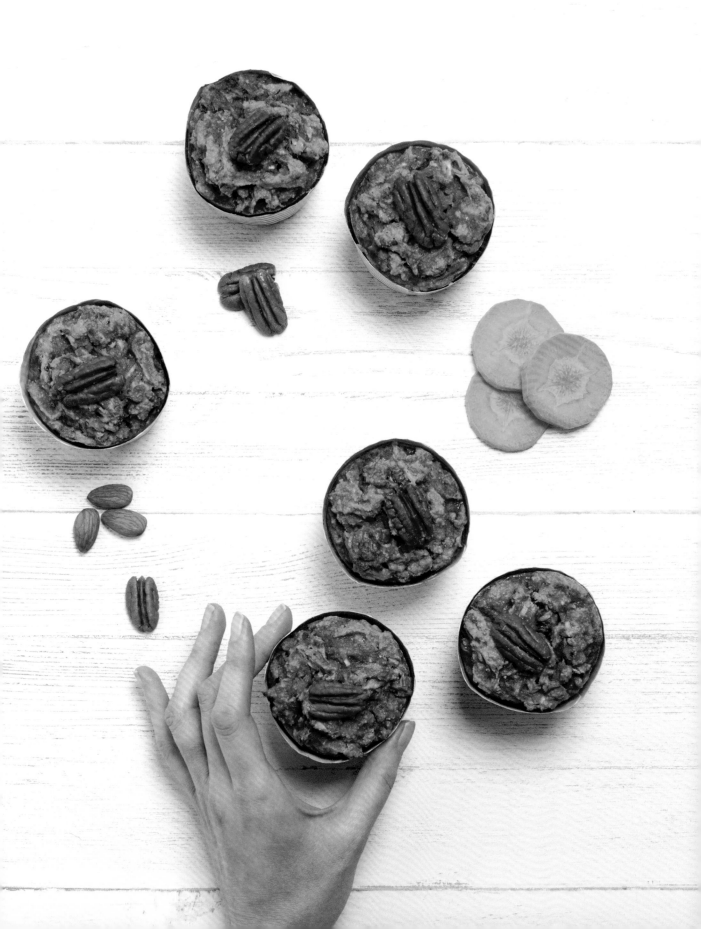

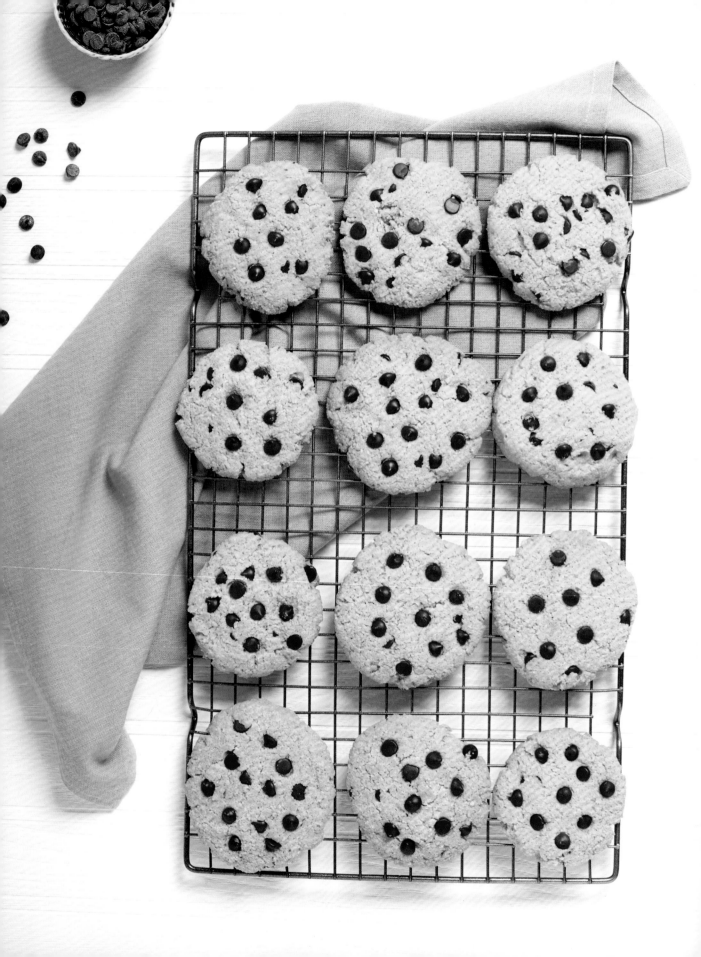

Chippy Chocolate Cookies

       Makes 14 large or 18 small cookies

OPTION   OPTION   OPTION

These cookies are the real deal. They are chewy on the inside and crispy on the outside. You won't believe they are healthy. The alternative flours make these cookies high in fibre, unlike conventional cookies made with refined white flour. The monk fruit erythritol crystals create a crispy texture similar to that of cookies made with refined sugar but without the blood sugar spike. When combined with Sweet Potato Ice Cream (page 282), these make a fantastic ice cream sandwich.

⅓ cup coconut oil or vegan butter, room temperature (see Tip)

¾ cup monk fruit erythritol crystals or coconut sugar (see Tip)

⅓ cup natural nut or seed butter, room temperature

2 teaspoons pure vanilla extract

2 large eggs (or flax or chia egg; see Tip)

1 cup almond, hazelnut or sunflower seed flour (extra fine flour is best; see Tip)

⅓ cup coconut flour

1 teaspoon baking powder

¼ teaspoon unrefined pink salt

½ cup stevia-sweetened chocolate chips (or ¾ cup cranberries or chopped nuts) (optional)

1. Combine the coconut oil, monk fruit erythritol crystals and nut butter in the bowl of a stand mixer. Mix at medium speed until well combined. (Alternatively, you can use an electric hand mixer and beat the mixture in a medium bowl.)

2. Mix in the vanilla and eggs at low speed until well incorporated.

3. In a large bowl, stir together the almond flour, coconut flour, baking powder and salt.

4. Stir the dry ingredients into the wet ingredients until well combined. If there is time, place the bowl in the refrigerator for 30 minutes to firm up the dough and make it easier to roll into balls.

5. Meanwhile, preheat the oven to 350°F. Line a baking sheet or two with unbleached parchment paper.

6. Using your hands, roll the dough into 14 large or 18 small balls and arrange them on the prepared baking sheets spaced 2 inches apart. Press the cookies down lightly with the palm of your hand, then gently press the chocolate chips (if using) into the dough. Avoid adding the chocolate chips before this step because it makes the cookies crumble.

7. Bake for 12 minutes for a chewy cookie or 14 minutes for a crispier cookie (for large cookies, add 1 minute to the baking time). The cookies will be very soft but continue to cook as they cool.

Recipe continues

8. Let cool completely on the baking sheets. Store in an airtight container on the countertop for up to 4 days or in the freezer for up to 3 months.

Tips:

1. If you live in a hot climate, place the coconut oil in the fridge for 15 minutes to firm it to the consistency of soft butter. If you use slightly melted coconut oil, the dough will be greasy and the chocolate chips (if using) will be hard to incorporate.

2. Coconut sugar is permitted if you are on the slow breakup plan and can tolerate sucrose.

3. To make the flax or chia egg, in a small bowl, whisk together 2 tablespoons ground flaxseed or chia seeds and 5 tablespoons hot water until well combined. Set aside to soak for 10 minutes so that the flaxseed can swell and absorb the liquid.

4. Sunflower seed flour can work as a substitute but will change the flavour.

No Sugar Added Option: Use monk fruit erythritol crystals.

Vegan Option: Use flax or chia egg substitute.

Wee Sunny Cheesecakes

OPTION   OPTION   **Makes 9 individual cheesecakes**

I know there are many cashew cheesecake recipes out there, so I wanted to push myself to create a sunflower seed version. Now there is a treat for those following a low-carb lifestyle and also avoiding nuts. My Scottish grandma often used the word *wee* to describe the tiny things in her life. She was so thrifty that she taught me a lot about how to save money wherever we could. Sunflower seeds are the most inexpensive seed in the store and are often grown locally, so I think this cake would make her proud. When I saw how cute these mini cheesecakes were, I heard her adorable voice ring out, "What a wee sunny cheesecake, Jules!" Here is a dish to make for your granny who is striving to get healthy but still loves a good treat.

Filling

2 cups raw sunflower seeds (see Tip)

3 cups water, for soaking

1 teaspoon pure monk fruit extract + ½ cup coconut cream (see Tip; or ½ cup raw honey)

⅔ cup coconut butter or oil

½ cup full-fat coconut milk

2 tablespoons lemon juice

2 teaspoons pure vanilla extract

½ teaspoon unrefined pink salt

½ teaspoon cinnamon

¼ teaspoon ground turmeric (or a few drops yellow natural food colouring) (optional)

Crust

1 cup unsweetened shredded coconut

1 cup raw pecans

¼ cup ground chia seeds or flaxseed

Pinch of unrefined pink salt

¼ cup coconut cream (see Tip)

½ teaspoon liquid stevia (or 1 teaspoon pure monk fruit extract)

1. To start making the filling, in a large bowl, soak the sunflower seeds in the water for 24 hours to soften them completely. Make sure to rinse and drain the seeds well in a mesh colander. Using a clean kitchen towel, pat dry the top and bottom of the colander to remove any excess moisture from the seeds.

2. To make the crust, combine the coconut, pecans, ground chia seeds, salt, coconut cream and stevia in a food processor. Pulse until a crumb-like mixture forms. Press the crust mixture into 3-inch tart pans or small ramekins. Clean the bowl of the food processor.

3. To finish making the filling, combine the soaked and drained sunflower seeds, monk fruit and coconut cream, coconut butter, coconut milk, lemon juice, vanilla, salt, cinnamon and turmeric (if using) in the food processor and blend until smooth. Divide the filling evenly among the tart pans or ramekins, smoothing the tops with the back of a spoon. Cover and place in the fridge for 1 hour to set. Clean the bowl of the food processor.

Recipe continues

Salty Caramel Sauce

6 large Medjool dates, pitted and soaked in 1 cup warm water for 30 minutes (reserve 2 tablespoons soaking liquid)

¼ cup unsweetened creamy nut or seed butter

3 tablespoons coconut oil

½ teaspoon pure vanilla extract

¼ teaspoon pure monk fruit extract (or 2 tablespoons yacón syrup or honey)

¼ to ½ teaspoon unrefined pink salt

Fresh berries (such as blueberries or raspberries) or edible flowers (such as violets, pansies or daisy and rose petals), for garnish (optional)

4. Meanwhile, make the salty caramel sauce. Combine the dates, nut butter, coconut oil, vanilla, monk fruit, salt and reserved soaking liquid into the food processor. Blend until completely smooth.

5. When ready to serve, top the cheesecakes with the salty caramel sauce and berries or edible flowers (if using) just before serving. Store the cheesecakes, without the sauce or garnishes, in an airtight container in the freezer until ready to serve.

Tips:

1. If you can tolerate nuts, this is decadent with cashews instead of sunflower seeds. You'll need to soak the cashews, too.

2. For coconut cream, place a 14-ounce can of full-fat coconut milk in the fridge overnight. Scoop out the solid coconut cream. Use the coconut water in smoothies and other recipes.

3. For low carb, omit the Salty Carmel Sauce.

No Sugar Added Option: Use pure monk fruit extract.

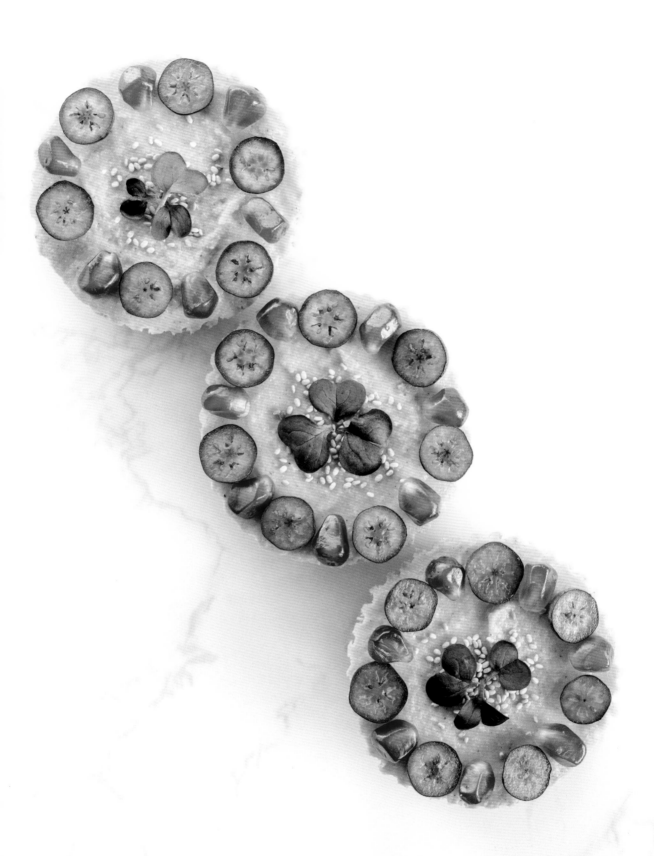

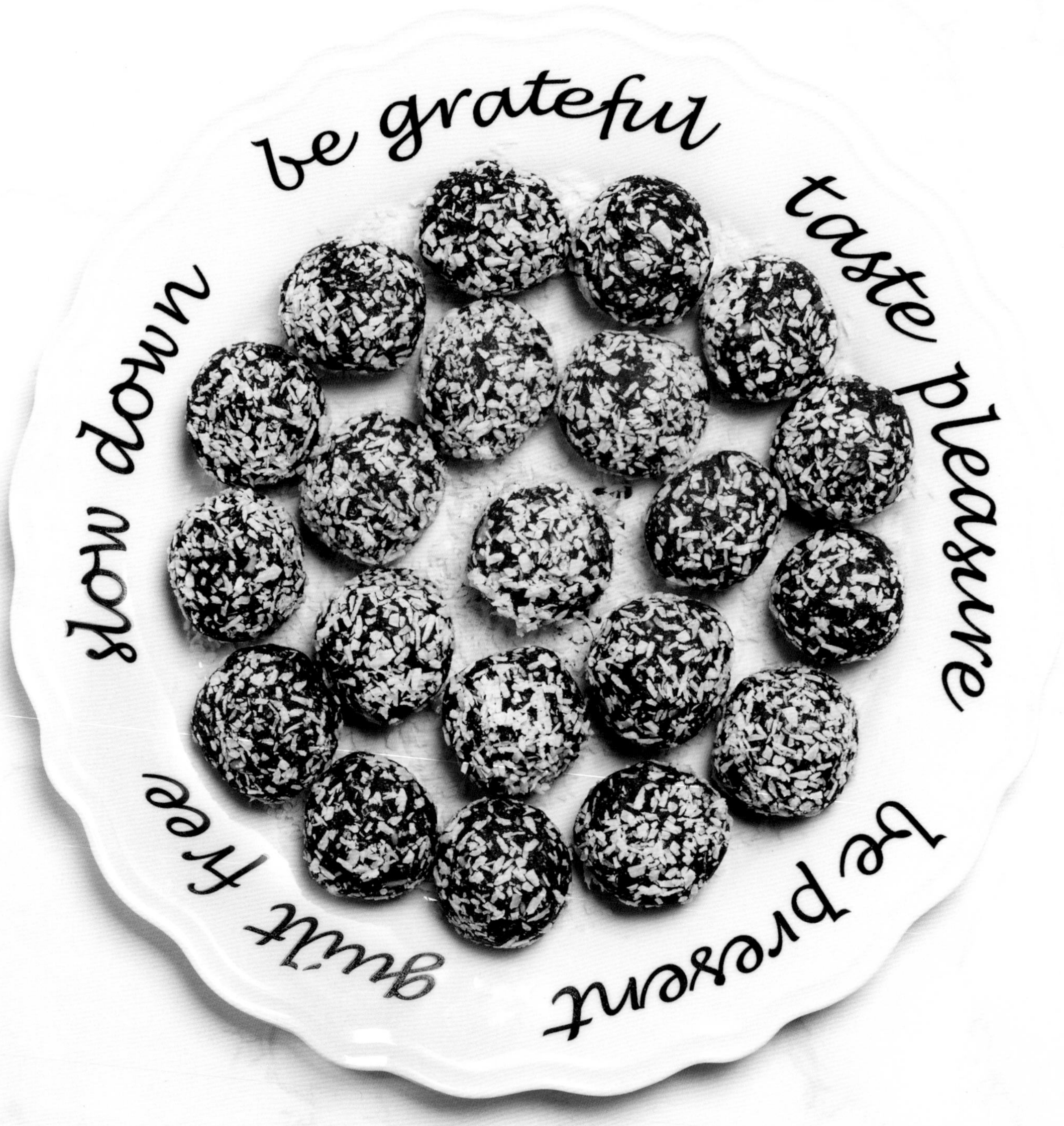
be grateful
taste pleasure
be present
guilt free
slow down

LynnBits

         Makes 24 energy balls

These energy balls look so much like Timbits® that my husband, Alan, named them LynnBits after my sister, Lynn, who created the recipe. They are nut- and egg-free, so they are perfect for bringing to gatherings or to school. I love to take these with me when I travel because they are so portable, keep nicely in my purse or computer bag and don't break apart easily.

1 cup raw sunflower seeds

2 tablespoons flax seeds

½ cup coconut flour

1 cup cocoa or cacao powder

1 teaspoon baking soda

½ teaspoon unrefined pink salt

3 tablespoons softened coconut oil (not melted)

½ cup raw honey (or ⅔ cup Faux Maple Syrup, page 225, + 3 tablespoons monk fruit erythritol powder)

¼ cup unsweetened flaked coconut

1. Position a rack in the upper third of the oven. Preheat the oven to 325°F. Line a baking sheet with unbleached parchment paper.

2. Grind the sunflower seeds into a flour in a clean coffee grinder or small food processor. Transfer to a small bowl.

3. Grind the flax seeds into a flour in a clean coffee grinder.

4. Combine the sunflower seed flour, ground flaxseed, coconut flour, cocoa powder, baking soda and salt in the bowl of a stand mixer. With the mixer running on low speed, slowly add the coconut oil, 1 tablespoon at a time, and then slowly add the honey. The resulting dough should be firm and easy to form into a ball.

5. Place the flaked coconut in a small bowl. Using your hands, roll 1 tablespoon of dough into a ball. Roll the ball in the flaked coconut and place it on the prepared baking sheet. Repeat with the remaining dough.

6. If you are using honey, bake for 10 minutes to create a stiff outer shell. Let cool completely on the pan. If you are making the low-carb version using the Faux Maple Syrup mixture, enjoy them raw out of the fridge.

7. For the baked version, store in an airtight container on the countertop for up to 2 weeks or in the freezer for up to 3 months.

No Sugar Added Option: Use Faux Maple Syrup and monk fruit erythritol powder mixture.

Vegan Option: Omit the honey.

T-Bars

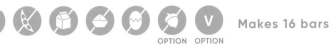

Makes 16 bars

These bars are sweet and satisfying for kids of all ages. My athletic nephew Taevan loves them so much that I decided they should be called T-bars. They make excellent energy bars for athletes and people on the run. I developed these when I was training for my first 5K charity race for Camp Ooch, which supports kids undergoing cancer treatment. The dates provide B vitamins, fibre and energy for running while avoiding the sugar crash. The unrefined pink salt gives you extra electrolyte minerals, and the cacao boosts energy. I love that you can make these in advance for events and parties.

2 cups pitted Medjool dates
(about 13 dates; see Tip)
1 cup chopped raw nuts
(walnuts, almonds, pecans)
or raw seeds (pumpkin or
sunflower)
¼ cup collagen, gelatin or
pumpkin seed protein
powder
2 tablespoons cocoa or cacao
powder
1 teaspoon pure vanilla extract
Pinch of unrefined pink salt

Optional Toppings
¼ cup hemp hearts, chia seeds,
raw pumpkin seeds,
unsweetened shredded
coconut, goji berries or
sugar-free chocolate chips
½ cup melted sugar-free
chocolate chips

1. Line an 11- × 7-inch baking dish with unbleached parchment paper.

2. Combine the dates, nuts, collagen, cocoa powder, vanilla and salt in a food processor. Process until a fine crumble forms.

3. Transfer the mixture to the prepared baking dish. Evenly spread and press the mixture into the dish to 1-inch thickness. Place in the fridge for 20 minutes.

4. Slice into bars using a butter knife. If using optional toppings or chocolate, press them into the unsliced bars or pour an even layer of melted chocolate over the bars before slicing. Store in an airtight container in the fridge for up to 1 month or in the freezer for up to 6 months.

Tip: Medjool dates are ideal because they are soft and easy to process. If unavailable, you can soften regular pitted dates by soaking them in hot water for a few minutes and draining them well. The water will shorten the life of the bars, so store them in the freezer once made.

Vegan Option: Use pumpkin seed protein powder. Check chocolate chips for traces of dairy.

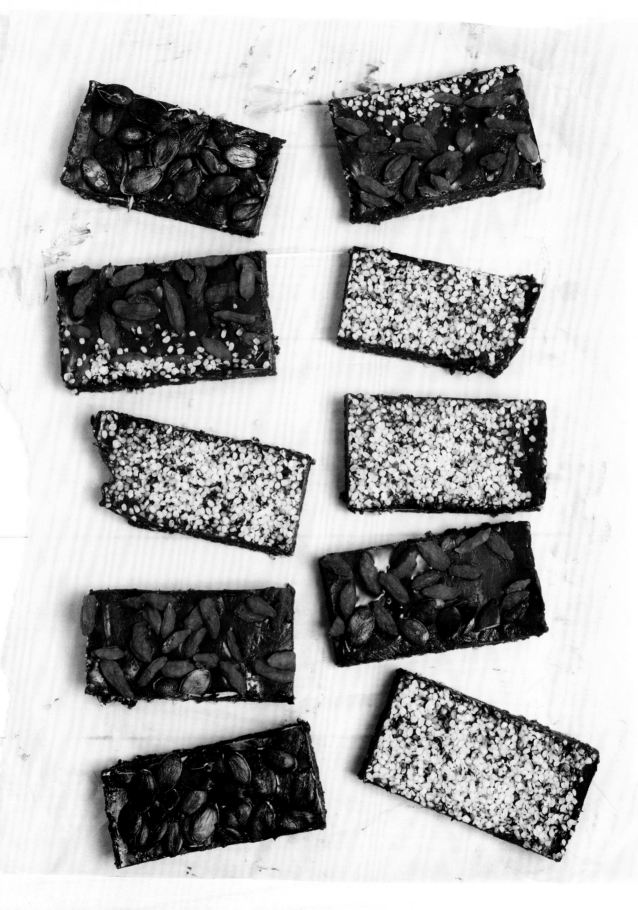

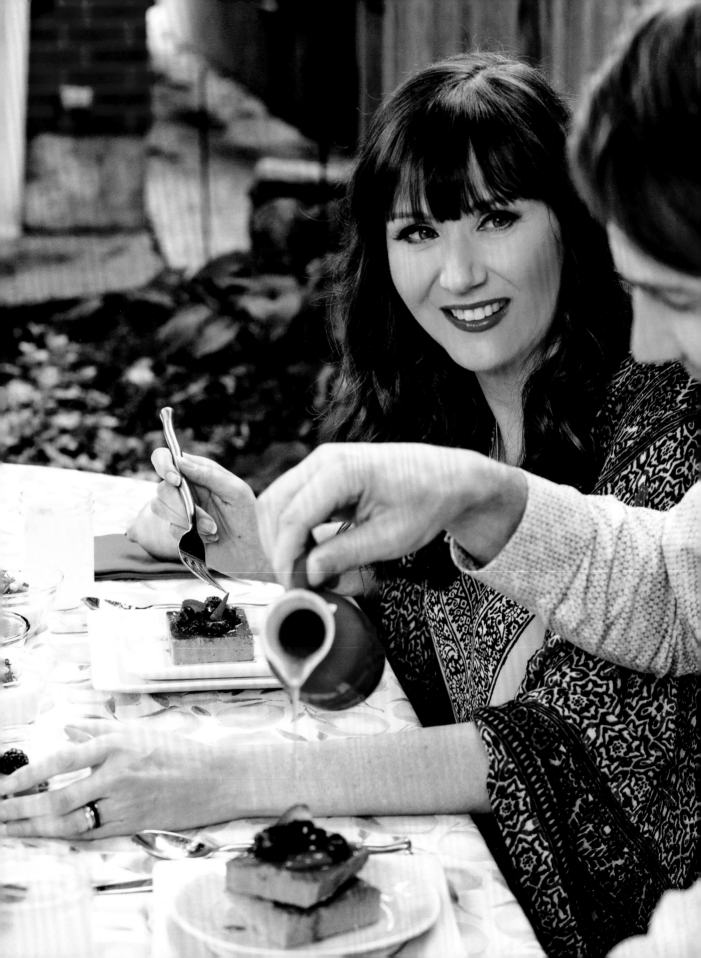

Jams, Dressings and Sauces

Avocado Mayonnaise

      Makes 1¼ cups

Real mayonnaise can be made healthfully, but the commercial brands may have terrible ingredients, including genetically modified and refined soybean or canola oil, high-fructose corn syrup, refined white sugar and modified corn starch. Once you realize that making sugar-free mayo is as easy as making a smoothie, you'll make this recipe weekly to use in dozens of recipes and improvised dishes. I love making this mayo with an immersion blender and mason jar because I don't waste any precious mayo in the bottom of a standard blender. Avocado oil has a delicate, neutral taste and heart-healthy omega-9 fatty acids. You can easily adapt this recipe to make a garlic or basil aioli (see Tips).

2 extra-large eggs, room temperature (organic and as fresh as possible)

1 cup avocado oil, divided

2 teaspoons lemon juice

½ teaspoon Dijon or stone-ground mustard

½ teaspoon unrefined pink salt

1 to 2 drops pure monk fruit extract (optional)

1. Bring a small pot of water to 160°F. (Use a candy thermometer to gauge the temperature, if you have one.) Using a slotted spoon, lower and completely submerge the eggs in the water for 2 minutes. Remove the eggs from the water and immediately plunge them into cold water. Some people choose to skip this step of pasteurization if they have access to very fresh organic eggs, but I advise you not to skip this step.

2. Crack the eggs and combine them with 2 tablespoons of the avocado oil, lemon juice, mustard, salt and monk fruit (if using) in a small food processor. With the motor running, very slowly drizzle the remaining avocado oil into the food processor. Do not rush adding the oil or the mayonnaise could split. You want the mayonnaise to be stiff and spreadable.

Tips:

1. To make a garlic aioli, add 1 crushed garlic clove and blend with the ingredients in step 2.

2. To make a basil aioli, add 1 teaspoon dairy-free pesto and blend with the ingredients in step 2.

Bold Barbecue Sauce

      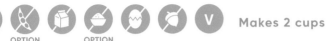

OPTION   OPTION

Makes 2 cups

My dad is a huge fan of HP Sauce, so when he gave up refined sugar, I worked hard to find a tasty replacement. The fibre in the dates and citrus thickens this sauce, so it does not need to be reduced on the stove unless you want a thicker sauce. (For a thicker sauce, simmer over medium heat for about 10 minutes.) To make a lower carb version, substitute the apple cider with fruit-flavoured herbal tea, such as an apple-flavoured herbal tea that is calorie-free but tastes strongly of apple.

½ cup tomato paste

½ cup apple cider

2 small clementines or 1 large orange, peeled

½ teaspoon pure monk fruit extract (or ⅓ cup pitted chopped dates)

3 tablespoons coconut sauce or wheat-free tamari

1 tablespoon smoked paprika

2 teaspoons onion powder

2 teaspoons yellow mustard

1½ teaspoons garlic powder

½ teaspoon pure vanilla extract

½ teaspoon unrefined pink salt

Optional Add-Ins (use up to 3)

1 tablespoon mesquite powder

2 teaspoons tamarind paste

½ to 1 teaspoons hot sauce, to taste

¼ teaspoon black pepper

1 tablespoon apple cider vinegar

¼ teaspoon organic clementine or orange zest

1. Combine all ingredients, and any add-ins, in a blender and blend on high speed until smooth, scraping down the sides as needed. Transfer to a mason jar and store in the fridge for up to 3 weeks. The sauce will thicken when refrigerated.

No Sugar Added Option: Use pure monk fruit extract.

Cheery Chimichurri   Makes ⅔ cup

Chimichurri sauce is an easy dairy-free substitute for basil pesto that can be made with parsley or cilantro (also known as coriander). It is used in many cuisines around the world and has powerful anti-inflammatory properties. The essential oil in cilantro helps reduce a type of yeast in the body called *Candida albicans*. It is important to reduce candida because when it overgrows in the body, it causes excessive sugar cravings and digestive trouble. If you don't like cilantro, just swap it out for basil.

3 cups fresh cilantro leaves (about 1 bunch)
2 cloves garlic, chopped
¼ teaspoon unrefined pink salt
2 tablespoons lemon or lime juice
3 tablespoons extra-virgin olive oil

1. Combine the cilantro, garlic, salt and lemon juice in a food processor or high-speed blender and blend until the desired consistency is reached, scraping down the sides as needed.

2. With the motor running, slowly add the olive oil until a creamy sauce forms. Transfer to a mason jar and seal tightly with a lid to avoid oxidation. Store in the fridge for up to 1 week.

Cranberry Sauce   Makes 1½ cups

In Ayurveda (the medicinal system of India), cranberries are used to stop diarrhea, relieve inflammation and strengthen the liver. In the West, cranberries are shown to prevent urinary tract infections (UTIs), flush out toxins and excess fluid, promote regularity and provide relief from bloating. A typical 2-tablespoon serving of a store-bought cranberry sauce can have up to 13 grams of sugar, compared to the 2 grams found in this recipe if you use monk fruit or stevia.

2 cups fresh or frozen cranberries
½ cup water
1 tablespoon finely ground chia seeds
½ teaspoon cinnamon
1 teaspoon pure monk fruit extract (or ¾ teaspoon stevia liquid or ¼ cup raw honey)

Vegan Option: Omit the honey.

1. In a medium saucepan, combine the cranberries and water over medium heat. Cook for 8 to 10 minutes, stirring occasionally until the cranberries burst and break down.

2. Remove from the heat and whisk in the chia seeds, cinnamon and monk fruit.

3. Transfer to a blender and blend until smooth.

4. Set aside to cool, then place in a serving bowl or transfer to a mason jar. Cover and refrigerate until ready to serve. Store in a mason jar, covered, in the fridge for up to 2 weeks.

No Sugar Added Option: Use pure monk fruit extract or liquid stevia.

Hoisin Sauce

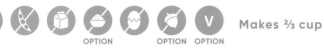

Makes ⅔ cup

This sugar-free hoisin sauce is easy to make and so much healthier than the store-bought versions, which can contain more than a teaspoon of sugar per tablespoon of sauce. In my version, the combination of the salty coconut sauce, the fat, the nut butter and the sweetness of the monk fruit will have you hitting the bliss point. I use this sauce in stir-fries and as a dipping sauce for simple mains that need a splash of pizzazz.

⅓ cup water

2 tablespoons unsweetened nut or seed butter, such as cashew or tahini

¼ cup coconut sauce or wheat-free tamari

⅛ teaspoon pure monk fruit extract (or 1 tablespoon raw honey)

2 teaspoons red wine vinegar

1 clove garlic, minced (or ⅛ teaspoon garlic powder)

2 teaspoons toasted sesame oil

2 tablespoons avocado oil

1. In a small saucepan, mix together all ingredients over low heat. Simmer until smooth and completely combined, about 10 minutes.

2. Let cool and transfer to a blender. Blend until smooth, then transfer to a mason jar. Store, covered, in the fridge for up to 1 month.

No Sugar Added Option: Use pure monk fruit extract.

Vegan Option: Omit the honey.

Honey Mustard Sauce

     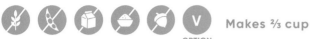 **Makes ⅔ cup**

This delicious honey mustard sauce has less than one carb per serving, making it a great substitute for similar store-bought sauces. Studies have demonstrated that mustard seed may be beneficial in reducing damage caused by oxidative stress associated with diabetes. It also aids in glucose metabolism. Perfect for dipping, as a condiment and even as a salad dressing, this sauce may find a special place in your heart and on your table.

½ cup Avocado Mayonnaise (page 218) or store-bought sugar-free vegan mayonnaise
1 tablespoon yellow mustard
2 teaspoons Dijon or stone-ground mustard
1 teaspoon garlic powder
½ teaspoon smoked paprika
¼ teaspoon pure monk fruit extract
Pinch of unrefined pink salt

1. Add all ingredients to a mason jar and shake to combine. Store, covered, in the fridge for up to 3 weeks.

Vegan Option: Use sugar-free vegan mayonnaise.

Keto Ketchup

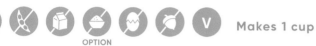 Makes 1 cup

OPTION

Ketchup can be one of the greatest sources of hidden sugar in the condiment aisle, as it is essentially a tomato jam. I love this sugar-free version because it adds a zesty pop to your favourite dishes. My version has only one naturally occuring carbohydrate (from the tomatoes) per tablespoon compared to five carbohydrates (from the sugar and tomatoes) per tablespoon found in standard ketchup. The cooked tomatoes are a wonderful source of lycopene, an antioxidant that protects both women's breast tissue and men's prostates. Kids use so much ketchup that I encourage you to mix up a batch once or twice a month to help them develop a taste for healthier choices.

¾ cup tomato paste

¾ cup water

½ to 1 teaspoon pure monk fruit extract (or ¼ cup date paste), more to taste

2 tablespoons apple cider vinegar

1 teaspoon unrefined pink salt, more to taste

¾ teaspoon onion powder

½ teaspoon garlic powder

¼ teaspoon sweet paprika

Optional (use 1)
Pinch of ground cloves
Pinch of mustard powder

1. In a small saucepan, whisk together all ingredients until well combined.

2. Simmer uncovered over low heat for 10 to 15 minutes, stirring occasionally, until the ketchup reduces slightly. (Time will vary widely depending on the size of your pan.)

3. Adjust the salt and monk fruit, to taste. For an improved texture, purée in a high-speed blender until smooth. Store in a mason jar with a lid in the fridge for up to 3 weeks.

No Sugar Added Option: Use pure monk fruit extract.

Fast in a Flash Relish

    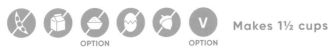 Makes 1½ cups

My husband, Alan, adores relish, but the standard store-bought versions are jammed full of refined sugar. It might surprise you that sweet relish can have more sugar than ketchup. This recipe takes less than ten minutes to make and tastes incredible. You can spice it up or keep it simple, depending on your taste preference. Sugar-free dill pickles are one of the lowest-calorie snack foods at just five to seven calories per serving. When you turn them into relish sweetened with monk fruit, you'll have a low-carb option that will add great flavour to your meal.

5 medium sugar-free dill pickles

⅛ teaspoon pure monk fruit extract (or 1 teaspoon raw honey or coconut nectar; see Tip)

2 teaspoons stone-ground mustard

1 teaspoon apple cider vinegar

Optional

1 teaspoon organic onion powder

½ teaspoon cinnamon

1 clove pickled garlic

¼ cup minced red sweet pepper

1. Add the pickles to a food processor or to a blender. Pulse for just a few seconds until you get a rough crumble.

2. Add the monk fruit, mustard, apple cider vinegar and any optional ingredients. Pulse for another 2 to 3 seconds until a lightly coarse relish texture forms. Adjust flavourings as desired.

3. Using a spatula, transfer the relish to a mason jar. Stir well, cover and let sit at room temperature for 1 hour. Check the seasoning again and adjust if necessary. Store, covered, in the fridge for up to 1 month.

Tip: Coconut nectar is permitted if you are on the slow breakup plan and can tolerate sucrose.

No Sugar Added Option: Use pure monk fruit extract.

Vegan Option: Omit the honey.

Faux Maple Syrup   Makes 1 cup

Do you need syrup to put on your low-carb pancakes and crepes? This keto maple or vanilla syrup is exactly what you're looking for and can be made in less than five minutes. Instead of raising your blood sugar (and fat-storing hormone insulin), this syrup substitute will keep your blood sugar in check. Talk about a sweet fix that gives back! You can also use this to make mocktails and sweeten smoothies. It might become your new friend in the battle against sugar. Xanthan gum is a popular alternative to starch-based thickeners and can be found in most health food stores or online.

1 cup warm water

2 tablespoons monk fruit erythritol powder (or ¾ teaspoon pure monk fruit extract)

1½ teaspoons pure maple or vanilla extract

¼ teaspoon xanthan gum

Pinch of unrefined pink salt

1. Combine all ingredients in a small blender and pulse at slow intervals to avoid excess foaming. Don't worry if it foams up too much; the bubbles should break down over time. Store in a mason jar with a lid in the fridge for up to 1 month.

Tip: To make a maple or vanilla cream version, add 2 tablespoons vegan butter or 2 tablespoons coconut oil + 1 teaspoon sunflower lecithin.

Jumbleberry Jam   Makes 2 cups

Soft fruits, such as black or red currants, raspberries, blackberries, blueberries or strawberries, are fantastic in this recipe, so choose your own adventure and mix it up or stick to one variety for a pure taste. Instead of all the cooking and pectin, I like to keep the berries raw and use ground chia seed to thicken the jam. Chia is a member of the mint family and contains rich amounts of fibre that further bind the natural sugar in the fruit to brilliantly stabilize your blood sugar.

3 cups fresh or thawed frozen organic berries (raspberries, blackberries, blueberries, strawberries)

2 tablespoons chia seeds

½ teaspoon pure monk fruit extract (or ¼ teaspoon liquid stevia or 2 tablespoons raw liquid honey)

1. Place the berries, chia seeds and monk fruit in a food processor and process until smooth.

2. Transfer to a mason jar, cover and refrigerate for a few hours to thicken. Store, covered, in the fridge for up to 2 weeks or in the freezer for up to 6 months. The jam will separate when thawed, so be sure to mix well before serving.

No Sugar Added Option: Use pure monk fruit extract or stevia.

Vegan Option: Omit the honey.

Sunny Anti-Inflammatory Dressing

      Makes 1½ cups

This dressing is my personal favourite for cooked vegetables. I put it on cooked spinach, kale, rapini and even sweet potatoes. It has a creamy dairy-like texture, and the warming spices will wrap your tummy in a big hug. Tahini (sesame paste) contains a compound called sesamin, which prevents omega-6 fats from becoming inflammatory. The bright yellow turmeric will cheer up any plate and reduce inflammation throughout the body.

½ cup tahini

⅔ cup water

3 tablespoons lemon juice

2 tablespoons sesame or olive oil

¼ to ½ teaspoon pure monk
  fruit extract (or 1 teaspoon raw
  honey or 2 teaspoons fruit
  juice-sweetened marmalade)

½ teaspoon unrefined sea salt

1 teaspoon ground turmeric

½ teaspoon ground ginger
  (optional)

1 clove garlic (optional)

2 tablespoons coconut sauce
  (optional)

1. Combine all ingredients in a blender or food processor and process until smooth. Transfer to a mason jar with a lid and store in the fridge for up to 4 weeks. It will thicken as it sits, so you can thin it out with warm water if desired.

No Sugar Added Option: Use pure monk fruit extract.

Vegan Option: Omit the honey.

Coconut Whipping Cream

    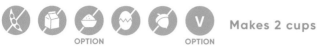   Makes 2 cups

Whenever I serve this to a new friend, I neglect to mention that it is dairy-free, and they don't even notice, as the coconut whipping cream creates the perfect consistency. I often use this as an icing on cakes or atop fruit salad, with rave reviews from my guests. It is now possible to find pre-made canned coconut whipping cream that just needs to be whipped with a bit of alternative sweetener. If you can't find coconut whipping cream, you can skim the top off of two refrigerated cans of coconut milk.

1 can (14 ounces) unsweetened full-fat coconut whipping cream (or 2 cans, 14 ounces each, full-fat coconut milk, chilled overnight in the fridge)

¼ teaspoon pure monk fruit extract (or 1 to 2 tablespoons raw honey or coconut nectar; see Tip)

Pinch of unrefined pink salt

Optional

1 teaspoon beet or raspberry powder (for a pink colour)

1 teaspoon Blue Majik algae powder (for a blue colour)

½ teaspoon arrowroot starch (or ¼ teaspoon xanthan gum if the canned coconut whipping cream doesn't contain it; check the package ingredient list)

1. Add the coconut whipping cream to a large bowl. (Alternatively, if using coconut milk, scoop out the solid coconut cream. Use the coconut water in smoothies and other recipes.)

2. Add the monk fruit, salt, colouring powder (if using) and arrowroot starch (if using) to the coconut cream. Using an electric mixer fitted with the whisk attachment, whisk until a thick texture forms. Store in a mason jar with a lid in the fridge for up to 1 week.

Tip: Coconut nectar is permitted if you are on the slow breakup plan and can tolerate sucrose.

No Sugar Added Option: Use pure monk fruit extract.

Vegan Option: Omit the honey.

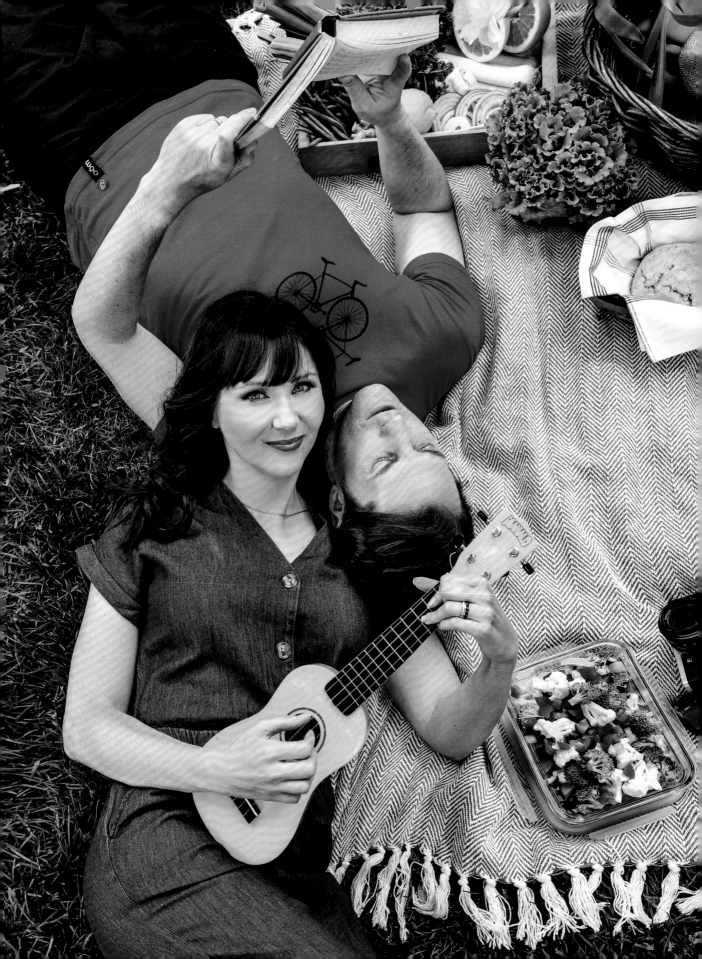

Crave-Busting Mains and Sides

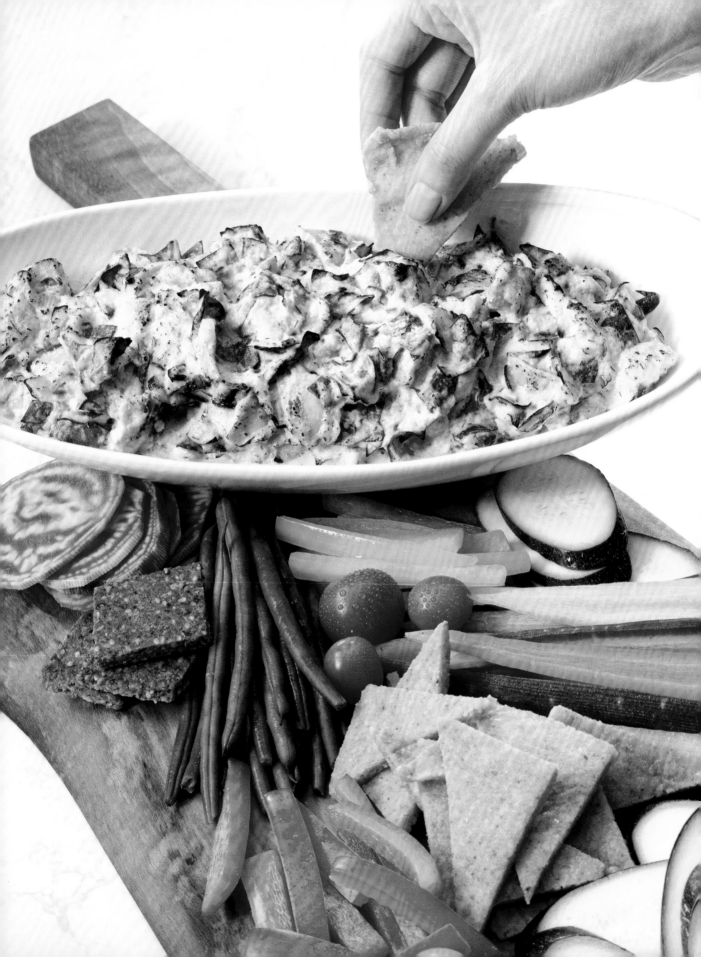

Crave-Busting Artichoke Dip or Casserole

 OPTION OPTION   Serves 10

Artichokes have a superpower of being able to make something you eat or drink alongside them taste sweeter than it is, which seriously helps you curb cravings for sugar. One of the phytochemicals in artichokes, called cynarin, latches on to sweet receptors on your tongue without activating them. This simulates a sensation of slight sweetness on your taste buds so that anything you eat or drink after this dip will taste sweeter. This recipe is very low carb and packed with fibre that helps keep you feeling full, and I love the flexibility of it. You can skip the spinach and serve it as a cold dip or add in some sustainable fish and make it a main dish.

½ cup raw cashew pieces or hemp hearts

1 cup hot water, for soaking

1½ cups cooked cauliflower, well drained

2 tablespoons lemon juice

½ cup canned full-fat coconut milk

⅓ cup nutritional yeast

2 cloves garlic

1 tablespoon fresh dill

1 tablespoon fresh oregano

½ cup Avocado Mayonnaise (page 218) or sugar-free vegan mayonnaise

½ teaspoon unrefined pink salt

4 cups packed fresh baby spinach

2 cups marinated artichokes, drained and diced

1 can (5 ounces) sustainable fish such as tuna or salmon (if making a main dish casserole) (optional)

For serving

Keto Seed Crackers (page 191)

Corn-Free Tortilla Chips (page 195)

Fresh vegetable sticks (celery, carrot, zucchini, sweet pepper, cucumber)

1. In a glass jar or measuring cup, soak the cashews in the hot water for about 20 minutes, or until softened. Drain and discard the water. (If using hemp hearts instead of cashews, do not presoak them.)

2. Meanwhile, preheat the oven to 350°F.

3. In a food processor, combine the drained cashews, cauliflower, lemon juice and coconut milk and blend into a smooth and creamy consistency.

4. Add the nutritional yeast, garlic, dill, oregano, Avocado Mayonnaise and salt and blend until combined. Transfer to a large bowl and stir in the spinach, artichokes and fish, if using.

5. Transfer to an 8-inch square baking dish. Bake for about 30 minutes until golden on top. Serve with Keto Seed Crackers, Corn-Free Tortilla Chips or vegetable sticks. Store, covered, in the fridge for up to 3 days.

Vegan Option: Use sugar-free vegan mayonnaise (also egg-free) and omit the fish.

Onion Ring Chips

     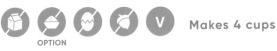   Makes 4 cups

Onions are naturally sweet and a wonderful tool in your fight against sugar. If you like onion rings, you are going to love these chips because they are sweet, salty and crispy—the perfect combo to satisfy your munchies when watching a movie with family. You might find yourself making double batches, as they taste as good as any salty snack you may find at the store. Plus, red onions help fight inflammation and allergies with a special phytonutrient called quercetin. For ease and precise slices, I like to use a mandoline to slice the onions for this recipe.

6 cups thinly sliced red onion (about 4 small onions)

⅓ cup tahini

2 tablespoons coconut sauce or wheat-free tamari

2 tablespoons lemon juice

¼ teaspoon pure monk fruit extract (or 1 tablespoon coconut nectar)

½ cup sesame seeds

½ teaspoon garlic powder

½ teaspoon ground cumin

¼ teaspoon ground turmeric

½ teaspoon unrefined pink salt

1. Preheat the oven to 275°F. Line 2 large baking sheets with unbleached parchment paper.

2. Place the sliced onions in a large bowl.

3. In a small bowl, mix together the tahini, coconut sauce, lemon juice, monk fruit, sesame seeds, garlic powder, cumin, turmeric and salt. Pour the mixture over the onions and, using tongs, toss until the onions are evenly coated.

4. Arrange the onion slices on the prepared baking sheets. Make sure to separate the onions as much as possible to ensure that they dry correctly. Bake for 2 hours or, if time permits, dehydrate in the oven at 170°F for 6 hours or in a dehydrator at 120°F for 8 hours. Whatever temperature or timing you choose, once the baking time is complete, leave them in the closed oven to dry completely as they cool. This ensures that they are bone dry and will last much longer. Store in an airtight container on the countertop for up to 3 months.

No Sugar Added Option: Use pure monk fruit extract.

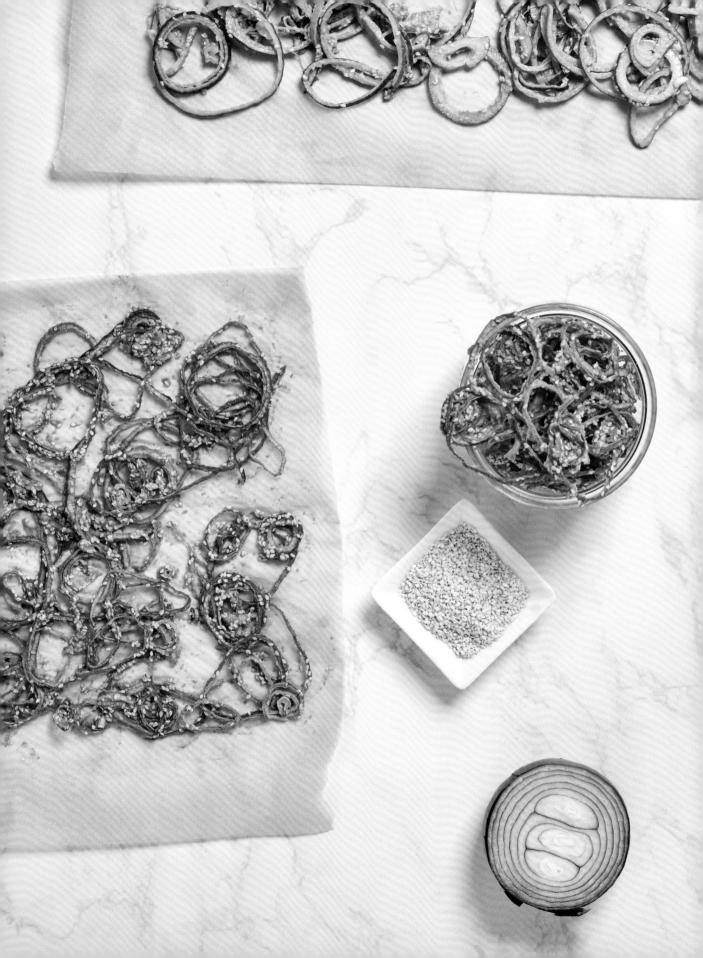

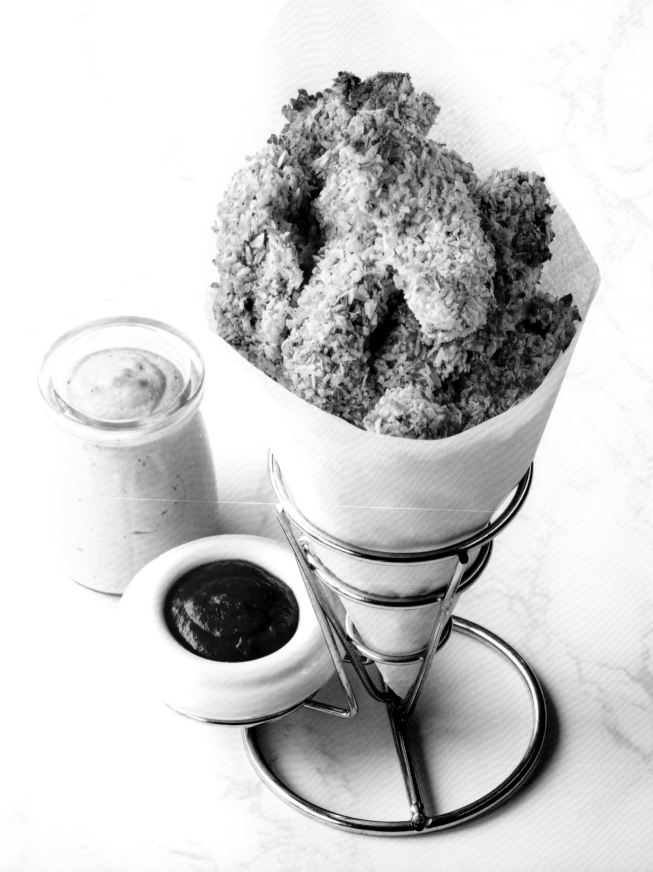

Baked Avocado Fries

OPTION   OPTION   **Serves 6, makes about 18 fries**

Avocados might be one of the most perfect foods on the planet, delivering incredible amounts of good fat and vitamin B6, which helps with hormonal balance. I suggest inviting friends over so that you have a bit of portion control. You may be surprised at how fast these fries can slide past your lips.

3 large firm, ripe avocados, peeled and pitted
½ cup coconut flour
¾ teaspoon unrefined pink salt, divided
2 large eggs (or flax or chia egg; see Tip)
1 cup unsweetened shredded coconut
½ teaspoon garlic powder
½ teaspoon onion powder
½ teaspoon sweet paprika

Dipping Sauce Options
Keto Ketchup (page 223)
Avocado Mayonnaise (page 218)

1. Preheat the oven to 450°F. Line a baking sheet with unbleached parchment paper and place a wire rack on top.

2. Slice the avocados in half lengthwise. Then cut each half into 3 wedges. You should have 18 wedges.

3. Set up 3 bowls in a row.

4. In the first bowl, mix together the coconut flour and ¼ teaspoon of the salt.

5. Crack the eggs into the second bowl and beat lightly.

6. In the third bowl, mix together the coconut, garlic powder, onion powder, paprika and remaining ½ teaspoon salt and stir to combine well.

7. One at a time, dredge the avocado slices in the coconut flour, then in the beaten egg, and then coat thoroughly with the coconut mixture and place on the wire rack.

8. Bake for 10 minutes, until the coconut flakes are lightly browned. Serve immediately with Keto Ketchup or Avocado Mayonnaise.

Tip: To make the flax or chia egg, in a small bowl, whisk together 2 tablespoons ground flaxseed or chia seeds and 5 tablespoons hot water until well combined. Set aside to soak for 10 minutes so that the flaxseed can swell and absorb the liquid.

Vegan Option: Use flax or chia egg substitute.

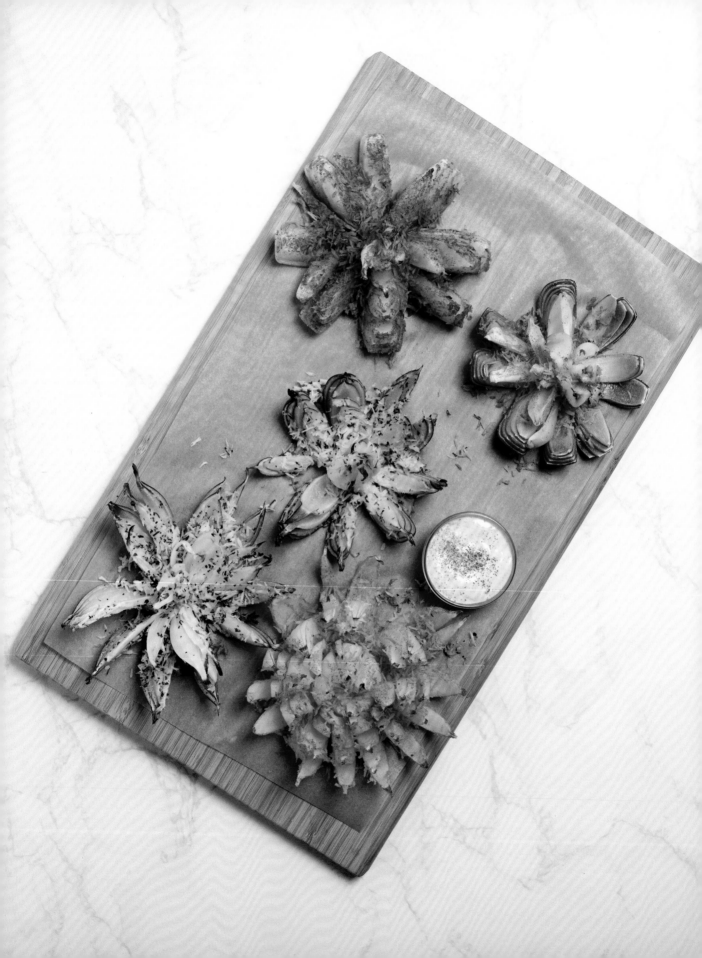

Baked Blooming Onions and Dipping Sauce

      V OPTION   **Makes 2 to 4 blooming onions**

When I first saw this recipe at my local country fair, I thought that maybe a magician had dropped into town and created a culinary trick. But the onions were deep-fried in wheat dough, so I set out on a mission to make a recipe just as pretty but also healthy. Onion is naturally sweet, so it helps keep your sweet tooth in check. It also offers many great health benefits, including being a rich source of allergy-busting quercetin.

Blooming Onions

4 medium onions (white, yellow or red) or 2 Spanish onions

½ cup unsweetened shredded coconut

1 tablespoon curry powder, ground turmeric or Italian seasoning

¼ teaspoon unrefined pink salt

2 large eggs (or flax or chia egg; see Tip)

Smoked Paprika Aioli (makes ⅔ cup)

½ cup Avocado Mayonnaise (page 218) or sugar-free vegan mayonnaise

2 tablespoons sugar-free salsa

¼ teaspoon unrefined pink salt

¼ teaspoon smoked paprika

⅛ teaspoon garlic powder

⅛ teaspoon dried oregano

1. Preheat the oven to 350°F. Line a baking sheet with unbleached parchment paper.

2. To make the blooming onions, cut the top (not the root) off each onion until a few of the inside layers are exposed (about ¼ inch off the top). Peel and discard the outermost layer of the onions, leaving the roots intact.

3. If time permits, soak the sliced onions in cold water overnight, as it will help the layers of the onions loosen and open up naturally.

4. Lay each onion on a cutting board with the flat top facing downward (the intact root of the onion should be on top).

5. Use a knife to slice each onion into 16 sections. Beginning with your knife ⅛ inch away from the root, cut vertically straight down. After each cut, move clockwise around the root until all cuts are completed.

6. Set the onions, root side down, on the prepared baking sheet. Then use your fingers to gently spread apart the petals. If any of your cuts did not go all the way through, use a paring knife to be sure that each onion is cut into 16 sections.

7. In a small bowl, mix together the coconut, curry powder and salt.

8. In another small bowl, whisk the eggs.

Recipe continues

9. Beginning with the lowest (bottom) layers of the onions, brush the top of each petal with the egg mixture until well coated, then immediately sprinkle with the coconut mixture. Repeat until all petals are coated. (The coconut will not stick completely when the egg is wet, so be liberal with your sprinkle.)

10. Bake for 25 to 30 minutes until the onion is soft and the petal tips are lightly crisped.

11. Meanwhile, make the smoked paprika aioli. In a small bowl, stir together all ingredients until smooth and well combined. Use immediately or transfer to an airtight container and refrigerate for up to 10 days.

12. Serve the blooming onions with the dipping sauce.

Tip: To make the flaxseed or chia egg, in a small bowl, whisk together 2 tablespoons ground flaxseed or chia seeds and 5 tablespoons hot water until well combined. Set aside to soak for 10 minutes so that the flaxseed can swell and absorb the liquid.

Vegan Option: Use flax or chia egg substitute and sugar-free vegan mayonnaise.

Cauliflower Gnocchi

     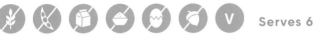 **Serves 6**

These homemade gnocchi are healthy and delicious. Although it takes some time to make, it's a great dish for cooking with a friend and is such a pleasing dish to serve to loved ones. The creamy sauce will have you dreaming of the next time you can enjoy the wonderful doughy texture of this Italian classic, reinvented to keep your blood sugar balanced. Cassava flour is made from a fibrous root vegetable and is low on the glycemic index (only 46 versus white potato, which is 96). This makes it the perfect way to bust your cravings for pasta. If you are in a hurry, just boil the gnocchi and serve it chewy, but if you want an extra-decadent treat, bake them for a crispy outside and a chewy inside.

Gnocchi
5 cups minced or riced cauliflower
¾ to 1¼ cups cassava flour
½ teaspoon unrefined pink salt
2 tablespoons avocado or olive oil, divided

Sauce (makes 2 cups)
1 cup diced red onion
2 cloves garlic, minced
1 tablespoon avocado or olive oil
1½ cups canned full-fat coconut milk
1 tablespoon cassava flour
Unrefined pink salt, to taste
6 cups packed baby spinach

¼ cup hemp hearts, for serving (optional)

1. Line a baking sheet with unbleached parchment paper.

2. To make the gnocchi, steam the cauliflower until soft, about 5 minutes. Carefully transfer the cauliflower to a clean kitchen towel. Let cool enough to touch. Place the towel into a colander over the sink, then roll the towel up tightly, squeezing out the excess water. The cauliflower should measure about 2½ cups.

3. In a food processor, combine the squeezed cauliflower, cassava flour (starting with ¾ cup and adding more until desired texture is reached) and salt and blend until smooth and dough-like. I provide a range for the flour because the amount used depends on the humidity of your environment and how much moisture you managed to extract from the cauliflower.

4. Divide the dough into 5 equal portions. On a flat surface lightly dusted with cassava flour, roll out each portion of dough into a ¾-inch-diameter log. Cut each log of dough into ½-inch pieces.

5. Bring a large pot of lightly salted water to a boil. When the water is boiling, drop in half of the gnocchi. Once the gnocchi rise to the surface, use a slotted spoon to transfer them to the prepared baking sheet. Drizzle with 1 tablespoon of the avocado oil. Repeat to cook the remaining gnocchi. You can serve the gnocchi soft and gooey or bake them for a crispy outside shell. Follow step 6 if you are baking the gnocchi. If not, skip to step 7.

Recipe continues

6. If baking, preheat the oven to 400°F, then bake for 15 minutes. Turn over the gnocchi and bake for another 15 minutes until golden.

7. Meanwhile, make the sauce. In a medium saucepan, cook the onion, garlic and avocado oil over medium heat until the onion is translucent. Add the coconut milk, cassava flour and salt. Mix with a whisk, stirring constantly to avoid clumping, or transfer the sauce to a blender and blend until smooth and thick, then transfer back to the pot. Be careful not to overheat the sauce or it will become too thick and gooey from the flour. Remove from the heat, stir in the spinach to wilt, then stir in the gnocchi. Serve warm with hemp hearts (if using) sprinkled on top.

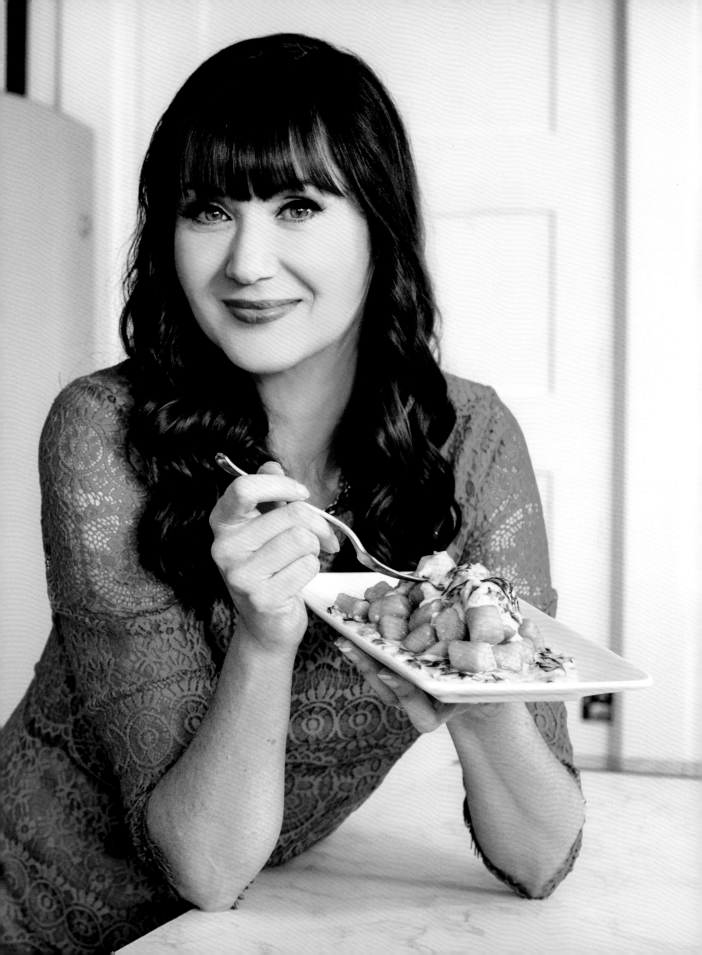

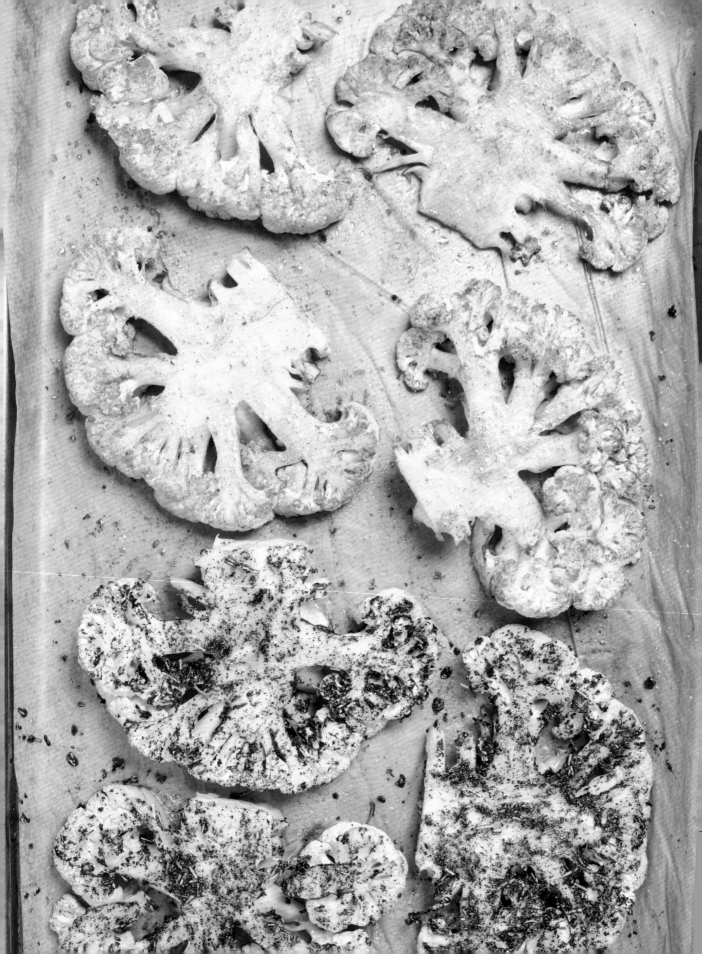

Cauliflower Steaks

OPTION   OPTION

Makes 4 to 6 steaks

This dish will impress and is easier than making steamed cauliflower! By pairing the cauliflower with protein-rich seeds, it can be served as a main dish, especially for your vegetarian friends. Cauliflower is awesome to cook healthy dishes with, as it has a neutral flavour yet is packed with hormone-balancing benefits. If you want to be economical, you can season the smaller pieces of cauliflower that are inevitable when making thick steaks and cook them in the same pan, or you can rice them and store in the fridge to be used in other recipes such as Cauliflower Gnocchi (page 239) or Cauliflower Keto Hummus (page 249).

1 large head cauliflower

2 tablespoons coconut or avocado oil

1 to 2 teaspoons curry powder or Italian seasoning

¼ teaspoon unrefined pink salt

Optional (use 1 to 4)

1 tablespoon coconut sauce or wheat-free tamari

1 tablespoon lemon juice

⅛ teaspoon pure monk fruit extract (or 1 tablespoon coconut nectar)

¼ teaspoon garlic powder

Toppings

¼ cup hemp hearts or raw pumpkin seeds

Freshly chopped flat-leaf parsley

1. Preheat the oven to 375°F. Line a baking sheet with unbleached parchment paper.

2. Remove the leaves and trim the end of the cauliflower, ensuring that you leave the stem intact so that the steaks hold together.

3. Slice the cauliflower so that you end up with four to six ½-inch steaks. You can roast the remaining bits of cauliflower alongside the steaks or keep them for another dish. Place the steaks on the prepared baking sheet.

4. In a small bowl, mix together the coconut oil, curry powder, salt and any optional ingredients. Using a pastry brush, a spoon or your fingers, gently rub the steaks with the mixture until evenly coated on both sides.

5. Bake for 20 minutes until browned. Flip carefully and bake for another 10 to 15 minutes until tender and browned. Serve immediately. For added protein, serve sprinkled with hemp hearts or pumpkin seeds and fresh parsley.

No Sugar Added Option: Use pure monk fruit extract.

Dill Pickle Rolls

     Makes 12 rolls

If you crave the classic taste of store-bought condensed mushroom soup (a comfort food for many), this recipe will hit the spot. Mushrooms are very filling and provide a lot of nutrition with few calories. My mother-in-law made these rolls for my husband's birthdays using ground moose meat when he was young, and he literally dreams about this dish. The combination of the dill, and mushrooms makes an irresistible taste sensation. My mother-in-law can never make enough of these rolls for our family gatherings, so she makes them ahead of time since they freeze well.

2 pounds ground turkey or beef

1 large egg, beaten

1 teaspoon dry mustard (or 2 teaspoons yellow mustard)

1½ teaspoons unrefined pink salt

2 large sugar-free dill pickles, drained and patted dry

1 tablespoon avocado oil

2 cups Creamy Mushroom Soup (condensed version, page 251)

¼ cup canned coconut cream or unsweetened coconut whipping cream

¼ cup pickle juice

Optional Garnishes (use 1 to 4)

½ cup finely chopped dill pickles

2 cups sautéed mushrooms (cremini, shiitake, portobello)

4 sprigs fresh dill

1 cup diced red onion

1. In a large bowl, mix together the ground turkey, egg, mustard and salt. Divide the mixture into 12 portions.

2. Slice each dill pickle lengthwise into 6 strips. Shape each portion of the meat mixture around a pickle strip until it is surrounded completely with meat.

3. In a heavy 10-inch frying pan, heat the avocado oil over medium-high heat. Place the rolls in the pan and sear on all sides until golden brown. You might need to cook the rolls in batches.

4. Meanwhile, preheat the oven to 350°F.

5. In a small bowl, mix together the condensed Creamy Mushroom Soup, coconut cream and pickle juice until smooth.

6. Place the cooked rolls in a shallow baking dish and spoon the mushroom mixture over the rolls. Bake for 30 minutes.

7. To serve, garnish with chopped pickles, sautéed mushrooms, sprigs of dill, and diced red onion, if desired. Store, covered, in the fridge for up to 2 days or in the freezer for up to 1 month.

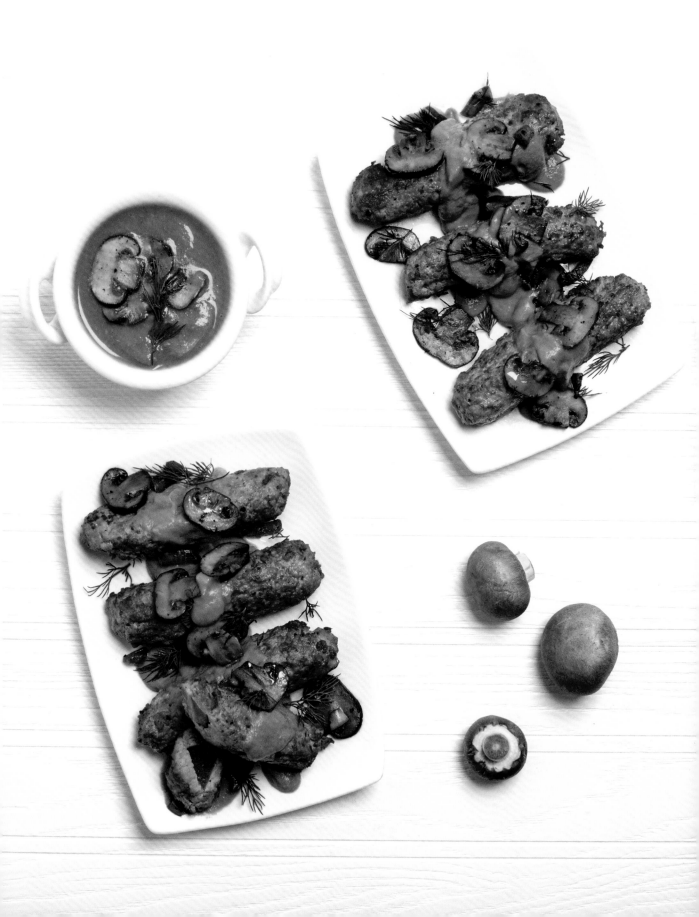

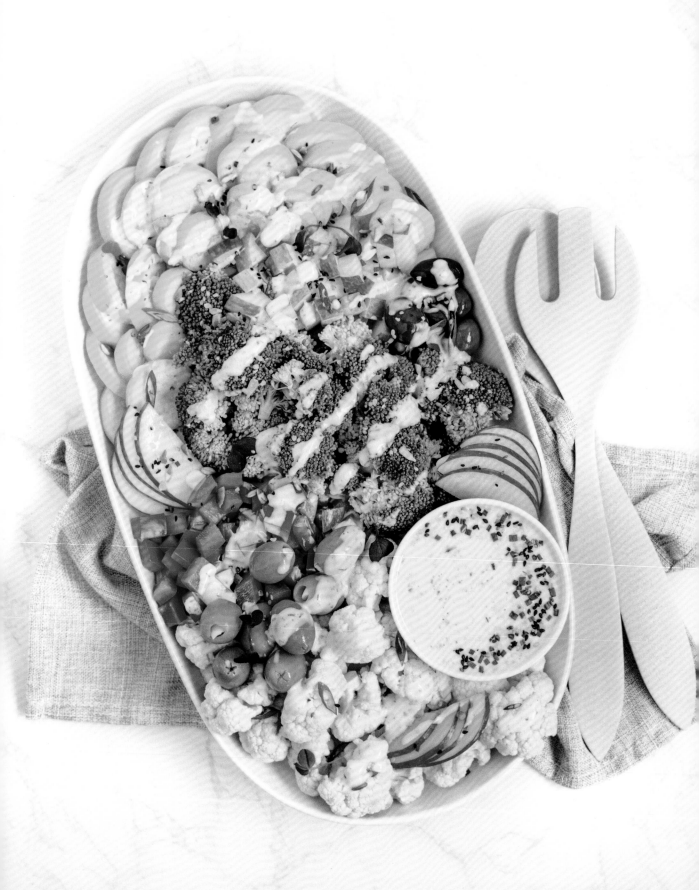

Crunchy Cruciferous Salad

      Makes 10 to 12 cups

OPTION OPTION OPTION

My sister, Lynn, started making broccoli salads back in college. Since then, our family has evolved her basic salad recipe in ten different ways because it is my dad's favourite way to eat raw vegetables. If you want to get kids of all ages to eat more vegetables, keep them crunchy and serve them with a dip or creamy dressing like the one in this recipe. This salad gets more delicious over time, so it is great for buffet meals.

To make this salad a main meal, add 4 ounces of protein, such as cooked cubed chicken, hard-boiled egg, tempeh, or flaked cooked fish, per person or ½ cup of hemp hearts.

Dressing
¾ cup Avocado Mayonnaise (page 218) or sugar-free vegan mayonnaise
2 tablespoons extra-virgin olive oil
1 to 2 tablespoons lemon juice or red wine vinegar
1 teaspoon Italian seasoning
¼ to ½ teaspoon unrefined pink salt
2 to 3 drops pure monk fruit extract (or 1 teaspoon raw honey)
1 clove garlic, minced (optional)

Salad
3½ cups chopped broccoli (about 1 head)
3½ cups chopped cauliflower (about ½ head)
2 cups cored and cubed apple or pear
1 cup sliced dill pickles or green or black pitted olives

Optional (add some or all)
1 to 2 green onions (white and light green parts only), chopped
1 to 2 cups diced English cucumber

1 to 2 cups diced zucchini
1 large red sweet pepper, diced

Optional Toppings
½ cup coarsely chopped raw nuts or seeds
Sprouts, chopped fresh chives or chopped fresh curly parsley

1. To make the dressing, in a small bowl, combine all ingredients and mix well. Taste and adjust the seasoning if desired. Store in a mason jar in the fridge for up to 2 weeks.

2. To make the salad, in a large bowl, mix together all ingredients and any options you desire. Drizzle the salad with enough dressing to coat it when tossed. Add any toppings you wish.

3. Serve immediately or store, with the dressing, in the fridge for up to 3 days.

No Sugar Added Option: Use pure monk fruit extract.

Vegan Option: Use sugar-free vegan mayonnaise and pure monk fruit extract.

Sweet Potato Latke Waffles

     Serves 2 to 4

OPTION

These sweet potato waffles are ready in ten minutes. They are a good source of vitamin A, which improves skin, eye and lung health. Although sweet potatoes taste sweeter than white potatoes, they are lower on the glycemic index. They are also higher in fibre, which helps reduce your insulin response and keep your blood sugar balanced. If you don't own a waffle iron, simply form them into small patties and cook them gently in a cast-iron pan over medium heat. These waffles taste great topped with applesauce to make a quick breakfast or used as the "bread" for a savoury sandwich.

4 cups grated sweet potato

3 large eggs

¼ cup almond, cassava or coconut flour (helps to bind the waffles; optional)

2 teaspoons cinnamon, for sweet waffles; or 1 tablespoon Italian seasoning (or 2 teaspoons curry powder), for savoury waffles

½ teaspoon unrefined pink salt

1 teaspoon avocado oil, divided, for the waffle iron

1. Preheat the waffle iron on medium heat (about 355°F). Preheat the oven to 200°F. Line a baking sheet with unbleached parchment paper.

2. In a large bowl, whisk together the sweet potato, eggs, almond flour (if using), cinnamon (for sweet waffles) or Italian seasoning (for savoury waffles) and salt.

3. Brush both sides of the waffle iron with ¼ teaspoon of the avocado oil. Pour about ½ cup of batter per waffle into the centre of the waffle iron, gently spreading it evenly before closing.

4. Cook until golden and crispy, about 5 minutes. Transfer to the prepared baking sheet and keep warm in the oven. Repeat with the remaining batter. Store any leftover waffles in an airtight container in the fridge for up to 1 week.

Cauliflower Keto Hummus

      V Makes 3 cups

OPTION

Cauliflower is brimming with isothiocyanates, plant compounds that are converted to sulforaphane when chopped or chewed. Sulforaphane is a powerful anti-inflammatory molecule that is being studied for its power to balance hormones by increasing liver function. Tahini (sesame seed butter) delivers a healthy dose of magnesium, which is shown to be particularly helpful in fending off type 2 diabetes and muscle cramps. Store this hummus in small mason jars and serve with zucchini and cucumber sticks. It is a fun way to transport your food and reduces plastic in the environment.

3 cups cauliflower florets

¼ cup water

¾ cup tahini

1 clove garlic, minced (or 1 teaspoon garlic powder)

⅓ cup fresh lemon juice

2 tablespoons extra-virgin olive oil, more for drizzling

1 teaspoon unrefined pink salt

2 teaspoons ground turmeric or curry powder (optional)

¼ cup hemp hearts, sesame seeds or pine nuts (optional)

1. In a medium saucepan over medium-high heat, add the cauliflower and water and cover with a lid to let steam for 7 to 10 minutes until fork-tender. Drain well and, using a clean kitchen towel, pat dry the cauliflower.

2. When cooled slightly, place the cauliflower in a food processor. Add the tahini, garlic, lemon juice, olive oil, salt and turmeric (if using) and blend until very smooth, about 5 minutes.

3. Scrape the hummus into a medium bowl, top with the hemp hearts (if using) and drizzle with more olive oil, if desired. Store in an airtight container in the fridge for up to 6 days.

Easy Coconut Cream of Broccoli Soup

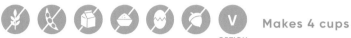 Makes 4 cups

OPTION

I once needed to make a meal in ten minutes before work and I had only a few things in my refrigerator. They say necessity is the mother of invention, and I would have to agree! The result of my slim pickings was a surprisingly delicious soup that is faster to make than a breakfast smoothie. You can top the soup with some protein-rich seeds or thin it out with some broth to your liking. I love it for its simplicity and heart-warming flavour.

1 bunch broccoli (about 4 cups roughly chopped broccoli)

2 cups vegetable or chicken broth (see Tip)

1 to 1½ cups canned full-fat coconut milk

2 to 3 tablespoons non-dairy pesto (or ½ batch Cheery Chimichurri, page 220)

½ teaspoon unrefined pink salt

Hemp hearts or toasted pumpkin seeds, for garnish (optional)

1. Remove the thick stem from the broccoli, leaving 1 to 2 inches beyond the base of each floret, and roughly chop.

2. In a large pot, add the broccoli and broth and bring to a boil over medium heat. Cook until the broccoli is soft, about 8 minutes. Carefully add the broccoli and broth mixture, coconut milk, pesto and salt to a high-speed blender and purée until smooth.

3. Serve in bowls and top with seeds, if using. Store in an airtight container in the fridge for up to 5 days.

Tip: You can use water instead of broth. Just add 1 teaspoon of apple cider vinegar or lemon juice for flavouring.

Vegan Option: Use vegetable broth.

Creamy Mushroom Soup

      V OPTION   Makes 10 to 14 cups

You can use any type of mushroom for this soup, but I recommend shiitakes because they are flavourful and healing. Between its meaty texture and delicious flavour, this recipe brings something special to every meal it visits. Umami, called the fifth taste sensation, roughly translates from Japanese to "deliciousness in flavour." If you are making this to enjoy with the Dill Pickle Rolls (page 244) or Green Bean Casserole (page 261), be sure to reduce the broth by half to make a condensed soup.

1 tablespoon avocado or
   coconut oil
2 cups medium-diced red or
   yellow onion
2 cloves garlic, minced
½ teaspoon unrefined pink salt
10 cups (about 2 pounds) sliced
   fresh mushrooms,
    assorted varieties (shiitake,
   oyster, portabello)
2 tablespoons apple cider
   vinegar
4 to 8 cups vegetable or
   chicken broth (use 4 cups if
   making condensed soup)
1 teaspoon dried thyme
½ teaspoon dried oregano
½ teaspoon dried basil
1 bay leaf

Optional Boosters

1 teaspoon medicinal mushroom
   powder
⅓ cup unsweetened full-fat
   coconut whipping cream (see
   Tip)

1. In a large pot, heat the avocado oil over medium heat. Add the onion, garlic and salt and cook, stirring frequently, until the onion is soft and translucent, about 3 minutes.

2. Add the mushrooms and cook, stirring occasionally, until most of the liquid released from the mushrooms has been absorbed, about 5 minutes.

3. Deglaze the pot with the apple cider vinegar and cook off the liquid. Add the broth, thyme, oregano, basil and bay leaf and stir.

4. Bring to a gentle boil, then reduce the heat to low and simmer for about 30 minutes until the mushrooms are tender.

5. Remove the bay leaf and discard. Add the mushroom powder and coconut whipping cream (if using) and stir to combine. Blend a third of the mixture at a time in a high-speed blender or use an immersion blender until the mixture is smooth.

6. Taste and adjust the seasoning if desired. Serve immediately or store in a mason jar with a lid in the fridge for up to 3 days.

Tip: If you only have canned coconut milk, place a 14-ounce can of full-fat coconut milk in the refrigerator overnight. Scoop out the solid coconut cream and add enough coconut water to equal ⅓ cup. Use the leftover coconut water in smoothies and other recipes.

Vegan Option: Use vegetable broth.

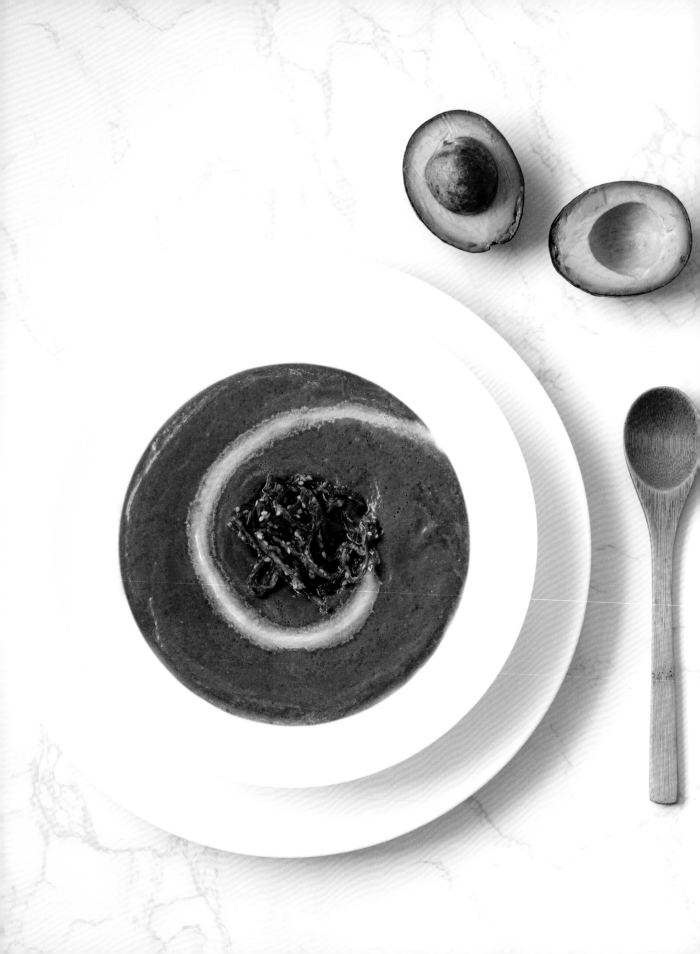

Dreamy Crave-Busting Soup

    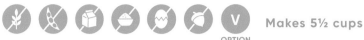 **Makes 5½ cups**

If you love guacamole, you will love this soup. It is delightfully filling, and the ingredients are packed with nutrients that help you break up with sugar cravings. If you don't like cilantro, just swap it for parsley. The spices help soothe digestion, so sip a mug of this soup the next time you feel out of sorts. I often make this soup when doing a cleanse, as it is easy to transport in a thermos when on the go.

3 to 4 cups vegetable or
   chicken broth (see Tip)
2 medium ripe avocados,
   peeled and pitted
2 to 3 tablespoons lemon juice
1 cup fresh cilantro or flat-leaf
   or curly parsley
1 clove garlic, minced (or
   ¼ teaspoon garlic powder)
½ to 1 teaspoon ground cumin
1 teaspoon dried basil
1 teaspoon dried thyme
½ teaspoon unrefined pink salt
   (reduce if using salted broth)
¼ cup canned full-fat coconut
   milk (or ½ cup if extra
   creaminess is desired)

Onion Ring Chips (page 232),
   for garnish

1. In a large pot, heat the broth over medium heat until warm.

2. Add the broth and the remaining ingredients to a high-speed blender and blend until smooth. Serve cold or return to the pot and heat over medium heat until warm before serving. Store in a mason jar with a lid in the fridge for up to 2 days.

Tip: You can use water instead of broth. Just add 1 teaspoon apple cider vinegar or lemon juice for flavouring. Garnish with the Onion Ring Chips.

Vegan Option: Use vegetable broth.

Fennel Apple Stir-Fry

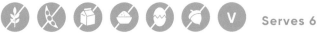 Serves 6

My sister, Lynn, came up with this elegant side dish. It has become a family favourite, as it tastes fancy yet is so easy to make. It's easy to fall in love with fennel; its crisp, crunchy texture and aromatic taste have endeared it to many culinary cultures. Fennel has the distinct ability to leave your mouth feeling fresh and has even been used for centuries as a digestive remedy. Many folks will say that it tastes like licorice crossed with celery. The slight licorice taste mellows completely when cooked. At only twenty-eight calories a cup and with good amounts of vitamins A, B and C, fennel may become your new best vegetable friend.

2 tablespoons avocado oil

4 cups sliced red or yellow onions

4 cups sliced fennel bulb (see Tip)

4 cups apples, sliced (about 2 large apples)

2 teaspoons Italian seasoning

¼ to ½ teaspoon unrefined pink salt

2 cups fresh sprouts such as broccoli, sunflower, or alfalfa (optional)

1. In a large pot, heat the avocado oil over medium heat. Add the onion and cook, stirring often, until soft and translucent, about 5 minutes.

2. Add the fennel, apple, Italian seasoning and salt and stir-fry until softened but still retaining a firm texture, about 10 minutes. Top with sprouts (if using) and serve.

Tip: Reserve the fennel fronds and use them when making homemade broth or as a salad topper (finely chopped).

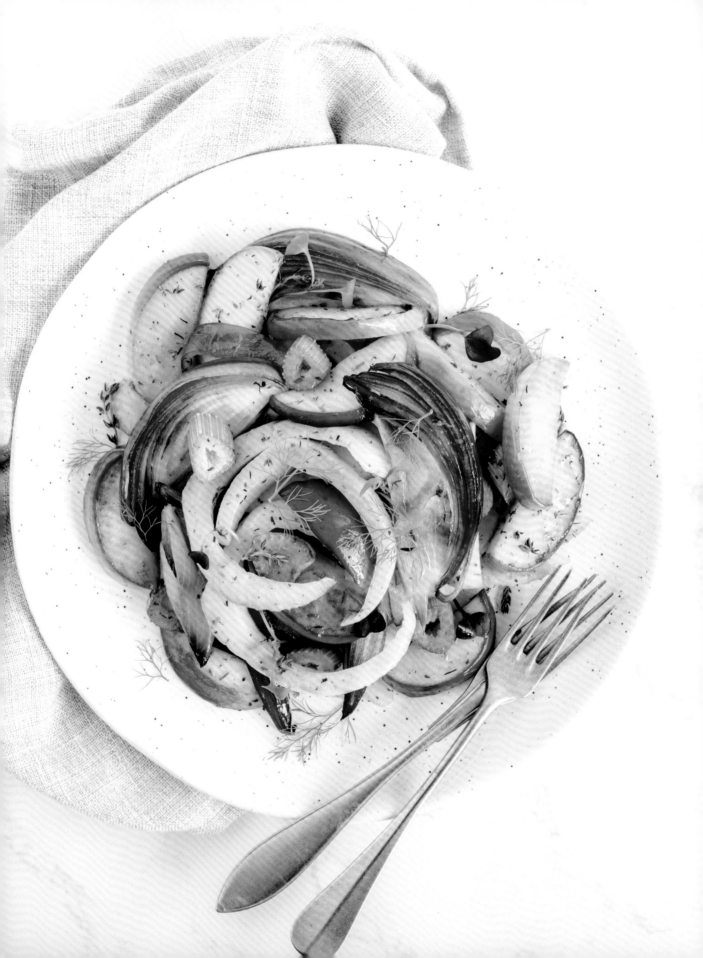

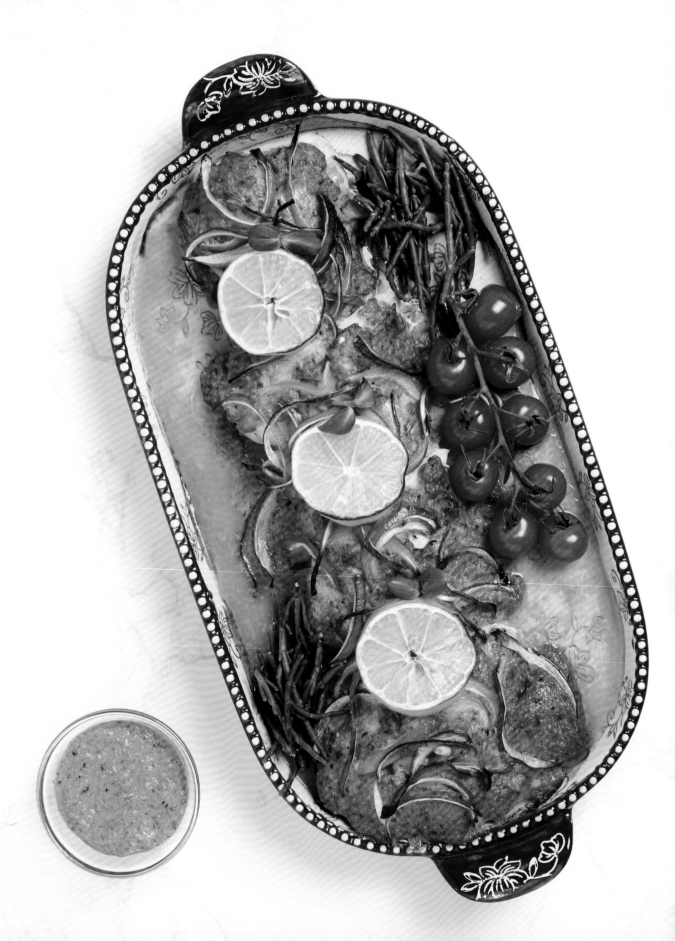

Red Pepper Pesto Fish

    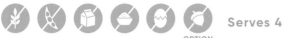 **Serves 4**
OPTION

Red sweet peppers are one of the vegetable world's highest sources of vitamin C. This pesto can be made in a flash by skipping the roasting of the peppers, but if time allows, roasting enhances the sweetness of the peppers and adds a smoky flavour. This pesto is good for saucing up main dishes, and you can thin it out with some oil and lemon to enjoy as a salad dressing. You can use any whitefish for this recipe, but my favourite is halibut. It is delicious and packed with magnesium, crave-busting omega-3 fatty acids and vitamins B6, B9 and B12, nutrients that help balance hormones and reduce inflammation. Serve this dish alongside vine-ripened tomatoes and steamed green beans or sea asparagus.

Red Pepper Pesto

2 red sweet peppers

2 cloves garlic

¼ to ½ teaspoon sweet paprika or sugar-free hot sauce (optional)

½ teaspoon ground ginger (optional)

¾ teaspoon unrefined pink salt

3 tablespoons hemp hearts or pine nuts

3 tablespoons extra-virgin olive oil

2 tablespoons lemon juice

Halibut

1 pound fresh halibut fillet

¼ teaspoon unrefined pink salt

Lemon juice

2 shallots (or ½ red onion), thinly sliced

1 organic lemon, sliced

Fresh parsley or sprouts, for garnish

1. To make the red pepper pesto, preheat the broiler on the lowest setting, about 400°F. Line a baking sheet with unbleached parchment paper.

2. Cut the sweet peppers lengthwise and trim away the stem and seeds. Blot dry and arrange on the prepared baking sheet, skin side up. Broil for 20 to 25 minutes, or until the skins start to wrinkle. Transfer to a plate to cool. When the peppers are cool, remove and discard the skin.

3. Place the roasted peppers, garlic, paprika (if using), ginger (if using), salt, hemp hearts, olive oil and lemon juice in a blender and pulse to desired consistency (less time for chunky, more time for smooth). Store in an airtight container in the fridge for up to 2 weeks.

4. To bake the fish, preheat the oven to 400°F. Cut the fillet into 4 portions. Spread a thin layer of red pepper pesto over the bottom of a 13- × 9-inch baking dish. Place the fish on top of the pesto. Sprinkle with the salt and a squeeze of fresh lemon juice. Cover each fillet with ¼ cup of the pesto, followed by the sliced shallots and then the sliced lemon. Bake until the fish is firm, 25 to 30 minutes depending on the thickness of the fillets. Check that the thickest part of the fish is flaky to ensure that it is done. The fish will continue to cook in the dish, so it is best not to overcook it in the oven. Serve immediately topped with fresh parsley or sprouts.

Friendly Fried Rice

       OPTION   Serves 6

Once I discovered cauliflower rice, I wondered why it took so long for the world to catch on to this amazing innovation. It is simply delicious and incredibly low in carbohydrates. If you add in the protein-rich mushrooms or eggs, this recipe can become a hearty main dish that travels well to work or school. For those enjoying a higher carb menu, the pineapple adds a nice sweetness to the dish.

2 tablespoons avocado oil, coconut oil or vegan butter

1½ cups chopped red or yellow onion (about 1 medium onion)

1½ cups mushrooms or small broccoli florets (optional)

1 to 2 cloves garlic, chopped (or ½ teaspoon garlic powder)

½ teaspoon unrefined pink salt

2 to 3 teaspoons mild curry powder or spice blend (see Tip)

3 tablespoons coconut sauce or wheat-free tamari (optional)

3 cups cauliflower rice (about 1 medium head)

1 cup fresh or frozen sweet peas

1 tablespoon grated fresh ginger (or ½ teaspoon ground ginger)

1 cup chopped fresh pineapple (optional)

1 to 2 large eggs, whisked (optional)

Fresh flat-leaf or curly parsley or cilantro, for garnish

Hoisin Sauce (page 221), to taste

1. In a large saucepan or pot, heat the avocado oil over medium heat. Add the onion, mushrooms (if using) and garlic and cook, stirring frequently, until the onion is soft and translucent, about 3 minutes.

2. Add the salt, curry powder and coconut sauce (if using) and cook for an additional 2 to 3 minutes until fragrant.

3. Add the cauliflower rice, sweet peas, ginger and pineapple, if using. Cook until completely warmed through, about 5 minutes.

4. Add the whisked egg (if using) and cook for 1 minute more.

5. Adjust the seasoning to taste. Top with the chopped parsley or cilantro and add Hoisin Sauce, if desired.

Tip: If you want to make your own spice blend, mix together 1 teaspoon turmeric, 1 teaspoon ground cumin, ½ teaspoon ground ginger and ½ teaspoon cinnamon.

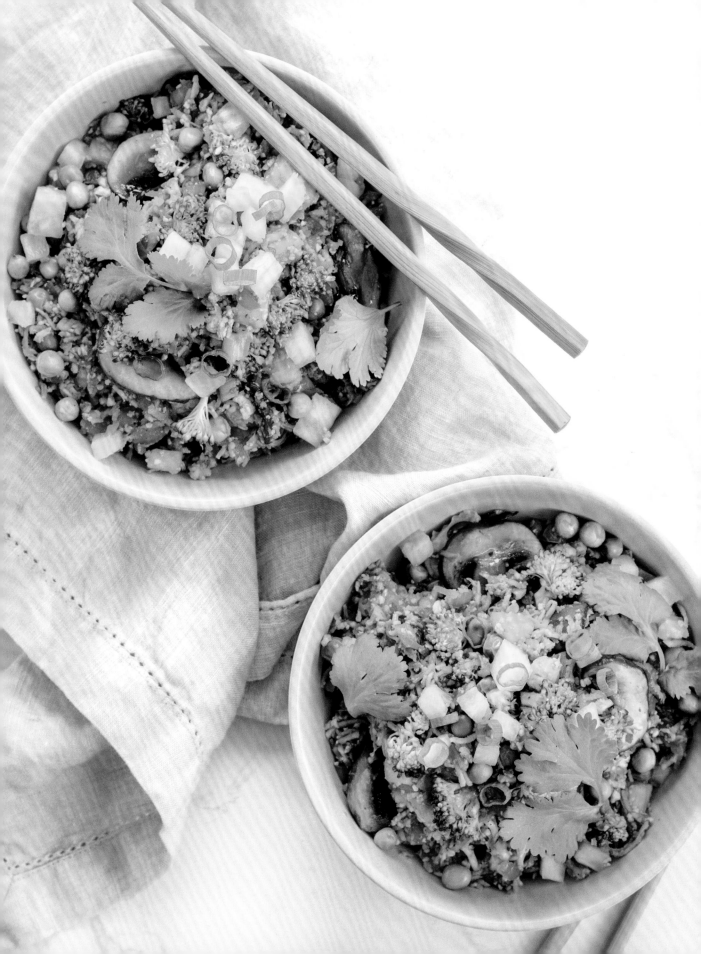

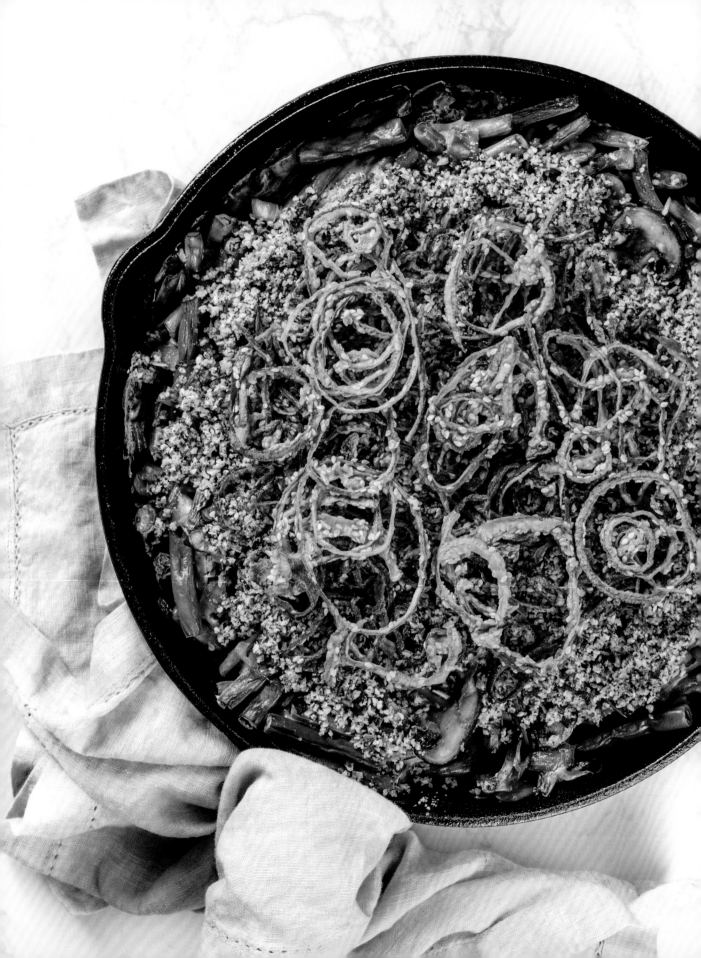

Green Bean Casserole

      V   Makes 4 mains or 8 sides

OPTION

I just love this vegan main dish because it satisfies most people, even picky eaters. The sweetness of the onions and the meaty flavour of the mushrooms provide a "stick to your ribs" casserole that is perfect for buffets and brunches. Did you know that five small mushrooms provide 3 grams of quality protein? Make sure to keep this recipe on hand for Meatless Mondays. One cup of green beans contains 33 mcg of vitamin B9 (folate), which not only protects the heart but also plays a role in mental health.

1 tablespoon avocado or coconut oil

2 cups chopped red or yellow onion

1½ cups sliced mushrooms (cremini, shiitake, portobello)

4 cups fresh French green beans, trimmed and cut into 3-inch pieces

3 cups Creamy Mushroom Soup (condensed version, page 251)

2 tablespoons whole tiger nuts, chopped (optional)

Topping

½ cup finely ground raw almond, hazelnut or sunflower seed flour

2 tablespoons onion flakes

2 tablespoons sesame seeds

1 tablespoon avocado oil

1 to 2 cups Onion Ring Chips (page 232; optional)

1. Preheat the oven to 375°F.

2. In a 12-inch cast-iron skillet, heat the avocado oil over medium heat. Add the onion and cook, stirring frequently, for 2 minutes. Add the mushrooms and cook, stirring occasionally, until lightly browned, 7 to 10 minutes. Remove from the heat.

3. Meanwhile, in a large pot, cover the green beans with water and boil until tender-crisp, 3 to 5 minutes. Drain well.

4. To assemble the casserole, place the cooked green beans, onion and mushroom mixture, condensed Creamy Mushroom Soup and tiger nuts (if using) in a 3-quart oven-safe casserole dish. Stir together until well combined.

5. To make the topping, in a small bowl, combine the almond flour, onion flakes and sesame seeds. Stir in the avocado oil until a crumble forms, then spread it evenly over the casserole. Bake until the topping is golden, 18 to 20 minutes. Serve immediately as is or with Onion Ring Chips on top, if using.

Low-Carb Pecan Stuffing

    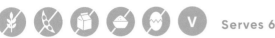   Serves 6

This stuffing is great for family dinners. It pairs nicely with a roasted chicken or vegetarian loaf, making it perfect for the holidays. Celery is a key ingredient in this recipe, and its fresh taste lends an amazing flavour to this dish. Celery is low in calories, as it is made almost entirely of water. It is a good source of vitamin K, which aids in binding calcium in your bones.

2 tablespoons avocado oil

1½ cups chopped red onion

2 cups chopped celery

1 teaspoon poultry seasoning

½ teaspoon dried thyme

½ teaspoon dried rubbed sage (optional)

½ teaspoon unrefined pink salt

1 cup roughly chopped raw pecans

½ cup chopped fresh curly parsley

Optional

1 cup cauliflower rice (or 2 slices Baba's Bread, cut into ½-inch cubes, page 187)

1 cup chopped apple or ¼ cup dried apple juice–infused cranberries

1. In a large skillet, heat the avocado oil over medium-high heat. Add the onion and celery and cook, stirring occasionally, until soft, about 4 minutes.

2. Reduce the heat to medium and stir in the poultry seasoning, thyme, sage (if using) and salt.

3. Add the pecans and parsley and the cauliflower rice or apple (if using) and cook for about 3 minutes to allow the pecans to absorb the flavour of the herbs. Taste and adjust the seasoning as desired. If using Baba's Bread, add it once the dish is fully cooked, just before serving. Store in an airtight container, without the bread, in the fridge, for up to 7 days.

Tip: Note that adding the optional apple or dried apple-juice infused cranberries will increase the amount of carbohydrates in this recipe.

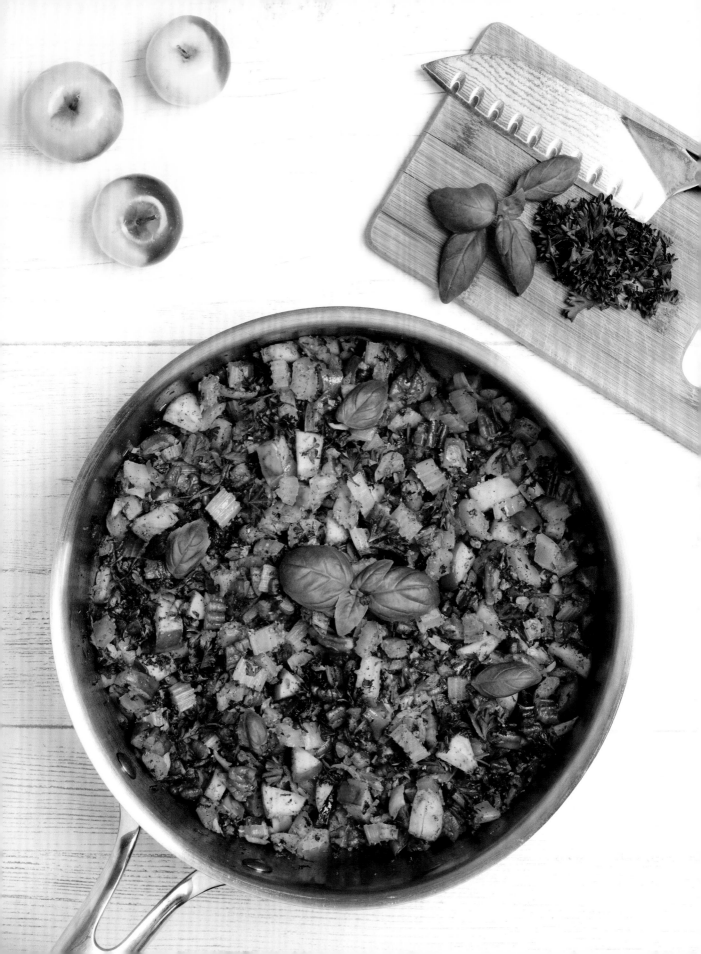

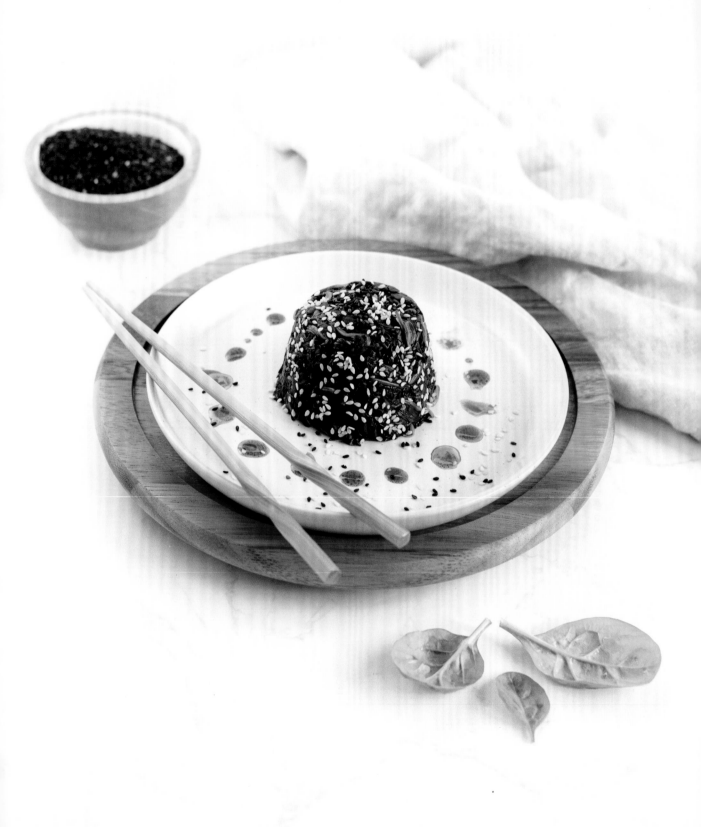

Oshitashi

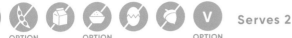

OPTION   OPTION   OPTION   Serves 2

Oshitashi, a delicious and flavourful Japanese spinach side, is my favourite dish to order in a Japanese restaurant. It not only tastes divine, but I love knowing that it contains large amounts of iron and B vitamins, as it is essentially a large amount of greens condensed into a small tasty package. Research shows that spinach has the power to stop cravings in its tracks. One study showed that women who consumed 5 grams of spinach extract per day reduced cravings for chocolate and high-sugar foods by more than 87 percent. This steamed spinach also pairs nicely with the Sunny Anti-Inflammatory Dressing (page 226), if you prefer a creamy dressing. Bonito flakes, also known as katsuobushi, are little wisps of dried, fermented skipjack tuna. They're available in many Asian stores or can be ordered online.

¼ teaspoon unrefined pink salt, divided
10 ounces fresh spinach, washed and stems removed
2 teaspoons coconut sauce or wheat-free tamari
2 teaspoons toasted sesame oil
1 drop pure monk fruit extract (or ¼ teaspoon honey) (optional)
1 teaspoon lemon juice
2 teaspoons black or white sesame seeds

Optional
1 tablespoon pickled ginger, for garnish
Bonito flakes, for garnish

1. Add ⅛ teaspoon of the salt to a large pot or saucepan of water and bring to a boil. When the water is boiling, add the spinach. Using a slotted spoon, remove the spinach as it starts to wilt slightly, about 30 to 60 seconds, and submerge it in a bowl of ice water. This stops the cooking process.

2. Transfer the spinach to a colander over the sink and squeeze out as much water as possible by pressing the spinach against the colander with a spoon.

3. Place the spinach in a large bowl. Add the coconut sauce, sesame oil, monk fruit (if using), remaining ⅛ teaspoon salt, lemon juice and sesame seeds.

4. Mix until well coated, then pack into a short glass or small ramekin. Transfer to a plate by tipping and tapping the glass to make a densely packed tower of spinach.

5. Garnish with pickled ginger and bonito flakes, if using. Serve warm or cold.

No Sugar Added Option: Use pure monk fruit extract.

Vegan Option: Omit the honey and bonito flakes.

Pizza Cheese

      Makes 2½ cups

This cheese has all of the flavour notes of pizza without all of the refined flour or dairy and is an impressive cheese to make for your guests at parties. Enjoy it as a cream cheese, or if you want a block of cheese, you can dehydrate it slightly and create a harder cheese.

2 cups raw cashew pieces
½ cup soft sun-dried tomatoes
2 cups water, for soaking
¼ cup dried basil
3 tablespoons lemon juice
1 to 2 cloves garlic (or 1 teaspoon
    garlic powder)
½ teaspoon unrefined pink salt

For serving
Fresh cut vegetables (carrot,
    celery, sweet pepper, zucchini)
Keto Seed Crackers (page 191)

1. In a small bowl, soak the cashews and sun-dried tomatoes in the water for 30 minutes. Drain well, discarding the soaking water.

2. In a blender or food processor, combine all ingredients and blend until a smooth paste forms, scraping down the sides as needed. If using a blender, you will need to spend more time scraping and blending until the ingredients blend together well.

3. Enjoy with fresh cut vegetables or Keto Seed Crackers. Store in an airtight container in the fridge for up to 2 weeks.

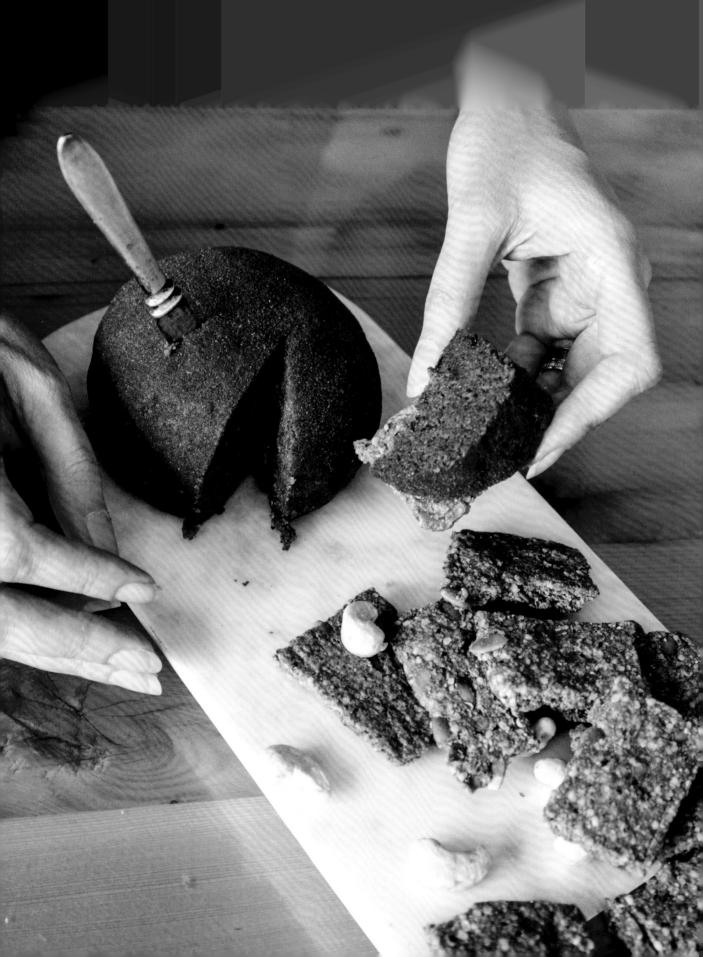

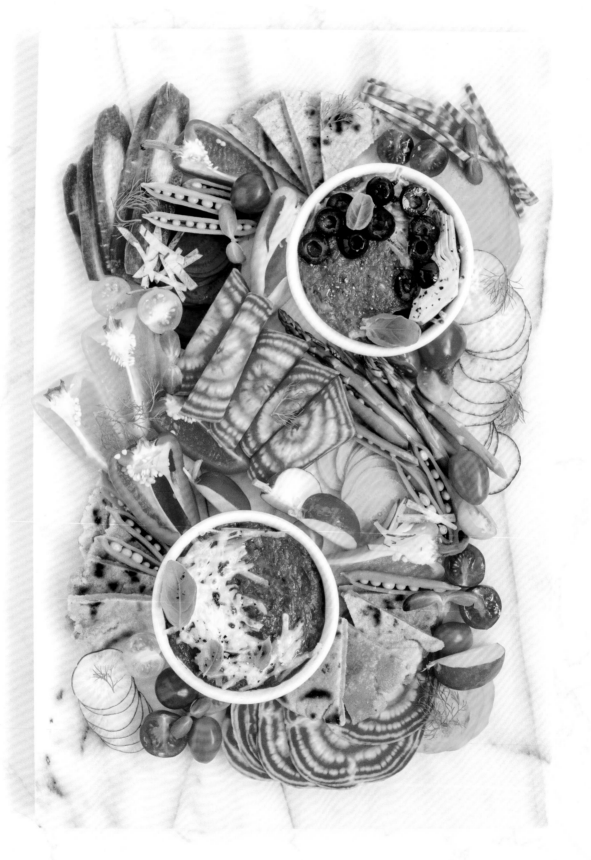

Pizza Dip and Vegetables

 Serves 8

Imagine all of the tasty flavours of a pizza baked into a deliciously warmed dip. If you don't have a sensitivity to the nightshade family of plants (and can tolerate tomatoes), these nutritional superstars will benefit you with their impressive antioxidant profile. Although raw tomatoes are delicious, it is best to consume them after they have been cooked to maximize the availability of the antioxidant carotenoids beta-carotene, lutein, zeaxanthin and lycopene. My family likes to pair this dip with Baba's Bread (page 187), Chewy Baguette (page 188) or Corn-Free Tortilla Chips (page 195) or use it as a sauce to create a Cassava Tortilla pizza (page 184).

Pizza Dip
2 tablespoons extra-virgin olive oil
1 cup finely chopped red or yellow onion
2 cloves garlic, minced
1 can (28 ounces) crushed tomatoes (see Tip)
2 tablespoons tomato paste (see Tip)
1 tablespoon Italian seasoning
2 teaspoons dried basil
3 drops pure monk fruit extract (if you like a sweet sauce; optional)
½ teaspoon unrefined pink salt

Optional
½ cup crumbled vegan cheese
¼ cup sliced pitted black or green olives or capers
½ cup sliced marinated artichoke hearts
12 fresh basil leaves, for garnish

Vegetables
3 green zucchini, sliced into sticks
3 yellow zucchini, sliced into sticks
1 bunch asparagus, trimmed and sliced into sticks
1 red sweet pepper, seeded and sliced into sticks
2 cups snap peas

Tip: To save time, you can use sugar-free organic tomato sauce as a substitute for the crushed tomatoes and tomato paste, but you may have to simmer it for longer (up to 45 minutes, depending on how watery your sauce choice is) before adding the toppings and baking.

1. In a 12-inch cast-iron skillet or oven-safe saucepan, heat the olive oil over medium heat. Add the onion and garlic and cook, stirring occasionally, until softened, about 5 minutes. Add the tomatoes and their juice, tomato paste, Italian seasoning, basil, monk fruit (if using) and salt. Stir to combine, then simmer for 30 minutes until the sauce thickens.

2. Meanwhile, preheat the oven to 350°F. Remove the pan from the heat and top the sauce with the vegan cheese, olives and artichoke hearts, if using. Bake for 10 minutes, until the cheese is melted and the toppings are warmed through. Garnish with the fresh basil (if using) and serve with the vegetables for dipping.

Reggae Roots Slaw

     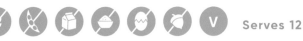 **Serves 12**

This salad was created for a steel drum band on my TV show, *Healthy Gourmet*, and is packed with anti-inflammatory goodness. Puréed avocado is the secret to this slaw's creamy richness. Beets are brilliant for detoxification, as they contain phytonutrients called betalains that are powerfully anti-inflammatory and assist in hormonal balance. If you don't own a food processor, a hand grater works well to prepare the slaw ingredients. The naturally occurring sugars in the fruit and beets will assist in satisfying a sweet tooth so that you are more likely to stay away from dessert.

Slaw

2 cups thinly sliced mango or apple

1 cup grated golden, candy stripe or red beets

1 cup julienned kale leaves or green cabbage, stems removed

2 cups grated carrot

1 tablespoon grated fresh ginger

1 cup chopped fresh flat-leaf parsley or cilantro

2 cups packed baby spinach or sprouts

Dressing

¾ cup diced ripe avocado

¼ cup lemon juice

3 tablespoons chopped fresh chives

½ teaspoon unrefined pink salt

⅓ cup extra-virgin olive oil

1. To make the slaw, in a large bowl, combine all ingredients, except the spinach or sprouts.

2. To make the dressing, in a high-speed blender, combine all ingredients and blend until smooth.

3. Toss the dressing with the slaw. Serve on a bed of baby spinach and/or top with sprouts. Store the dressed slaw in an airtight container in the fridge for up to 3 days.

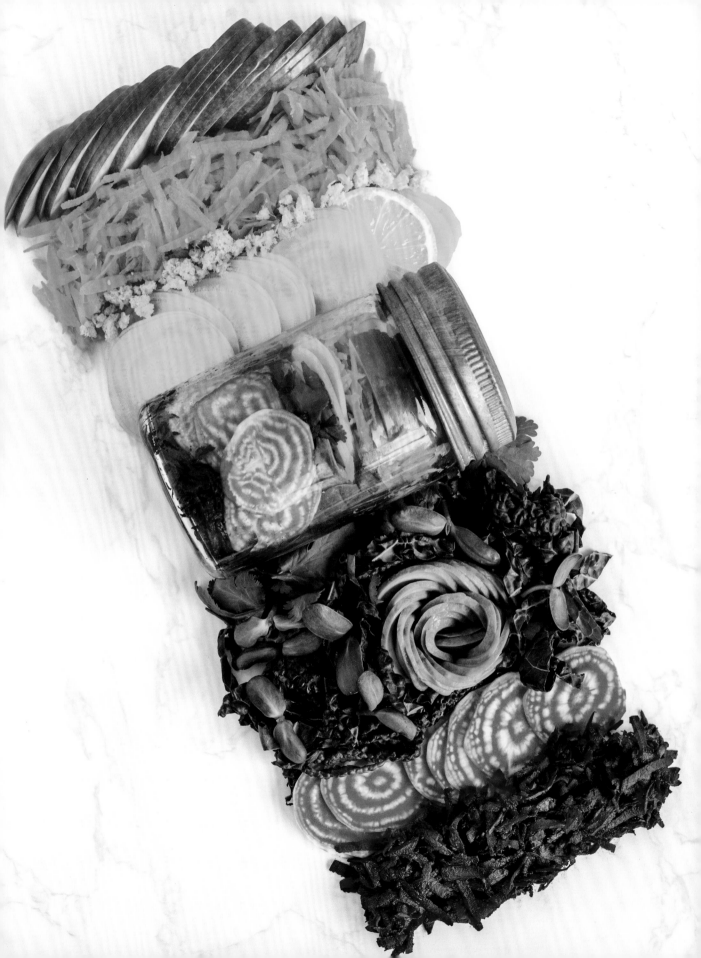

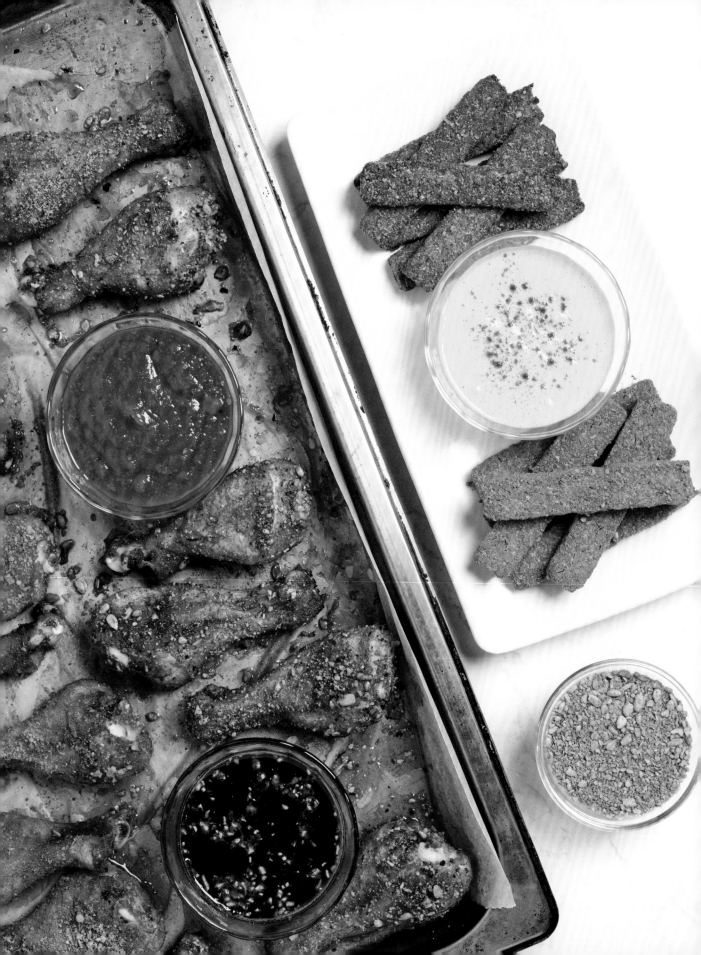

Shake and Bake Chicken or Tempeh

      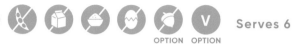 Serves 6

OPTION   OPTION

This main dish takes about ten minutes to prepare, which is amazing on busy weeknights when you have too many activities to juggle and palates to satisfy. Commercially sold ready mixes include sugar, maltodextrin (sugar), modified food starch (breaks down to sugar), partially hydrogenated soybean and cottonseed oil, brown sugar, caramel colour and sodium silicoaluminate as an anticaking agent. I provide two seasoning choices in this recipe, as well as protein options to suit whatever lifestyle you follow. With this recipe in your back pocket, I hope you never need to buy a ready mix again.

½ cup almond, hazelnut or sunflower seed flour or unsweetened shredded coconut

2 teaspoons unrefined pink salt

3 pounds organic skin-on chicken drumsticks (or two 8-ounce packages of tempeh, cut into twenty-four 1- × 3-inch slices)

1 tablespoon avocado oil, if using tempeh

Classic Seasoning Mix

2 teaspoons sweet paprika

1 teaspoon ground cumin

1 teaspoon dried basil

½ teaspoon garlic powder

½ teaspoon onion powder

1 teaspoon dried rosemary (optional)

½ teaspoon dried thyme or oregano (optional)

Curry Seasoning Mix

2 teaspoons unrefined pink salt

2 teaspoons turmeric

1 teaspoon ground cumin

½ teaspoon ground ginger

½ teaspoon cinnamon

½ teaspoon garlic powder

½ teaspoon onion powder

½ teaspoon ground cardamom (optional)

1. Preheat the oven to 400°F. Line two baking sheets with unbleached parchment paper.

2. In a large bowl, combine the almond flour, salt, and seasoning mix of choice.

3. If using tempeh, coat the slices with the avocado oil.

4. Evenly coat each chicken drumstick or tempeh slice with the flour mixture, then place them on the prepared baking sheets.

5. If using chicken drumsticks, bake, uncovered, for 30 minutes, then turn them over and bake for an additional 15 to 20 minutes. If using tempeh, bake for 30 minutes total (no need to flip halfway through). Serve immediately or store in an airtight container in the fridge for up to 3 days for the chicken or up to 1 week for the tempeh.

Vegan Option: Use tempeh.

Vegan Curry Casserole

       Serves 10 to 12

This is a gentle and soothing main dish that tastes so comforting that even your picky meat-eater friends will enjoy it. The psyllium husk binds the dish together and balances your blood sugar. The beta-carotene in the sweet potato converts to vitamin A, which assists in boosting your immune system and protecting your digestive lining. This recipe makes a great lunch as well, so you will be happy with the leftovers, if there are any!

3 tablespoons avocado oil, divided

4 cups grated unpeeled sweet potato

2 cups chopped green onions (white and light green parts only) or diced red onion

1 cup chopped celery

1 cup almond, hazelnut or sunflower seed flour

½ cup raw cashew pieces

½ cup hemp hearts (see Tip)

2 tablespoons psyllium husks

2 teaspoons ground turmeric

1 teaspoon cinnamon

1 teaspoon ground cumin

½ teaspoon ground ginger

¼ cup vegetable broth or canned full-fat coconut milk

1 tablespoon lemon juice

½ teaspoon unrefined pink salt, or to taste

1. Preheat the oven to 350°F. Grease an 8- × 11-inch baking dish with 1 tablespoon of the avocado oil.

2. Place the sweet potato in a large bowl.

3. In a food processor fitted, combine the green onion, celery, almond flour, cashews, hemp hearts, psyllium, turmeric, cinnamon, cumin, ginger, vegetable broth, the remaining 2 tablespoons avocado oil, lemon juice and salt. Pulse until well mixed but with some texture remaining. You don't want to overprocess the mixture and make a paste.

4. Transfer the mixture to the bowl with the sweet potato and toss to combine.

5. Press the mixture into the prepared baking dish. Bake for 50 minutes, or until the top edges begin to appear golden and the centre is dry.

Tips:

1. If you tolerate spicy food, you can swap the individual spices for 1½ tablespoons curry powder.

2. Hemp hearts provide the protein in this recipe. If not available, you can use sunflower seeds, but they are much lower in protein.

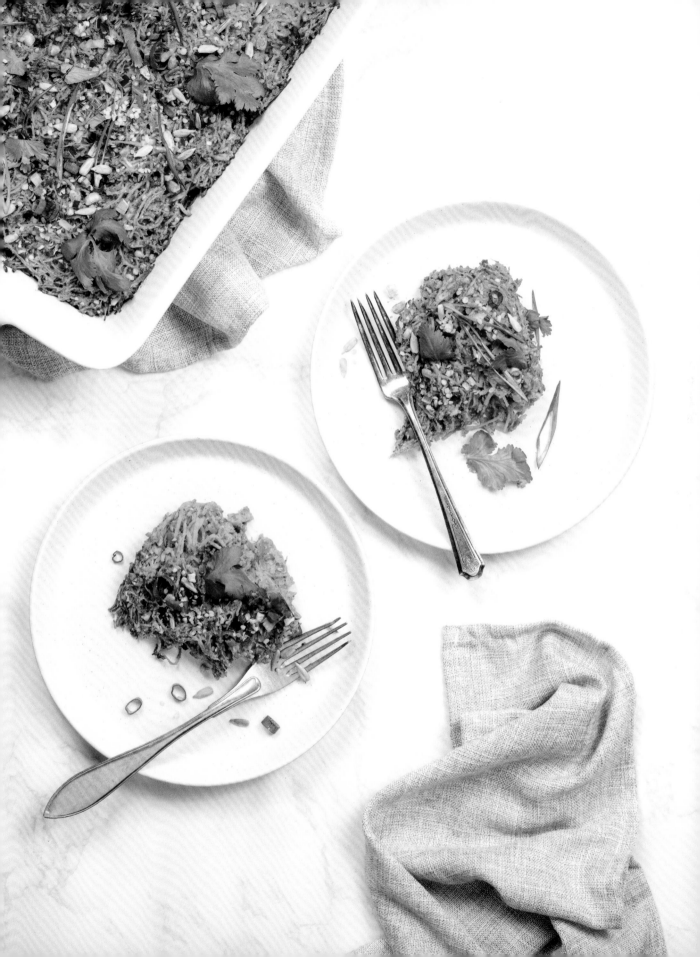

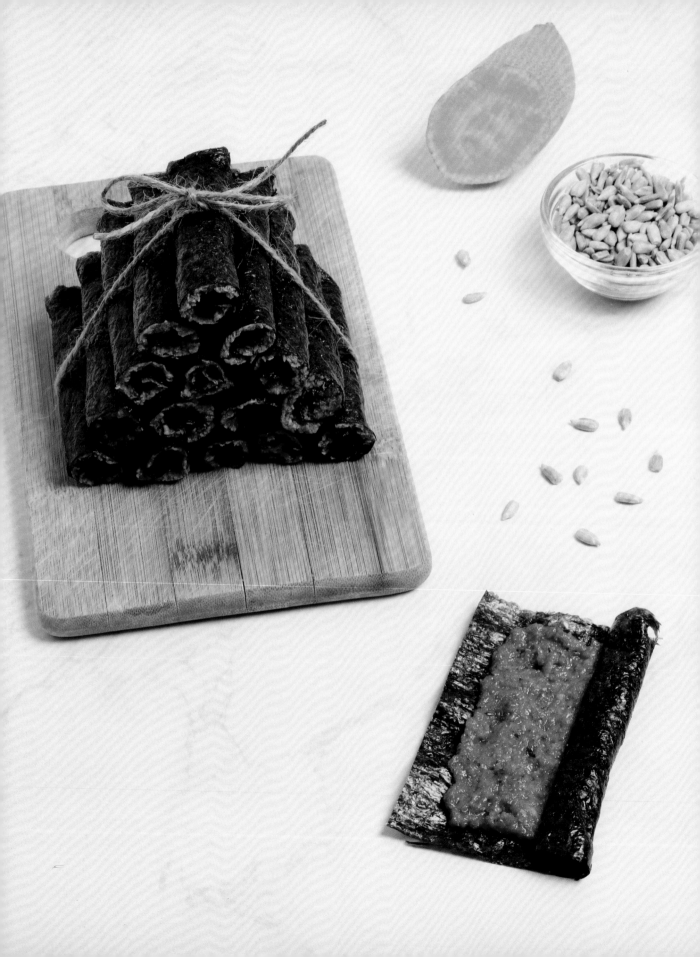

Vegan Pepperoni Stix

OPTION   OPTION   Makes 52 stix

Are you tired of the sugar- and flour-filled snacks available in convenience stores, cafes and gas stations? I love these salty stix, as I consider them a vegan pepperoni. It is my dream that our sugar-free movement will grow big enough that savoury and sugar-free snacks are available everywhere, so that you won't have to stress out when you're "hangry." Until we change the world, start by carrying snacks in your purse, bag or car.

2½ cups raw sunflower seeds,
2½ cups grated sweet potato
1½ cups hemp hearts or
  cashews
½ cup coconut sauce or wheat-
  free tamari
⅓ cup apple cider vinegar
¼ teaspoon unrefined pink salt
1 tablespoon turmeric
1 teaspoon ground ginger
1 teaspoon garlic powder
½ teaspoon sugar-free hot
  sauce (optional)
Pinch of black pepper (optional)
1 teaspoon sweet paprika
  (optional)
13 sheets nori paper

1. Soak the sunflower seeds in 3 cups of warm water for 20 minutes. Drain well and discard the water. Make sure the sunflower seeds are well drained so that no extra liquid is added to the recipe. In a food processor fitted, combine the sunflower seeds, sweet potato, hemp hearts, coconut sauce, apple cider vinegar, salt, turmeric, ginger, garlic powder, hot sauce, black pepper and paprika (if using) and blend until a paste forms.

2. Cut each sheet of nori into 4 equal squares. Using a spatula, evenly spread about 1½ tablespoons of the paste onto the rough side of each square, leaving ¼ inch of space at one end to allow for a strong seal. Roll into a cigar shape.

3. If using an oven, preheat the oven to 170°F. Line a baking sheet with unbleached parchment paper. Place the rolls, seam side down, on the prepared baking sheet and dehydrate for 6 hours. Leave them in the oven overnight to continue to dry, then transfer them to an airtight container in the morning. They should have the texture of a pepperoni stick. If using a dehydrator, add in a single layer and dehydrate at 120°F for 8 hours. Store in an airtight container on the countertop for up to 1 month or in the freezer for up to 3 months.

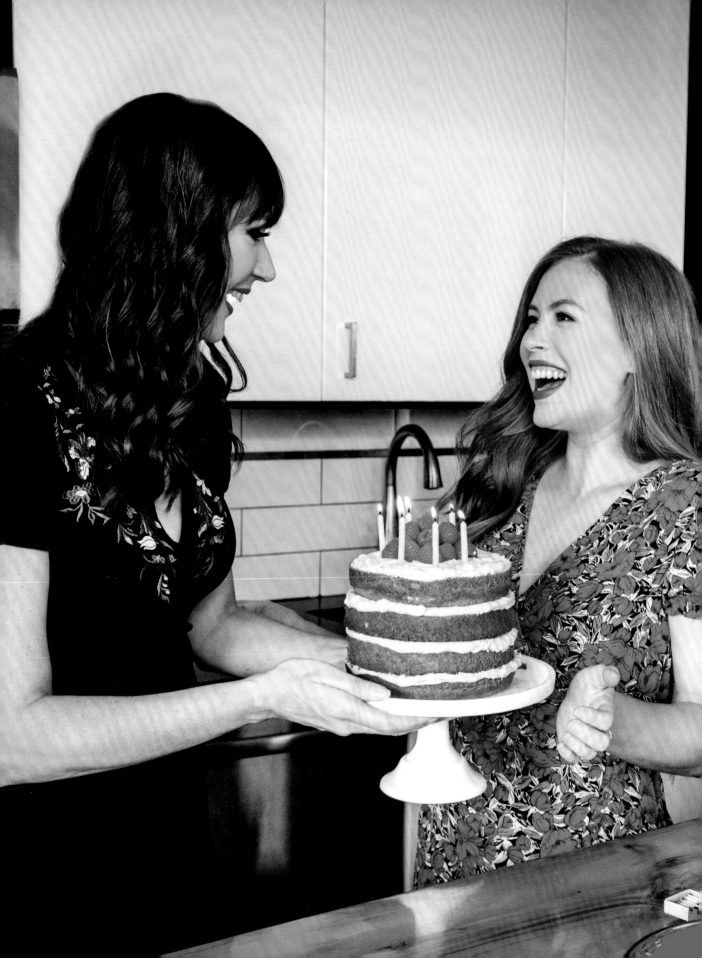

Special Occasions

Gummy Candy

 Makes 300 mini gummies

Who does not love a good gummy candy? This is a fun recipe to share around the office and school. I wanted to create a fun activity for my nephews and nieces, so I made sure that the recipe had only a few ingredients and no added sugar. It was a smash hit, and they did not even know that it sported a lot of collagen to help them grow and recover from snowboarding. I use silicone moulds in the shape of the classic gummy bear (about ½ inch in size), which you can purchase online.

2 cups unsweetened organic fruit juice of choice, divided
⅓ cup unflavoured gelatin powder
1 teaspoon lemon juice
¼ teaspoon pure monk fruit extract

Optional
Pinch of unrefined pink salt
1 teaspoon beet powder (for colour)
½ teaspoon pure vanilla or orange extract

1. Pour 1 cup of the juice into a medium glass bowl. Sprinkle the gelatin over the juice and let sit to bloom.

2. Pour the remaining 1 cup juice into a medium saucepan and heat over medium heat for 5 to 7 minutes until warm but not boiling.

3. Whisk the warm juice, lemon juice, monk fruit, salt (if using), beet powder (if using) and vanilla (if using) into the bloomed gelatin until dissolved.

4. Carefully pour the gummy liquid into the moulds, or use a turkey baster for easier transfer. Place the moulds in the refrigerator and chill for 2 hours or until fully set.

5. If using smaller moulds with intricate designs, briefly plunge the bottom of the moulds into warm water to make releasing the shapes easier. Store in the fridge for up to 2 weeks until ready to serve. If packing these as a portable snack, include an ice pack to keep them cool.

Tummy Gummies

       Makes 250 mini or 50 small square gummies

These bite-size, anti-inflammatory, lemon drop gummies are easy to prepare and full of health benefits. I recommend that you buy some silicone moulds so that you can enjoy some cute bear-shaped gummies, especially if you have children nearby. If you are following a lower carb menu, you will appreciate that there are almost no carbs in this recipe. The fibre I typically use in this recipe is a hydrolyzed guar gum that helps regulate the digestive system and is recommended for people who suffer from irritable bowel syndrome (IBS) and other digestive complaints.

1 cup water
½ cup lemon juice
½ teaspoon turmeric
1 teaspoon pure monk fruit extract (or ½ teaspoon liquid stevia)
⅓ cup unflavoured gelatin powder
Pinch of unrefined pink salt

Optional Boosters
2 tablespoons soluble fibre (see Tip)
½ teaspoon vitamin C powder (used as a coating)

1. In a large pot, combine the water, lemon juice, turmeric and monk fruit and heat over medium-high heat until thoroughly warmed and mixed, about 3 minutes. Do not bring to a boil or the gelatin will split when you add it.

2. Remove the pot from the heat and sprinkle the gelatin over the liquid, mixing well to hydrate the gelatin. Return the pot to the heat and whisk until the gelatin is completely dissolved.

3. Remove the pot from the heat and mix in the soluble fibre, if using, and salt, stirring until dissolved.

4. Pour the mixture into an 8-inch square baking dish or, using a dropper, carefully fill silicone moulds. Chill in the refrigerator for at least 15 minutes or until firm.

5. Once fully chilled, slice into small cubes or extract the gummies from the moulds and place in a bowl or on a plate. Shake the vitamin C powder (if using) evenly over top if you want them to be sour. Store in an airtight container in the fridge for up to 2 weeks or they might melt and clump together.

Tip: Soluble fibre blends completely dissolve in water and leave no grit.

Sweet Potato Ice Cream

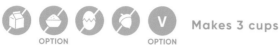 Makes 3 cups

My nephew Taevan is a huge fan of dairy-free coconut ice cream, but it can cost up to nine dollars a pint. I was determined to figure out a recipe that would keep him happy and keep our shopping budget in check. Chocolate is a source of phenylethylamine (PEA), which prevents the reuptake of dopamine and norepinephrine, similar to the mechanism of action provided by attention-deficit/hyperactivity disorder (ADHD) medications. In fact, some people report that enjoying sugar-free chocolate may decrease the symptoms of ADHD. As someone diagnosed with ADHD, I sure find it helpful!

1 cup mashed roasted sweet potato

1 cup full-fat coconut cream (see Tip)

½ cup coconut butter (or coconut oil if unavailable)

½ cup cocoa powder

¼ to ½ cup yacón, honey or coconut nectar (or ½ teaspoon chocolate-flavoured liquid stevia; see Tip)

1 teaspoon pure vanilla extract

¼ teaspoon unrefined pink salt

2 tablespoons chocolate collagen or other protein powder (optional)

1 tablespoon lucuma powder (optional)

½ teaspoon cinnamon (optional)

Fresh berries or unsweetened shredded coconut, for garnish

1. In a blender, combine the mashed sweet potato, coconut cream, coconut butter, cocoa powder, yacón, vanilla, salt and collagen, lucuma powder and cinnamon, if using. Blend until fully combined and smooth. Taste and adjust the sweetness, if desired.

2. Pour into a 4-cup container or bowl, cover and freeze for 2 hours or until completely frozen.

3. To serve, remove from the freezer and let come to room temperature. The ice cream will melt to a creamy soft serve texture, but don't let it melt too much.

4. Scoop into bowls and serve with fresh berries or shredded coconut, if desired.

Tips:

1. If using coconut milk, place a can (14 ounces) of full-fat coconut milk in the fridge overnight. Scoop out the solid coconut cream. Use the coconut water in smoothies and other recipes.

2. Coconut nectar is permitted if you are on the slow breakup plan and can tolerate sucrose.

No Sugar Added Option: Use liquid stevia.

Vegan Option: Use liquid stevia and vegan protein powder. Omit the honey.

Frozen Faux Chocolate Cups

 Makes 36 bite-size chocolate cups

Bone building, relaxing because of their high mineral content and with no added refined sugar, these cups can certainly help you break your chocolate addiction if using carob. These delicious treats were inspired by Jessica Tucker, a nutritionist at the Living Proof Institute. I adapted it to use monk fruit and nut butter, and the results taste like a peanut butter cup. Carob is caffeine-free, so these cups are the perfect after-dinner treat. Caffeine stays in your system for hours, so choose carob over chocolate if planning to indulge in the evening. Consider this like a high-power fat bomb that delievers more than just good fats.

1 cup unsweetened cashew butter (see Tip)

1 cup coconut oil

1 cup carob or cocoa powder (see Tip)

1 teaspoon pure peppermint extract (or 1 tablespoon pure vanilla extract)

¼ teaspoon unrefined pink salt

½ teaspoon pure monk fruit extract (or ¼ to ½ cup raw honey)

1 or 2 tablespoons collagen powder (optional)

1. In a food processor, combine all ingredients and process until completely smooth.

2. Divide the mixture among 1-inch-diameter silicone cups or chocolate moulds. Place in the freezer to set, about 30 minutes. Store in an airtight container in the freezer for up to 3 months. Serve and consume directly from the freezer, as these cups thaw quickly at room temperature.

Tips:

1. If you have nut allergies, you can replace the cashew butter with an additional cup of coconut oil.

2. If you want to use cocoa instead of carob, increase the monk fruit to 1 teaspoon or the raw honey to ½ cup.

No Sugar Added Option: Use pure monk fruit extract.

Vegan Option: Omit the collagen and honey.

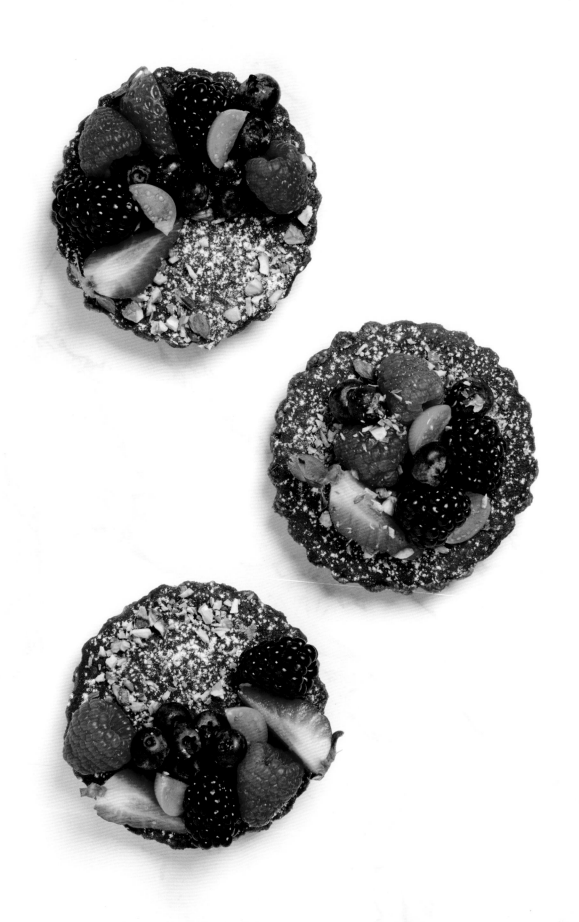

Decadent Chocolate Ganache Tarts

    Makes 6 individual tarts

This recipe is low carb and free of animal products, making it the perfect dessert for everyone at the table. I adore adding in the mint extract because it makes for a cool sensation on your tongue, but the vanilla option pairs beautifully with an assortment of fresh fruit.

Crust

1 cup chopped raw almonds or pecans
1 cup unsweetened shredded coconut
2 tablespoons melted coconut oil
1 tablespoon canned full-fat coconut milk
1 tablespoon cacao powder
2 tablespoons yacón, raw honey or coconut nectar (see Tip)
Pinch of unrefined pink salt

Filling

¾ cup coconut cream (top layer of canned coconut milk; see Tip)
7 ounces sugar-free dark chocolate, chopped into small pieces (about 2 bars)
Pinch of unrefined pink salt
2 teaspoons pure mint or vanilla extract (optional)
Raw cacao nibs, chopped nuts or seeds, fresh berries or mint leaves, for garnish

1. To make the crust, combine all ingredients in a food processer and blend until a chewy dough consistency forms.

2. Press the crust mixture into six 3-inch ramekins or tart pans and place in the fridge.

3. To make the filling, in a saucepan, heat the coconut cream over medium heat until very warm, but be careful not to bring it to a boil. Remove from the heat.

4. Add the chocolate, salt and mint or vanilla extract, if using. Let stand for a few minutes without stirring. Then stir gently until smooth, 1 or 2 minutes. If the chocolate is too thick to pour, gently warm it on the stove over the lowest heat possible and add a few teaspoons of the reserved coconut water.

5. Pour the chocolate mixture into the prepared ramekins and place in the fridge to set for at least 2 hours.

6. Serve topped with cacao nibs, nuts or seeds, fresh berries or mint leaves. Store, covered, in the fridge for up to 5 days.

Tips:

1. Coconut nectar is permitted if you are on the slow breakup plan and can tolerate sucrose.

2. For coconut cream, place a 14-ounce can of full-fat coconut milk in the fridge overnight. Scoop out the solid coconut cream. Reserve the coconut water to thin the chocolate if needed. Use any remaining coconut water in smoothies and other recipes.

Vegan Option: Omit the honey.

Chocolate Mint Cheesecake

   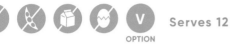 **Serves 12**

OPTION

My sister, Lynn, really outdid herself with this cheesecake. As a passionate environmentalist, I know she would want you to vote with your wallet and buy ethically traded, organic cacao powder and cashews, and I completely agree. It may cost a bit more, but it is worth it, as conventional chocolate is often produced with child labour and toxic pesticides that are harmful to farm workers. It is ideal if you look for raw cocoa (called cacao), as it has a higher amount of phytonutrients, which help protect the heart.

Crust

2 cups raw pecans

¼ cup raw honey or coconut nectar (see Tip)

¼ teaspoon unrefined pink salt

Filling

2 cups raw cashews, soaked in water for at least 4 hours or overnight

¼ cup melted coconut oil

½ cup raw honey (or 1 teaspoon pure monk fruit extract)

½ cup coconut cream (see Tip)

1 cup cacao powder

1 teaspoon pure peppermint extract

½ teaspoon unrefined pink salt

Topping

1 cup fresh or frozen raspberries

2 tablespoons raw honey (or ¼ teaspoon pure monk fruit extract)

1 teaspoon pure vanilla extract

Vegan Option: Omit the honey.

1. To make the crust, in a food processor, combine the pecans, honey and salt and grind into a coarse meal.

2. Press the pecan mixture into a 9-inch pie plate and up the sides to form a crust. Clean the bowl of the food processor.

3. To make the filling, drain the cashews and discard the water. Combine the cashews, melted coconut oil, honey, coconut cream, cacao powder, peppermint and salt. Process into a smooth paste, scraping down the sides as needed. This can take 10 to 15 minutes. The mixture will become warm.

4. Spoon the filling evenly into the crust and smooth the top. Let set in the refrigerator for about 1 hour.

5. Once the cheesecake is set, make the topping. In a small saucepan, mix together the raspberries, honey and vanilla. Bring to a gentle boil, then reduce the heat and simmer until the mixture is reduced by about half.

6. To serve, spoon the raspberry topping evenly over the cheesecake. Store, covered, in the fridge for up to 3 weeks or in the freezer for up to 3 months.

Tips:

1. Coconut nectar is permitted if you are on the slow breakup plan and can tolerate sucrose.

2. For coconut cream, place a 14-ounce can of full-fat coconut milk in the fridge overnight. Scoop out the solid coconut cream. Reserve the coconut water to thin the chocolate if needed. Use any remaining coconut water in smoothies and other recipes.

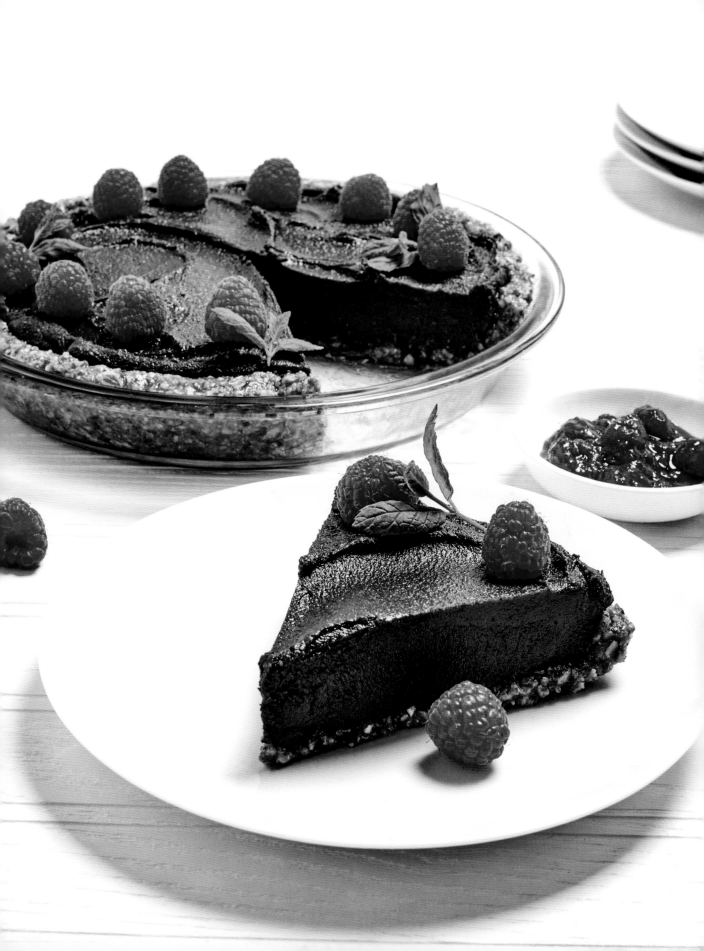

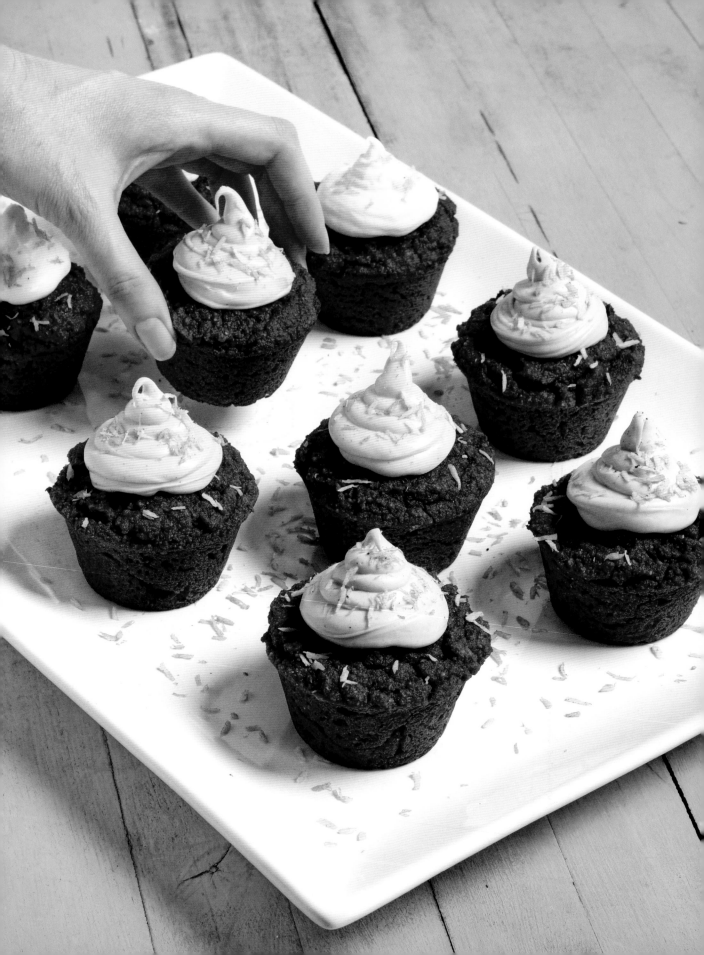

Red Velvet Cupcakes

Makes 9 large or 12 small cupcakes

These crimson gems not only will satisfy a sweet tooth, but also contain rich amounts of detoxifying ingredients that help achieve hormonal balance. Sunflower seeds contain good amounts of zinc, folate and iron, three nutrients that many people struggle to get enough of on a daily basis. Zinc is critical for both testosterone and estrogen metabolism, and folate is critical for liver detoxification. One in three women globally are anemic (iron deficient), and the beets in this recipe sport a good amount of bioavailable iron for optimal health.

1½ cups almond, hazelnut or sunflower seed flour

½ cup coconut flour

¼ cup cocoa powder

2 teaspoons baking powder

¼ teaspoon unrefined pink salt

1¼ cups red beet purée (about 2 cooked beets; see Tip)

⅓ cup coconut oil

½ cup raw honey or coconut nectar (see Tip)

3 large eggs (or flax or chia egg; see Tip)

1 teaspoon pure vanilla extract

2 tablespoons lemon juice

Vegan Option: Use flax or chia egg substitute. Omit the honey.

1. Preheat the oven to 350°F. Line a muffin tin with unbleached paper liners.

2. In a small bowl, combine the almond flour, coconut flour, cocoa powder, baking powder and salt.

3. Place the cooked beets in a blender and blend into a rough purée. If desired, measure the beet purée to ensure that you have the correct amount. Add the coconut oil, honey, eggs, vanilla and lemon juice to the blender and blend until smooth. Transfer to a large bowl.

4. Add the dry ingredients to the wet ingredients and mix until well combined.

5. Fill the muffin cups about three-quarters full. Bake for 32 to 35 minutes for small cupcakes or 45 to 50 minutes for large cupcakes, or until a toothpick inserted in the middle comes out clean.

6. Remove the cupcakes from the tins and let cool completely on a wire rack. Store in an airtight container in the fridge for up to 2 weeks or in the freezer for up to 3 months.

Recipe continues

Red Velvet Cupcakes continued

Tips:

1. To quickly cook the beets, slice them and steam for 20 minutes until soft when pierced with a fork. Alternatively, you can bake the beets, wrapped in parchment paper-lined foil, in a 350°F oven for 1 hour until soft.

2. Coconut nectar is permited if you can tolerate sucrose.

3. To make the flax or chia egg, in a small bowl, whisk together 3 tablespoons ground flaxseed or chia seeds and 7 tablespoons + 1½ teaspoons hot water until well combined. Set aside to soak for 10 minutes so that the flaxseed can swell and absorb the liquid.

Guilt-Free Vanilla Birthday Cake or Cupcakes

OPTION

Makes 12 cupcakes or one 4-layer cake (doubled recipe)

My niece Jade was brave enough to give up refined sugar shortly before her birthday, so we wanted to make something special for her so that she would feel supported in her decision. Instead of making cupcakes, I thought it would be fun to make a four-layer cake with pretty pink icing so that she did not miss a "beet." By hiding a whole zucchini in the cake and some beetroot powder in the icing, the princess in your life will have no idea she is getting her veggies in such a decadent treat. Be sure to use small zucchini to ensure that the taste is not bitter.

1 cup coconut flour
½ cup arrowroot flour
2 teaspoons baking powder (if unavailable, use baking soda)
½ teaspoon unrefined pink salt
½ teaspoon cinnamon
1½ cups peeled and finely chopped zucchini
¾ cup raw honey or ¾ cup Faux Maple Syrup (page 225) + 2 tablespoons monk fruit erythritol powder
8 large eggs
3 tablespoons coconut oil
1 tablespoon pure vanilla extract

1 batch Vegan Buttercream Icing (page 293); double batch if making a cake

1. Preheat the oven to 350°F. Line a muffin tin with unbleached paper liners.

2. In a blender, combine all ingredients except for the icing and blend until completely smooth.

3. Fill the muffin cups about three-quarters full. Bake for 26 to 28 minutes for muffins until golden on top, or until a toothpick inserted in the middle comes out clean.

4. Remove from the tin or pan and let cool completely before frosting with Vegan Buttercream Icing. Store in the fridge, covered, for up to 4 days.

VARIATION

Four-Layer Cake: To make a four-layer cake, double the recipe. Divide the batter evenly between two greased 9-inch round cake pans lined with parchment paper circles. Bake for 42 to 44 minutes until golden on top, or until a toothpick inserted in the middle comes out clean.

When the cakes are cool, using a long serrated knife cut each cake layer in half crosswise to create 4 layers. Frost the layers and top of the cake with Vegan Buttercream Icing. Store, covered, in the fridge for up to 4 days.

No Sugar Added Option: Use Faux Maple Syrup and pure monk fruit extract erythritol powder mixture.

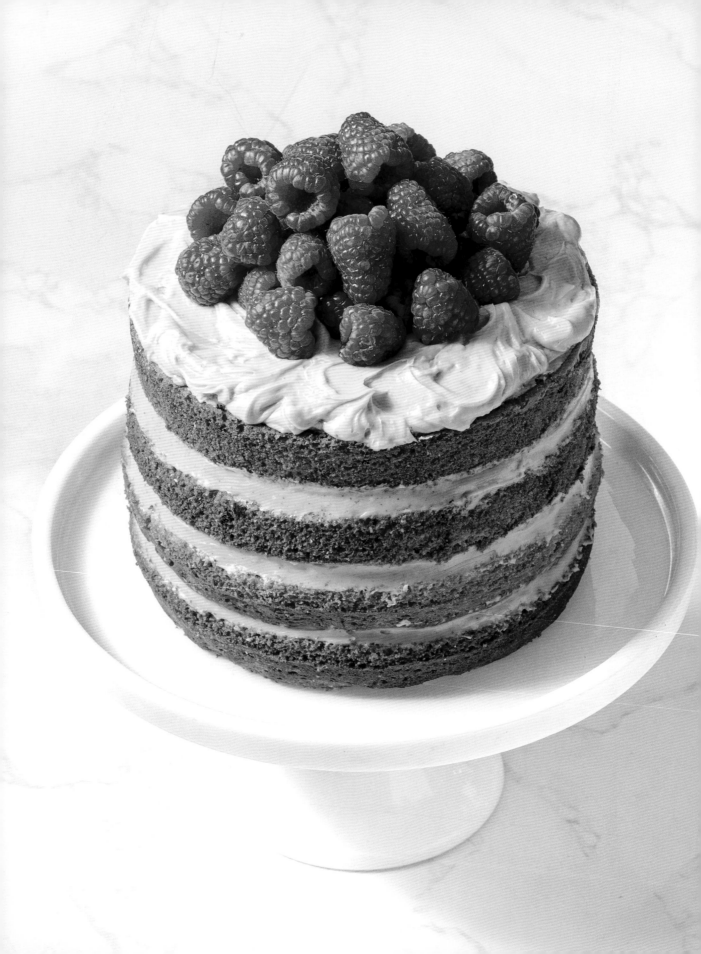

Vegan Buttercream Icing

 Makes 1½ cups

This buttercream is as smooth and silky as its classic counterpart, and you may wake up dreaming about it. Everyone loves frosting, but the conventional stuff is one of the most concentrated sources of sugar per serving you can find (it's full of confectioners powdered sugar). Crack out this healthier version for a birthday cake or cupcakes, like the Guilt-Free Vanilla Birthday Cake or Cupcakes (page 291). Take it easy on this recipe and bring it out only for special occasions because it is sweetened with the sugar alcohol erythritol.

2 cups vegan butter
⅛ teaspoon unrefined pink salt
1 teaspoon pure vanilla extract
2 cups monk fruit erythritol
   powder

Optional
½ teaspoon xanthan gum
   powder (or 1 teaspoon
   arrowroot flour)
½ teaspoon beetroot powder
   or raspberry powder (for a
   pink colour; see Tip)
¼ teaspoon Blue Majik algae
   powder (for a blue colour;
   see Tip)

1. Combine the vegan butter, salt, vanilla and any optional ingredients in the bowl of a stand mixer. Slowly add the monk fruit erythritol powder, starting at slow speed to avoid the powder becoming airborne and gradually increasing the speed until the icing becomes thick and smooth.

2. If the icing is too thick, add coconut milk, a drop at a time; if it's too thin, add another ¼ cup monk fruit erythritol powder. Spread onto cakes, pipe onto cupcakes or store in an airtight container in the fridge for up to 3 weeks until ready to use.

Tip: You can substitute the powders used for colouring with ⅛ teaspoon of liquid natural food colouring.

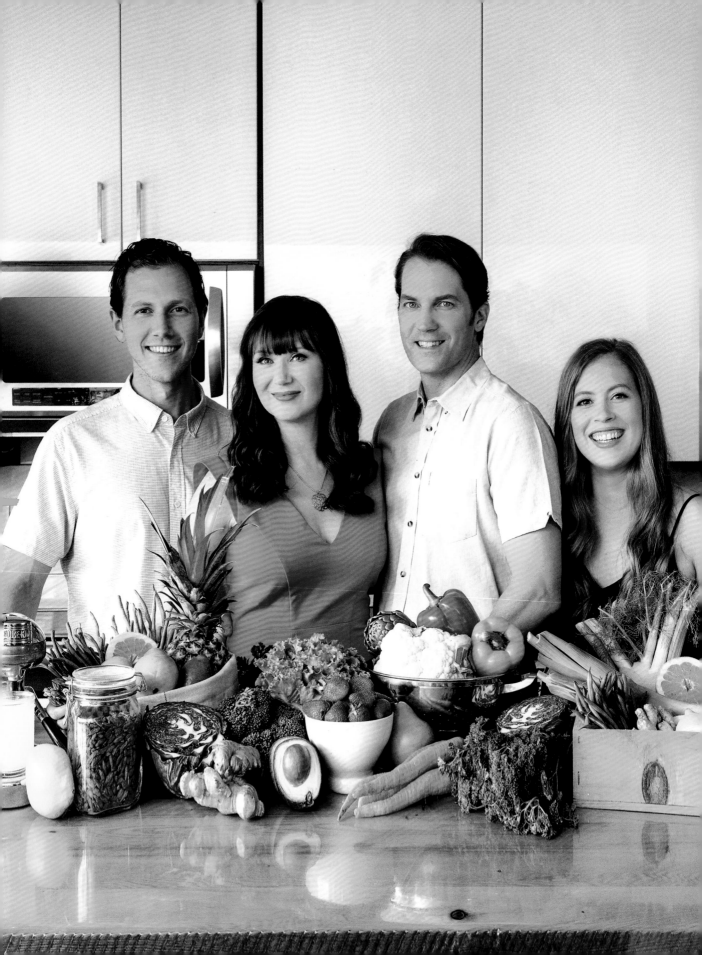

Acknowledgements

My gratitude overflows toward the team that worked tirelessly to ensure that this book is useful, beautiful and well researched:

Andrea Magyar, publishing director and my editor at Penguin Canada. Her unflappable calm was such an oasis in the creation of this book. She has great taste and a wealth of experience that made me feel that the project was in wonderful hands.

My naturopathic adviser, Dr. Lynne Racette, ND, helped to clarify and fact-check information and contributed to content on sweeteners, keto and fasting. She also did a great job of making sense of the hundreds of references we collected to ensure we could back up the book with solid science.

Illustrators Katie Stewart and Taevan Gangnier created the lovely infographics for the book. Their visual talents were such a fresh and insightful contribution.

Katie Mitton captured some of my thoughts via dictation, which allowed me to teach and share more organically. Her joyful work ethic made sure we could hit our deadline.

My husband, Alan Smith, became the lead photographer on this book, and I am so proud of his determination and talents. Thanks to Bethany Bierema and Nat Caron for additional photos and to Joanna Wojewoda and Mike Rees for teaching us new skills in food photography. I'm very grateful to makeup artist Voula Zisis for her ability to beautify our crew. Big kudos go out to my dear friend Tanya Scata, who was the lead food stylist along with Laura Ricci, Stuart Vaughan, Bethany Bierema and Carol Dudar.

Fellow nutritionist Daniella Rambaldini contributed important research and writing clarity for the sweeteners chapter. Katie Stewart, Sarah Dobec, Maureen Kirkpatrick and Cathy Hayashi, and the Standards Department of the Big Carrot Natural Food Market made contributions to the sweeteners chart. Thank you to fellow nutritionists Katie Stewart and Jessica Tucker, who each contributed a tasty recipe.

Lead recipe tester Laura Ricci added a wonderful calm energy to the recipe creation process, and she tested each recipe with precision and passion. Lynn Daniluk and Elaine Daniluk helped test some of our family favourites until they were perfect and made some fabulous contributions. Our Thrive Community members did a third test to see how these sugar-free recipes work in home kitchens. Thank you to Kandis Thompson, Jade Milot, Kim McNeill, Kim Naar, Morgan Bartolini, Stephanie Hutchinson, Stephanie Walker, Sue Keuhl, Susan Trautmanis and Sylvia Marusyk.

My literary agent and friend Rick Broadhead went to bat for this fourth book, and I don't know if it ever would have come to fruition without his determination.

References

For a full list of references, please visit www.JulieDaniluk.com

Introduction

Goyal, S.K. et al, 2010. Stevia (*Stevia rebaudiana*)... *Int J Food Sci Nutr.*

Johnson, R.K. et al, 2009. Dietary sugars intake... *Circulation.*

Ng, S.W. et al, 2012. Use of caloric and noncaloric sweeteners... *J Acad Nutr Diet.*

Phillips, K.M. et al, 2009. Total antioxidant content... *J Am Diet Assoc.*

Sigman-Grant, M. et al, 2003. Defining and interpreting... *Am J Clin Nutr.*

U.S. Food and Drug Administration, 2004. *How to Understand and Use the Nutrition Facts Label.*

U.S. Food and Drug Administration, 2012. Agency information collection... *Fed Regist.*

Part 1: Chapter 1

Anderson R.A. et al, 1990. Urinary chromium excretion... *Am J Clin Nutr.*

Avena N.M. et al, 2008. After daily bingeing … *Physiol Behav.*

Chazelas E. et al, 2019. Sugary drink consumption... *BMJ.*

Christakos S. et al, 2011. Vitamin D and intestinal... *Mol Cell Endocrinol.*

Danby F.W., 2010. Nutrition and aging... *Clin Dermatol.*

De la Monte S. et al, 2008. Alzheimer's disease is... *J Diabetes Sci Technol.*

D'Erasmo E. et al, 1999. Calcium homeostasis during... *Horm Metab Res.*

Djurhuus M.S. et al, 1995. Insulin increases renal... *Diabet Med.*

Douard V. et al, 2012. Dietary fructose inhibits... *FASEB J.*

Douard V. et al, 2013. Excessive fructose intake... *Am J Physiol Endocrinol Metab.*

Douard V. et al, 2014. Chronic high fructose... *PLoS One.*

Goren J.L., 2016. Brain-derived neurotrophic... *Ment Health Clin.*

Kim B. et al, 2012. Insulin resistance in... *Trends Endocrinol Metab.*

Knuppel A. et al, 2017. Sugar intake from... *Sci Rep.*

Kozlovsky A.S. et al, 1986. Effects of diets... *Metabolism.*

Langlois K. et al, 2010. Sugar consumption among... *Health Rep.*

Lemann J. et al, 1970. Evidence that glucose... *J. Clin Invest.*

Lennon E.J. et al, 1970. A comparison of... *J Clin Invest.*

Lennon E.J. et al, 1974. The effect of... *J Clin Invest.*

Molteni R. et al, 2002. A high-fat... *Neuroscience.*

Noble E. et al, 2017. Gut to brain dysbiosis... *Front Behav Neurosci.*

Paolisso G. et al, 1990. Magnesium and glucose... *Diabetologia.*

Pereira M. et al, 2018. Effect of dietary additives... *Dis Model Mech.*

Potter M. et al, 2016. The Warburg effect... *Biochem Soc Trans.*

Roth C.L. et al, 2012. Vitamin D deficiency... *Hepatology.*

Sanchez A. et al, 1973. Role of sugars... *Am J Clin Nutr.*

Swaminathan R., 2003. Magnesium metabolism and... *Clin Biochem Rev.*

Wilson J.X., 2005. Regulation of vitamin C... *Annu Rev Nutr.*

Wise P. et al, 2016. Reduced dietary intake... *Am J Clin Nutr.*

Chapter 2

Allison M. et al, 2014. 20 years of leptin... *J Endocrinol.*

Amin F. et al, 2013. Fiver-free white flour... *Lipids Health Dis.*

Avena N. et al, 2008. After daily bingeing... *Physiol Behav.*

Avena N. et al, 2008. Evidence for sugar addiction... *Neurosci Biobehav Rev.*

Bantle J.P., 2009. Dietary fructose and... *J Nutr.*

Bawa A. et al, 2013. Genetically modified foods... *J Food Sci Technol.*

Bonnardel-Phu E. et al, 2000. Advanced glycation end... *J Mal Vascul.*

Bron A. et al, 1998. The lens and... *Int Opthamol Clin.*

Considine R.V. et al, 1996. Serum immunoreactive-leptin... *N Engl J Med.*

Daghestani M., 2009. A preprandial and... *J King Saud Univ.*

Davis W., 2019. *Wheat Belly: Lose the Wheat...* Rosedale.

De Cabo R. et al, 2019. Effects of intermittent... *New Engl J Med.*

De Faria Maraschin J. et al, 2010. Diabetes mellitus classification... *Arq Bras Cardiol.*

Dos Santos Oliveria P. et al, 2019. Serum uric acid...*Bipolar Disorder.*

Faeh D. et al, 2005. Effect of fructose... *Diabetes.*

Fisher J.S. et al, 2002. Activation of AMP kinase... *Am J Physiol Endocrinol Metab.*

Fournet M. et al, 2018. Glycation damage...*Aging Dis.*

Galvan A. et al, 1995. Effect of insulin... *American Journal of Physiology Endocrinology and Metabolism.*

Gannon M.C. et al, 2011. Effect of a high-protein... *Metabolism.*

Gearhardt A. et al, 2011. Neural correlates of food addiction... *Arch Gen Psychiatry.*

Gholnari T. et al, 2018. The effects of coenzyme Q10... *J Am Coll Nutr.*

Goldin A. et al, 2006. Advanced glycation end... *Circulation.*

Gul A. et al, 2009. The role of fructose... *Graefes Arch Clinc Exp Opthalmol.*

Hellsten Y. et al, 2004. Effect of ribose... *Am J Physiol.*

Ho Do M. et al, 2018. High-glucose or -fructose diet... *Nutrients.*

Huerta A.E. et al, 2015. Effects of alpha-lipoic... *Obesity.*

Katta A. et al, 2009. Glycation of lens... *Biomed Res.*

Kim S. et al, 2012. Gestational diabetes and... *Curr Opin Obstet Gynecol.*

Klok M.D. et al, 2007. The role of leptin... *Obes Rev.*

Lenoir M. et al, 2007. Intense sweetness surpasses... *PLoS ONE.*

Leung C. et al, 2014. Soda and cell aging...*Am J Public Health.*

Logan K. et al, 2016. Development of early... *Diabetes Care.*

Ma X. et al, 2013. Ghrelin receptor regulates... *Nut Diabetes.*

Madani Z. et al, 2015. Sardine protein diet... *Mol Med Rep.*

Mahoney D. et al, 2018. Understanding D-ribose and... *Adv Biosci Clin Med.*

Mesarwi O. et al, 2013. Sleep disorders and... *Endocrin Metab Clin.*

Mofidi A. et al, 2012. The acute impact...*J Nutr Metab.*

Molfino A. et al, 2010. Caloric restriction and... *J Prenter Enteral Nutr.*

Monique P. et al, 2017. The healthfulness and... *Health Promot Chronic Dis Prev Can.*

Navale A. et al, 2016. Glucose transporters: physiological... *Biophys Rev.*

Ortiz R. et al, 2015. Purinergic system dysfunction... *Prog Neuropsychopharmacol Biol Psychiatry.*

Ortiz-Sanchez J. et al, 2013. Maize prolamins could... *Nutrients.*

Quiclet C. et al, 2019. Pancreatic adipocytes mediate... *Metab Clin Exp.*

Raygan F. et al, 2016. The effects of coenzyme Q10... *Eur J Nutr.*

Rippe J. et al, 2016. Relationship between added... *Nutrients.*

Sambeat A. et al, 2019. Endogenous nicotinamide riboside... *Nat Commun.*

Schoenthaler S.J. et al, 1997. The effect of randomized...*J Nutr Environ Med.*

Shoelson S. et al, 2006. Inflammation and insulin resistance. *J Clin Invest.*

Stanhope K.L. et al, 2013. Adverse metabolic effects... *Curr Opin Lipidol.*

Stubbs B.J. et al, 2018. A ketone ester... *Obesity.*

Szymczak I. et al, 2019. Analysis of association... *Nutrients.*

Tamez-Perez H. et al, 2015. Steroid hyperglycemia: prevalence... *World J Diabetes.*

Teitelbaum J.E. et al, 2006. The use of D-ribose... *J Altern Complement Med.*

Toyoli D. et al, 2017. Insulin stimulates uric acid... *American Journal of Physiology Renal Physiology*

Trammell S. et al, 2016. Nicotinamide riboside is... *Nat Commun.*

U.S. National Library of Medicine, 2020. *Lactose Intolerance.*

Wiss D. et al, 2018. Sugar addiction... *Front Psychiatry.*

Chapter 3

Raw Honey (*Apis mellifera* products)

Bilsel Y. et al, 2002. Could honey have... *Dig Surg.*

Bogdanov S. et al, 2008. Honey for nutrition... *J Am Coll Nutr.*

Cooper R., 2007. Honey in wound care... *GMS Krankenhhyg Interdiszip.*

Ezz El-Arab A.M. et al, 2006. Effect of dietary... *BMC Complem Altern M.*

Hamdy A.A. et al, 2009. Determination of flavonoid... *J Egypt Public Health Assoc.*

Molan P.C. et al, 2004. Clinical usage of... *J Wound Care.*

Münstedt K. et al, 2009. Effect of honey... *J Med Food.*

Pipicelli G. et al, 2009. Therapeutic properties of honey. *Health.*

Ruiz-Matute A.I. et al, 2010. Carbohydrate composition of... *J Agric Food Chem.*

Ruiz-Matute A.I. et al, 2010. Detection of adulterations... *J Food Compost Anal.*

Yaghoobi N. et al, 2008. Natural honey and... *Sci World J.*

Licorice (*Glycyrrhiza* spp.)

Al-Dujaili E.A.S. et al, 2011. Liquorice and glycyrrhetinic... *Mol Cell Endocrinol.*

Amabile C.M. et al, 2010. Keeping your patient... *Arch Intern Med.*

Choi H.J. et al, 2008. Hexane/ethanol extract... *Exp Biol Med.*

D'Angelo S. et al, 2009. Protective effect of... *J Med Food.*

Eu C.H.A. et al, 2010. Glycyrrhizic acid improved... *Lipids Health Dis.*

Fuhrman B. et al, 2004. Antiatherosclerotic effects of... *Nutrition.*

He J. et al, 2006. Antibacterial compounds from... *J Nat Prod.*

Hu C. et al, 2009. Estrogenic activities of... *J Steroid Biochem.*

Isobrucker R.A. et al, 2006. Risk and safety... *Regul Toxicol Pharmacol.*

Kim K.R. et al, 2010. Anti-inflammatory effects... *J Biomed Biotechnol.*

Ko B-S. et al, 2007. Changes in components... *Biosci Biotech Bioch.*

Oulomi M.M. et al, 2007. Healing potential of... *J Vet Res.*

Sato S. et al, 2004. The effects of... *Yakugaku Zasshi.*

Scientific Committee on Food, 2003. Opinion of the Scientific... European Commission Health and Consumer Protection Directorate-General.

Sena S.F., 2001. Licorice and laboratory tests. *Herbal Supplements: Efficacy, Toxicity, and...* John Wiley & Sons.

Størmer F.C. et al, 1993. Glycyrrhizic acid in... *Food Chem Toxicol.*

Tiger Nut (*Cyperus esculentus*)

Adejuyitan J.A., 2011. Tigernut processing... *Am J Food Technol.*

Arafat S.M. et al, 2009. Chufa tubers (*Cyperus...* *World Appl Sci J.*

Chukwuma E.R. et al, 2010. The phytochemical composition... *Pak J Nutr.*

Coskuner Y. et al, 2002. Physical and chemical properties... *J Sci Food Agric.*

Glew R.H. et al, 2006. Amino acid, mineral... *Plant Food Hum Nutr.*

Yang X. et al, 2006. Insulin-sensitizing and... *J Inorg Biochem.*

Yacón (*Smallanthus sonchifolius*)

Lachman J. et al, 2003. Yacon [*Smallanthus sonchifolia...* *Plant Soil Environ.*

Lobo A.R. et al, 2007. Effects of fructans-containing... *Br J Nutr.*

Mentreddy S.R., 2007. Medicinal plant species... *J Sci Food Agric.*

Valentová K. et al, 2003. *Smallanthus sonchifolius* and... *Biomed Pap Med Fac Univ Palacky Olomouc Czech Repub.*

Syrup from Maple (*Acer* spp.) and Other Trees

Ball D.W., 2007. The chemical composition... *J Chem Educ.*

Bassaganya-Riera J. et al, 2011. Treatment of obesity-related... *J Obes.*

Bruzzone S. et al, 2008. Abscisic acid is... *J Biol Chem.*

Davison R.M. et al, 1973. Abscisic-acid content of... *Planta.*

Guri A.J. et al, 2007. Dietary abscisic acid... *Clin Nutr.*

Li L. et al, 2011. Further investigation into... *J Agric Food Chem.*

Phillips K.M. et al, 2009. Total antioxidant content... *J Am Diet Assoc.*

U.S. Department of Agriculture, Agricultural Research Service, 2009. *USDA National Nutrient Database for Standard Reference.*

Coconut (*Cocos nucifera*) Sugar and Saps from Other Palm (*Arecaceae* spp.)

Ranasinghe C.S. et al, 2007. Photosynthetic assimilation, carbohydrates... *Cocos.*

Ranilla L.G. et al, 2008. Antidiabetes and antihypertension... *J Med Food.*

Brown Rice (*Oryza sativa*) Malt and Syrup

Banchuen J. et al, 2009. Effect of germinating... *Thai J Agric Sci.*

Liang J. et al, 2008. Effects of soaking... *Food Chem.*

Unrefined Sugarcane (*Saccharum* spp.)

Karthikeyan J. et al, 2010. Sugarcane in therapeutics. *J Herb Med Toxicol.*

Phillips K.M. et al, 2009. Total antioxidant content... *J Am Diet Assoc.*

Rice R.W. et al, 2010. Nutritional requirements for... Document SS-AGR-228. Agronomy Department, Florida Cooperative Extension Service, Institute of Food and Agricultural Sciences, University of Florida.

Savant N.K. et al, 1999. Silicon nutrition and... *J Plant Nutr.*

Singh N. et al, 2010. Adverse health effects... *Toxicol Appl Pharmacol.*

Molasses (*Saccharum* spp.)

Craig S.A.S., 2006. Betaine in human nutrition. *Am J Clin Nutr.*

Groetch M., 2008. Diets and nutrition. *Food Allergy: Adverse Reactions to Foods and Food Additives.* John Wiley & Sons.

Phillips K.M. et al, 2009. Total antioxidant content... *J Am Diet Assoc.*

U.S. Department of Agriculture, Agricultural Research Service, 2009. *USDA National Nutrient Database for Standard Reference.*

Wang B.-S. et al, 2011. Inhibitory effects of... *Food Chem.*

Date (*Phoenix dactylifera*) Sugar

Ahmed M.B. et al, 2008. Protective effects of... *Iran J Pharm Res.*

Ahmed S.H. et al, 2009. Antioxidant properties of... *Mod Appl Sci.*

Al-Qarawai et al, 2005. The ameliorative effect... *J Ethnopharmacol.*

Bnouham M. et al, 2002. Medicinal plants used... *Int J Diabetes Metab.*

Lin Y.-P. et al, 2009. Neural cell protective... *Phytochemistry.*

Majid A.S. et al, 2008. Neuroprotective effects... *Pak J Med Sci.*

Puri A. et al, 2000. Immunostimulant activity of... *J Ethnopharmacol.*

Ranilla L.G. et al, 2008. Antidiabetes and antihypertension... *J Med Food.*

Rock W. et al, 2009. Effects of date... *J Agric Food Chem.*

Tahraoui A. et al, 2007. Ethnopharmacological survey of... *J Ethnopharmacol.*

Vyawahare N. et al, 2009. Neurobehavioral effects of... *J Young Pharm.*

Monk Fruit aka Lo Han Quo (*Siraitia grosvenorii*)

Akihia T. et al, 2007. Cucurbitane glycosides from... *J Nat Prod.*

Chen W.J. et al, 2007. The antioxidant activities... *Int J Food Sci Nutr.*

Chen X.-B. et al, 2011. Potential AMPK activators... *Bioorg Med Chem.*

Hossen M.A. et al, 2005. Effect of lo han kuo... *Biol Pharm Bull.*

Kinghorn A.D. et al, 2002. Discovery of terpenoid... *Pure Appl Chem.*

Konoshima T. et al, 2002. Cancer-chemoprotective effects... *Pure Appl Chem.*

Lindley M., 2006. Other sweeteners. *Sweeteners and Sugar Alternatives in Food Technology.* Wiley-Blackwell

Lu F. et al, 2019. Phytochemicals from *Siraitia... EC Pharmacol Toxicol.*

Qi X.-Y. et al, 2008. Mogrosides extract from... *Nutr Res.*

Suzuki Y.A. et al, 2005. Triterpene glycosides of... *J Agric Food Chem.*

Suzuki Y.A. et al, 2007. Antidiabetic effect of... *Br J Nutr.*

Takasaki M. et al, 2003. Anticarcinogenic activity of... *Cancer Lett.*

Takeo E. et al, 2002. Sweet elements of... *J Atheroscler Thromb.*

Xiangyang Q. et al, 2006. Effect of a *Siraitia... Mol Nutr Food Res.*

Ying Z. et al, 2009. Insulin secretion stimulating... *Yao Xue Xue Bao.*

Lúcuma (*Pouteria lucuma*)

Da Silva Pinto M. et al, 2009. Evaluation of antihyperglycemia... *J Med Foods.*

Izquierdo J. et al, 1998. Under-utilized Andean... *Acta Hortic.*

Silva C.A.M. et al, 2008. Genus *Pouteria*: Chemistry... *Rev Bras Farmacogn.*

von der Linden U.M., 2005. "Functional fruits"—neglected potential? *Fruit Processing.*

Stevia (*Stevia rebaudiana*)

Abudula R. et al, 2004. Rebaudioside A potently stimulates... *Metab Clin Exp.*

Abudula R. et al, 2008. Rebaudioside A directly... *Diabetes Obes Metab.*

Badawi A.M. et al, 2005. Stevioside as a low... *Egypt J Hosp Med.*

Boonkaewwan C. et al, 2006. Anti-inflammatory and immunomodulatory... *J Agric Food Chem.*

Boonkaewwan C. et al, 2008. Specific immunomodulatory and secretory... *J Agric Food Chem.*

Brandle J.E. et al, 1998. *Stevia rebaudiana*: Its... *Can J Plant Sci.*

Carlsen M.H. et al, 2010. The total antioxidant... *Nutr J.*

Chang J.-C. et al, 2005. Increase of insulin... *Horm Metab Res.*

DuBois G.E. et al, 1984. Diterpenoid sweeteners... *J Med Chem.*

European Food Safety Authority (EFSA), 2010. Scientific opinion on the safety... *EFSA J.*

Ferreira E.B. et al, 2006. Comparative effects of... *Planta Med.*

Gardana C. et al, 2003. Metabolism of stevioside... *J Agric Food Chem.*

Geeraert, B. et al, 2010. Stevioside inhibits atherosclerosis... *Int J Obes (Lond).*

Goyal S.K. et al, 2010. Stevia (*Stevia rebaudiana*)... *Int J Food Sci Nutr.*

Gregersen S. et al, 2004. Antihyperglycemic effects of... *Metabolism.*

Huxtable R.J., 2002. Pharmacology and toxicology of... *Stevia: The Genus* Stevia. Taylor & Francis.

Jeppesen P.B. et al, 2000. Stevioside acts directly on... *Metabolism.*

Jeppesen P.B. et al, 2002. Stevioside induces antihyperglycaemic... *Phytomedicine.*

Jeppesen P.B. et al, 2003. Antihyperglycemic and blood... *Metabolism.*

Konoshima T. et al, 2002. Cancer-chemopreventive effects... *Pure Appl Chem.*

Kujur R.S. et al, 2010. Antidiabetic activity and... *Pharmacogn Res.*

Lindley M., 2006. Other sweeteners. *Sweeteners and Sugar Alternatives in Food Technology.* Wiley-Blackwell.

Michalik A. et al, 2010. Steviamine, a new indolizine... *Phytochem Lett.*

Mizushima Y. et al, 2005. Structural analysis of... *Life Sci.*

Prakash I.G.E. et al, 2008. Development of rebiana... *Food Chem Toxicol.*

Sehar I. et al, 2008. Immune up regulatory... *Chem Biol Interact.*

Takasaki M. et al, 2009. Cancer preventative agents... *Bioorg Med Chem.*

Carob (*Ceratonia siliqua*)

Ahmed M.M., 2010. Biochemical studies on... *Nature and Science.*

Al-Aboudi A. et al, 2011. Plants used for... *Pharm Biol.*

Awad A.B. et al, 2000. Phytosterols as anticancer... *J Nutr.*

Bates S.H. et al, 2000. Insulin-like effect of pinitol. *Br J Pharmacol.*

Dakia P.A. et al, 2007. Isolation and chemical... *Food Chem.*

Dang N.T. et al, 2010. D-Pinitol and *myo*-inositol... *Biosci Biotech Bioch.*

Gruendel S. et al, 2007. Increased acylated plasma... *Br J Nutr.*

Guimaraes C.M. et al, 2007. Antioxidant activity of... *J Food Sci.*

Klenow S. et al, 2009. Does an extract... *J Agric Food Chem.*

Milek dos Santos L. et al, 2015. Respuesta glucémica de Algarrobo... *Nutr Hosp.*

Rakib E.M. et al, 2010. Determination of phenolic... *J Nat Prod.*

Ramberg J.E. et al, 2010. Immunomodulatory dietary polysaccharides... *Nutr J.*

Saganuwan A.S., 2010. Some medicinal plants... *J Med Plant Res.*

Silanikove N. et al, 2006. Analytical approach and... *Livest Sci.*

Son D. et al, 2010. Glycemic index of... *J Ginseng Res.*

Ulbricht C., 2010. Gastrointestinal disorders... *Alternative and Complementary Therapies.*

U.S. Department of Agriculture, Agricultural Research Service, 2009. *USDA National Nutrient Database for Standard Reference.*

Wang B.-S. et al, 2011. Inhibitory effects of... *Food Chem.*

Mesquite (*Prosopis* spp.)

Bosha J.A. et al, 2004. Pharmacological effects of... *Nig Vet J.*

Brand J.C. et al, 1990. Plasma glucose and... *Am J Clin Nutr.*

Brionis-Labarca V. et al, 2011. Effect of high hydrostatic... *Food Res Int.*

Cardozo M.L. et al, 2010. Evaluation of antioxidant... *Food Res Int.*

Choge S.K. et al, 2007. *Prospois* pods as... *Water SA Special Edition.*

Da Silva Pinto et al, 2009. Evaluation of antihyperglycemia... *J Med Food.*

Felker P., 2005. Mesquite flour. New... *Gastronomica.*

Lamarque A.L. et al, 1994. Proximate composition and... *J Sci Food Agric.*

Odibo F.J.C. et al, 2008. Biochemical changes during... *J Ind Microbiol Biot.*

Pasiecznik N.M. et al, 2001. *The* Prosopis juliflora– Prosopis pallida *Complex: A Monograph.* HDRA.

Singh S. et al, 2011. Antibacterial properties of... *Int J Pharm Sci Res.*

U.S. Department of Agriculture, Agricultural Research Service, 2009. *USDA National Nutrient Database for Standard Reference.*

Vilela A. et al, 2009. Past, present and... *J Arid Environ.*

Oubli (*Pentadiplandra brazzeana*)

Faus I., 2000. Recent developments in... *Appl Microbiol Biotechnol.*

Hellekant G. et al, 2005. Brazzein a small... *Chem Senses.*

Mabeku L.B.K. et al, 2011. Screening of some... *Int J Biol.*

Ming D. et al, 1994. Brazzein, a new high-potency... *FEBS Lett.*

Nantia E.A. et al, 2009. Medicinal plants as... *Andrologie.*

Noumi E. et al, 2000. Medicinal plants used... *Fitoterapia.*

Pfeiffer J.F. et al, 2000. Modeling the sweetness... *Food Qual Prefer.*

Telefo P.B. et al, 2011. Ethnopharmacological survey of... *J Ethnopharmacol.*

Sugar Alcohols

Kearsley M.W. et al, 2008. Maltitol and maltitol syrups. *Sweeteners and Sugar Alternatives in Food Technology.* John Wiley & Sons.

Kearsley M.W. et al, 2008. Sorbitol and mannitol. *Sweeteners and Sugar Alternatives in Food Technology.* John Wiley & Sons.

Erythritol

Arrigoni E. et al, 2005. Human gut microbiota... *Br J Nutr.*

Bernt W.O. et al, 1996. Erythritol: a review... *Regul Toxicol Pharm.*

Bornet F.R.J. et al, 1996. Gastrointestinal response and... *Regul Toxicol Pharm.*

den Hartog G.J.M. et al, 2010. Erythritol is a sweet antioxidant. *Nutrition.*

European Commission, 2003. Opinion of the scientific committee... EU Health and Consumer Protection Directorate-General, Scientific Committee on Food.

European Food Safety Association (EFSA) Panel on Food Additives and Nutrient Sources (ANS), 2010. Statement in relation to the safety of erythritol... *EFSA J.*

Hiele M. et al, 1993. Metabolism of erythritol... *Br J Nutr.*

Horning E.C. et al, 1974. Gas phase analytical... *J Chromatogr.*

Ichikawa T. et al, 2008. The enhancement effect... *J Dent.*

Livesy G., 2003. Health potential of... *Nutr Res Rev.*

Mäkinen K.K., 2010. Sugar alcohols, carries... *Int J Dent.*

Moon H.-J. et al, 2010. Biotechnological production of... *Appl Microbiol Biotechnol.*

Munro I.C. et al, 1998. Erythritol: an interpretive... *Food Chem Toxicol.*

Oku T. et al, 1990. Influence of chronic... *Nutr Res.*

Oku T. et al, 1996. Laxative threshold of... *Nutr Res.*

Spencer N., 1967. Ion exchange chromatography... *J Chromatogr.*

Storey D. et al, 2006. Gastrointestinal tolerance of... *Eur J Clin Nutr.*

Yokozawa T. et al, 2002. Erythritol attenuates the... *J Agric Food Chem.*

Mannitol

Hayes M.L. et al, 1978. The breakdown of... *Arch Oral Biol.*

Kearsley M.W. et al, 2008. Maltitol and maltitol syrups. *Sweeteners and Sugar Alternatives in Food Technology.* John Wiley & Sons.

Kearsley M.W. et al, 2008. Sorbitol and mannitol. *Sweeteners and Sugar Alternatives in Food Technology.* John Wiley & Sons.

Livesey G., 2008. Glycaemic responses and toleration. *Sweeteners and Sugar Alternatives in Food Technology.* John Wiley & Sons.

Stowell J., 2008. Calorie control and weight management. *Sweeteners and Sugar Alternatives in Food Technology.* John Wiley & Sons.

Wisselink H.W. et al, 2002. Mannitol production by... *Int Dairy J.*

Sorbitol

Bhanuprakash Reddy G. et al, 2008. Erythrocyte aldose reductase... *Mol Vis.*

Fernández-Bañares F. et al, 2009. Fructose-sorbitol malabsorption. *Curr Gastroenterol Rep.*

Hagopian K. et al, 2009. Caloric restriction counteracts... *Biogerontology.*

Hayes M.L. et al, 1978. The breakdown of... *Arch Oral Biol.*

Hogg S.D. et al, 1991. Can the oral... *J Dent.*

Kearsley M.W. et al, 2008. Maltitol and maltitol syrups. *Sweeteners and Sugar Alternatives in Food Technology.* John Wiley & Sons.

Kearsley M.W. et al, 2008. Sorbitol and mannitol. *Sweeteners and Sugar Alternatives in Food Technology.* John Wiley & Sons.

Livesey G., 2008. Glycaemic responses and toleration. *Sweeteners and Sugar Alternatives in Food Technology.* John Wiley & Sons.

Maguire A., 2008. Dental health. *Sweeteners and Sugar Alternatives in Food Technology.* John Wiley & Sons.

Ouyang X. et al, 2008. Fructose consumption as... *J Hepatol.*

Xylitol

Bais R. et al, 1985. The purification and... *Biochem J.*

Brown C.L. et al, 2004. Xylitol enhances bacterial... *Laryngoscope.*

Burt B.A., 2009. The use of sorbitol-... *J Am Dent Assoc.*

Çaglar E. et al, 2007. Effect of chewing... *Clin Oral Investig.*

Carvalho W. et al, 2007. Semi-continuous xylitol... *Braz J Pharm Sci.*

Dunayer E.K., 2006. New findings on... *Vet Med.*

Ferreira A.S. et al, 2011. Xylitol inhibits J774A.1... *Braz Arch Biol Technol.*

Isokangas P. et al, 2000. Occurrence of dental... *J Dent Res.*

Karhumaa K. et al, 2007. Comparison of the... *Microb Cell Fact.*

Kurola P. et al, 2009. Xylitol and capsular... *J Med Microbiol.*

Ly K.A. et al, 2008. Xylitol gummy bear... *BMC Oral Health.*

Mäkinen K.K., 2000. The rocky road of... *J Dent Res.*

Milgrom P. et al, 2010. Xylitol pediatric topical... *Arch Pediat Adol Med.*

Sezen O.S. et al, 2008. Xylitol containing chewing... *Mediterranean Journal of Otology.*

Twetman S., 2009. The role of xylitol... *Oralprophylaxe und Kinderzahnheilkunde.*

Vernacchio L. et al, 2007. Tolerability of oral... *Int J Pediatr Otorhinolaryngol.*

Weissman J.D. et al, 2011. Xylitol nasal irrigation... *Laryngoscope.*

Artificial Sweeteners

Bian X. et al, 2017. The artificial sweetener... *PLoS ONE.*

Cong W.-N. et al, 2013. Long-term artificial sweetener... *PLoS ONE.*

Fowler S.P. et al, 2008. Fueling the obesity... *Obesity.*

Levine J. et al, 1995. Double-blind, controlled trial... *Am J Psychiatry.*

Mukai T. et al, 2014. A meta-analysis of... *Hum Psychopharmacol.*

Palatnik A. et al, 2001. Double-blind, controlled, crossover... *J Clin Psychopharmacol.*

Santamaria A. et al, 2012. One-year effects of myo-inositol... *Climacteric.*

Spender M. et al, 2016. Artificial sweeteners: A systematic... *J Neurogastroenterol Motil.*

Suez J. et al, 2014. Artificial sweeteners induce... *Nature.*

Zheng Y. et al, 2013. Effect of the artificial... *J Gastrointest Surg.*

Corn

Cabrera-Chavez F. et al, 2008. Transglutaminase treatment of... *J Agric Food Chem.*

Davidson I. et al, 1979. Antibodies to maize... *Clin Exp Immunol.*

Ortiz-Sanchez J. et al, 2013. Maize prolamins could... *Nutrients.*

Allulose

Chung Y.M. et al, 2012. Dietary D-psicose reduced... *J Food Sci.*

Hayashi N. et al, 2010. Study on the postprandial... *Biosci Biotechnol Biochem.*

Hayashi N. et al, 2014. Weight reducing effect... *J Funct Foods.*

Iida T. et al, 2008. Acute D-psicose administration... *J Nutr Sci Vitaminol.*

Matsuo T. et al, 2012. The 90-day oral... *J. Clin Biochem Nutr.*

Ochiai M. et al, 2014. D-psicose increases energy... *Int J Food Sci Nutr.*

Williamson P. et al, 2014. A single-dose, microtracer... *FASEB J.*

Yagi K. et al, 2009. The study on... *J Clin Biochem Nutr.*

Agave Nectar or Syrup (*Agave* spp.)

Bowen S. et al, 2009. Geographical indications, *terroir... J Rural Stud.*

Burwell T., 1995. Bootlegging on a... *Hum Ecol.*

Dalton R., 2005. Saving the agave. *Nature.*

Martínez-Salvador M. et al, 2007. Assessment of sustainability... *Int J Sustainable Dev World Ecol.*

Molina-Freaner F. et al, 2003. The pollination biology of... *Am J Bot.*

Patent Storm, 1998. US Patent 5846333. *Method of producing fructose syrup from agave plants.*

Scott P.E., 2004. Timing of *Agave palmeri*... *Southwest Nat.*

Slauson L.A., 2000. Pollination biology of... *Am J Bot.*

Tapioca Syrup (*Manihot esculenta*)

Ocloo F.C.K. et al, 2006. Physical, chemical and... *Afr J Biotechnol.*

Silva R. et al, 2008. Production of glucose... *Ciência Tecnol Aliment.*

Tonukari N.J., 2004. Cassava and the future... *Electron J Biotechn.*

Aspartame

Abdollahi M. et al, 2003. Mechanism of aspartame-induced... *Indian J Pharmacol.*

Alleva R. et al, 2011. *In vitro* effect of... *Toxicol In Vitro.*

AlSuhaibani E.S., 2010. *In vivo* cytogenetic... *Comp Funct Genomics.*

Belpoggi F. et al, 2006. Results of long-term... *Ann NY Acad Sci.*

Bergstrom B.P. et al, 2007. Aspartame decreases evoked... *Neuropharmacology.*

Burkhart C.G., 2009. "Lone" atrial fibrillation... *Int J Cardiol.*

Eigenmann P.A. et al, 2008. The respiratory tract... *Food Allergy: Adverse Reactions to Foods and Food Additives.* John Wiley & Sons.

Fernstrom J.D. et al, 2007. Tyrosine, phenylalanine... *J Nutr.*

Fountain S.B. et al, 1988. Aspartame exposure and... *Fund Appl Toxicol.*

Halldorsson T.I. et al, 2010. Intake of artificially... *Am J Clin Nutr.*

Holder M.D. et al, 1989. Behavioral assessment... *Pharmacol Biochem Behav.*

Humphries P. et al, 2008. Direct and indirect... *Eur J Clin Nutr.*

Ishii H., 1981. Incidence of brain... *Toxicol Lett.*

Kavet R. et al, 1990. The toxicity of... *Crit Rev Toxicol.*

Magnuson B.A. et al, 2007. Aspartame: a safety... *Crit Rev Toxicol.*

Maher T.J., 1987. Natural food constituents... *J Allergy Clin Immunol.*

O'Brien P.J. et al, 2005. Aldehyde sources, metabolism... *Crit Rev Toxicol.*

Portela G.S. et al, 2007. Effects of aspartame... *Int J Morphol.*

Rajasekar P. et al, 2004. Circadian variations of... *Pharm Biol.*

Ranney R.E. et al, 1979. A review of... *J Environ Pathol Tox.*

Simintzi I. et al, 2007. The effect of aspartame... *Pharmacol Res.*

Simintzi I. et al, 2008. *L*-Cysteine and glutathione... *Food Chem Toxicol.*

Smith J.D. et al, 2001. Relief of fibromyalgia... *Ann Pharmacother.*

Soffritti M. et al, 2005. Aspartame induces lymphomas... *Eur J Oncol.*

Soffritti M. et al, 2007. Life-span exposure to... *Environ Health Perspect.*

Soffritti M. et al, 2009. First experimental demonstration... *Environ Health Perspect.*

Soffritti M. et al, 2010. Aspartame administered in... *Am J Ind Med.*

Sturgeon S.R. et al, 1994. Associations between bladder... *Epidemiology.*

Teng S. et al, 2001. The formaldehyde metabolic... *Chem Biol Interact.*

Trocho C. et al, 1998. Formaldehyde derived from... *Life Sci.*

Vences-Mejía A. et al, 2006. The effect of aspartame... *Hum Exp Toxicol.*

Sucralose (Splenda™)

Abou-Donia M.B. et al, 2008. Splenda alters gut... *J Toxicol Environ Health.*

Binns N.M., 2003. Sucralose—all sweetness... *Nutr Bull.*

Brusick D. et al, 2009. Expert Panel report... *Regul Toxicol Pharmacol.*

Brusick D. et al, 2010. The absence of... *Food Chem Toxicol.*

Chattopadhyay S. et al, 2011. Artificial sweeteners—a review. *J Food Sci Technol.*

Finn J.P. et al, 2000. Neurotoxicity studies on... *Food Chem Toxicol.*

Ford H.E. et al, 2011. Effects of oral... *Eur J Clin Nutr.*

Grice H.C. et al, 2000. Sucralose—an overview... *Food Chem Toxicol*

Grotz V.L. et al, 2003. Lack of effect... *J Am Diet Assoc.*

Jang H. J. et al, 2007. Gut-expressed gustducin... *Proc Natl Acad Sci.*

Ma J. et al, 2010. Effect of the... *Br J Nutr.*

Mace O.J. et al, 2007. Sweet taste receptors... *J Physiol.*

McLean Baird I. et al, 2000. Repeated dose study... *Food Chem Toxicol.*

Memon M.Q. et al, 2011. Haemodynamic effects of... *J Liaquat Univ Med Health Sci.*

Molinary S.V. et al, 2008. Sucralose. *Sweeteners and Sugar Alternatives in Food Technology.* John Wiley & Sons.

Renwick A.G. et al, 2010. Sweet-taste receptors, low-energy... *Br J Nutr.*

Sasaki Y.F. et al, 2002. The comet assay... *Mutat Res Genet Toxicol Environ Mutagen.*

Scientific Committee on Food (SCF), 2000. Opinion of the... European Commission Health and Consumer Protection Directorate-General.

Sham C.W., 2005. Splenda—a safe... *Nutrition Bytes.*

Sims J. et al, 2000. The metabolic fate... *Food Chem Toxicol.*

Tandel K.R., 2011. Sugar substitutes: health... *J Pharmacol Pharmacother.*

Weber R.W., 2008. Neurological reactions to... *Food Allergy. Adverse Reactions to Foods and Food Additives.* John Wiley & Sons.

Worthley D.L. et al, 2009. A human, double-blind... *Am J Clin Nutr.*

Artichokes

Bundy R. et al, 2008. Artichoke leaf extract... *Phytomedicine.*

Loi B. et al, 2013. Reducing effect of... *Phytother Res.*

Lupattelli G. et al, 2004. Artichoke juice improves... *Life Sci.*

Nadova S. et al, 2008. Growth inhibitory effect... *Phytother Res.*

Salem M.B. et al, 2015. Pharmacological studies of... *Plant Food Hum Nutr.*

Trojan-Rodrigues M. et al, 2012. Plants used as... *J Ethnopharmacol.*

Chapter 4

How It Feels to React to Sugar

Aan het Rot M. et al, 2008. Bright light exposure... *Eur Neuropsychopharmacol.*

Abramson E, *Emotional Eating.*

Ahmed S.H. et al, 2013. Sugar addiction: pushing... *Curr Opin Clin Nutr Metab Care.*

Amodeo G. et al, 2017. Depression and inflammation... *Neuropsychiatry.*

Avena N. et al, 2008. After daily bingeing... *Physiol. Behav.*

Barral J.P. et al, 2009. Chapter 22: Vagus nerve. *Manual Therapy for the Cranial Nerves.* Elsevier.

Berg J.M. et al, 2002. *Biochemistry.* 5th Edition. W.H. Freeman.

Breit S. et al, 2018. Vagus nerve as... *Front Psychiatry.*

Brickman C., 1971. Hedonic relativism and... *Adaptation Level Theory: A Symposium.* Academic Press.

Cappelletti S. et al, 2015. Caffeine: cognitive and... *Curr Neuropharmacol.*

Chen C. et al, 2017. Association between omega-3... *J Diabetes Investig.*

Chepulis L.M. et al, 2009. The effects of long-term... *Physiol Behav.*

Corsica J. et al, 2008. Carbohydrate craving... *Eating Behaviors.*

Dinan T.G. et al, 2013. Psychobiotics: a novel class... *Biol Psychiatry.*

Easterbrook G., 2003. *The Progress Paradox.* Random House.

Evans et al, 2017. Acute ingestion of... *Int J Sport Nut Ex Met.*

Farzi A. et al, 2018. Gut microbiota and the... *Neurotherapeutics.*

Gangwisch J. et al, 2015. High glycemic index... *Am J Clin Nutr.*

Gareau M. et al, 2007. Probiotic treatment of... *Gut.*

Hajnal A. et al, 2002. Repeated access to... *Neuroreport.*

Hoon J. et al, 2015. Association between the... *Psychiat Genet.*

Jenkins T. et al, 2016. Influence of tryptophan... *Nutrients.*

Johnson R. et al, 2018. A review of vagus... *J Inflamm Res.*

Kjaer T.W. et al, 2002. Increased dopamine tone... *Brain Res Cogn Brain Res.*

Knuppel A. et al, 2017. Sugar intake from... *Sci Rep.*

Koekkoek L. et al, 2017. Glucose-sensing in the... *Front Neurosci.*

Laukkanen T. et al, 2015. Association between sauna... *JAMA Intern Med.*

Lenoir M. et al, 2007. Intense sweetness surpasses... *PLoS One.*

Lew L.C. et al, 2019. Probiotic *Lactobacillus plantarum*... *Clin Nutr.*

Liao Y. et al, 2019. Efficacy of omega-3... *Transl Psychiatry.*

Mooventhan A. et al, 2014. Scientific evidence-based effects... *N Am J Med Sci.*

Pase M. et al, 2017. Sugary beverage intake... *Alzheimers Dement.*

Patrick R. et al, 2014. Vitamin D hormone regulates... *FASEB J.*

Pepino M. et al, 2005. Sucrose-induced analgesia... *Pain.*

Rada P. et al, 2005. Daily bingeing on... *Neuroscience.*

Sabir M. et al, 2018. Optimal vitamin D spurs... *Genes Nutr.*

Salmon P., 2001. Effects of physical exercise... *Clin Psychol Rev.*

Sanchez M. et al, 2017. Probiotic *Bifidobacterium longum*... *Gastroenterology.*

Spangler R. et al, 2004. Opiate-like effects of... *Brain Res Mol Crain Res.*

St-Onge M.P. et al, 2016. Effects of diet on... *Adv Nutr.*

St-Onge M.P. et al, 2016. Fiber and saturated fat... *J Clin Sleep Med.*

Volkow N. et al, 2012. Evidence that sleep... *J Neurosci.*

Wallace C. et al, 2017. The effects of... *Ann Gen Psychiatry.*

Wansink B. et al, 2007. Mindless eating: the... *Environ Behav.*

Weinstein A., 2010. Computer and video... *Am J Drug Alcohol Abuse.*

Part 2

The Sugar Free Plan

Akbari M. et al, 2018. The effects of... *Metabolism.*

Anon, 2001. Vaccinium myrtillus (Bilberry)... *Altern Med Rev.*

Anton S. et al, 2008. Effects of chromium... *Diabetes Technol Ther.*

Arguin H. et al, 2012. Short- and long-term effects... *Menopause.*

Balk E. et al, 2007. Effect of chromium... *Diabetes Care.*

Bergamini E., 2006. Autophagy: a cell... *Mol Asp Med.*

Bhattacharyaa, 2003. Adaptogenic activity of... *Pharmacology, Biochemistry and Behavior.*

Chang W. et al, 2015. Berberine as a... *Biochem Cell Biol.*

Dannecker E.A. et al, 2012. The effect of fasting... *Exp Gerontol.*

DiMeglio D.P. et al, 2000. Liquid versus solid... *Int J Obes Relat Metab Disord.*

Efird J. et al, 2014. Potential for improved... *Int J Environ Res Public Health.*

Faris M.A. et al, 2012. Intermittent fasting during... *Nutr Res.*

Fedacko J. et al, 2016. Fenugreek seeds decrease... *World Heart J.*

Harber M.P. et al, 2010. Muscle protein synthesis... *Am J Physiol Regul Integr Comp Physiol.*

Harvie M.N. et al, 2011. The effects of intermittent... *Int J Obes.*

Hoggard N. et al, 2013. A single supplement... *J. Nutr Sci.*

Insil K. et al, 2011. Mitochondrial degradation by... *Am J Physiol Cell Physiol.*

Jamshidi N. et al, 2017. The clinical efficacy... *Evid Based Complement Alternat Med.*

Jayawardena R. et al, 2012. Effects of zinc... *Diabetol Metab Syndr.*

Johnson J.B. et al, 2009. Pretreatment with alternate... *Med Hypotheses.*

Knott E. et al, 2017. Fenugreek supplementation during... *Sci Rep.*

Mattson M.P. et al, 2003. Meal size and... *J Neurochem.*

McDougall G.J. et al, 2008. Current developments on... *Biofactors.*

Pang B. et al, 2015. Application of berberine... *Int J Endocrinol.*

Ranade M. et al, 2017. A simple dietary... *Ayu.*

Vallianou N. et al, 2009. Alpha-lipoic acid and... *Rev Diabet Stud.*

Williams K.V. et al, 1998. The effect of short... *Diabetes Care.*

Yin J. et al, 2008. Efficacy of berberine... *Metabolism.*

General References

Bantle J.P., 2009. Dietary fructose and... *J Nutr.*

Bawa A. et al, 2013. Genetically modified foods... *J Food Sci Technol.*

Faeh D. et al, 2005. Effect of fructose... *Diabetes.*

Hellsten Y. et al, 2004. Effect of ribose... *Am J Physiol Regul Integr Comp Physiol.*

Mahoney D. et al, 2018. Understanding D-ribose and... *Adv Biosci Clin Med.*

Rippe J. et al, 2016. Relationship between added... *Nutrients.*

Stanhope K.L et al, 2013. Adverse metabolic effects... *Curr Opin Lipidol.*

Teitelbaum J.E. et al, 2006. The use of D-ribose... *J Altern Complement Med.*

Supplements That Help You Break Up with Sugar

Fisher J.S. et al, 2002. Activation of AMP... *Am J Physiol Endocrinol Metab.*

Gholnari T. et al, 2018. The effects of coenzyme... *J Am Coll Nutr.*

Molfino A. et al, 2010. Caloric restriction and... *J Prenter Enteral Nutr.*

Raygan F. et al, 2016. The effects of coenzyme... *Eur J Nutr.*

Sambeat A. et al, 2019. Endogenous nicotinamide riboside... *Nat Commun.*

Trammell S. et al, 2016. Nicotinamide riboside is... *Nat Commun.*

Supplements for Reducing Cravings and Balancing Blood Sugar

Akbari M. et al, 2018. The effects of alpha-lipoic... *Metabolism.*

Anton S. et al, 2008. Effects of chromium... *Diabetes Technol Ther.*

Balk E. et al, 2007. Effect of chromium... *Diabetes Care.*

Chang W. et al, 2015. Berberine as a... *Biochem Cell Biol.*

Efird J. et al, 2014. Potential for improved... *Int J Environ Res Public Health.*

Fedacko J. et al, 2016. Fenugreek seeds decrease... *World Heart J.*

Hoggard N. et al, 2013. A single supplement... *J. Nutr Sci.*

Jamshidi N. et al, 2017. The clinical efficacy... *Evid Based Complement Alternat Med.*

Jayawardena R. et al, 2012. Effects of zinc... *Diabetol Metab Syndr.*

Knott E. et al, 2017. Fenugreek supplementation during... *Sci Rep.*

McDougall G.J. et al, 2008. Current developments on... *Biofactors.*

[no authors listed], 2001. *Vaccinium myrtillus* (Bilberry). *Altern Med Rev.*

Pang B. et al, 2015. Application of berberine... *Int J Endocrinol.*

Ranade M. et al, 2017. A simple dietary... *Ayu.*

Vallianou N. et al, 2009. Alpha-lipoic acid... *Rev Diabet Stud.*

Yin J. et al, 2008. Efficacy of berberine... *Metabolism.*

Zhang D. et al, 2013. Curcumin and diabetes... *Evid Based Complement Alternat Med.*

Ketogenic Diet

D'Andrea Meira I. et al, 2019. Ketogenic diet and... *Front Neurosci.*

McClernon F. et al, 2007. The effects of... *Obesity.*

McDougall A. et al, 2018. The ketogenic diet... *Brain Inj.*

Paoli A. et al, 2012. Ketogenic diet does... *J Int Soc Sports Nutr.*

Rhyu H. et al, 2014. The effects of... *J Exerc Rehabil.*

Samaha F. et al, 2003. A low-carbohydrate as... *N Engl J Med.*

Stafstrom C. et al, 2012. The ketogenic diet... *Front Pharmacol.*

Sumithran P. et al, 2013. Ketosis and appetite-mediating... *Eur J Clin Nutr.*

Volek J. et al, 2004. Comparison of energy-restricted... *Nutr Metab.*

Westman E. et al, 2005. The effect of... *Nutr Metab.*

Ketone Supplements

Ari C. et al, 2016. Exogenous ketone supplements...
Front Mol Neurosci.

Ciarlone S. et al, 2016. Ketone ester supplementation... *Neurobiol Dis.*

Gormsen L. et al, 2017. Ketone body infusion...
J Am Heart Assoc.

Henderson S., 2008. Ketone bodies as...
Neurotherapeutics.

Kephart W. et al, 2017. The 1-week and 8-month...
Nutrients.

Kesl S. et al, 2016. Effects of exogenous... *Nutr
Metab.*

Maalouf M. et al, 2007. Ketones inhibit mitochondrial... *Neuroscience.*

Mahendran Y. et al, 2013. Association of ketone...
Diabetes.

Pinckaers P. et al, 2017. Ketone bodies and... *Sports
Med.*

Poff A. et al, 2014. Ketone supplementation
decreases... *Int J Cancer.*

Poff A.M. et al, 2015. Non-toxic metabolic management... *PLoS One.*

Reger M. et al, 2004. Effects of B-hydroxybutyrate...
Neurobiol Aging.

Wallace D. et al, 2010. Mitochondrial energetics and
therapeutics *Annu Rev Pathol.*

White H. et al, 2011. Clinical review: ketones... *Crit
Care.*

Yin J.X. et al, 2016. Ketones block amyloid...
Neurobiol Aging.

Youm Y. et al, 2015 Ketone body
B-hydroxybutyrate... *Nat Med.*

Zou Z. et al, 2002. dl-3-hydroxybutyrate administration prevents... *Am J Physiol Heart Circ
Physiol.*

Inulin

Guess N. et al, 2016. A randomised crossover...*Ann
Nutr Metab.*

Shoaib M. et al, 2016. Inulin: properties, health...
Carbohydr Polym.

Your Brain on Sugar

Amodeo G. et al, 2017. Depression and inflammation... *Neuropsychiatry.*

Avena N. et al, 2008. After daily bingeing... *Physiol.
Behav.*

Gangwisch J. et al, 2015. High glycemic index... *Am
J Clin Nutr.*

Hajnal A. et al, 2002. Repeated access to...
Neuroreport.

Knuppel A. et al, 2017. Sugar intake from... *Sci Rep.*

Koekkoek L. et al, 2017. Glucose-sensing in the
reward system. *Front Neurosci.*

Pase M. et al, 2017. Sugary beverage intake...
Alzheimers Dement.

Spangler R. et al, 2004. Opiate-like effects of...
Brain Res Mol Crain Res.

St-Onge M.P. et al, 2016. Effects of diet on sleep
quality. *Adv Nutr.*

St-Onge M.P. et al, 2016. Fiber and saturated...
J Clin Sleep Med.

Warren J. et al, 2017. A structured literature... *Nutr
Res Rev.*

Part 3: Recipes

de Almeida Freires I. et al, 2014. *Coriandrum
sativum L.* (coriander)... *PLOs One.*

Eriksson N. et al, 2012. A genetic variant... *BMC.*

French J.M. et al, 1957. The effect of ... *QJM.*

He J. et al, 2010. Anthocyanins: natural colorants...
Annu Rev Food Sci Technol.

Kelley D. et al, 2018. A review of the health benefits
of cherries. *Nutrients.*

Liestianty D. et al, 2019. Nutritional analysis of...
IOP Conf Ser Mater Sci Eng.

Ma Z. et al, 2019. Goji berries as... *Oxid Med Cell
Longev.*

Montelius C. et al, 2014. Body weight loss...
Appetite.

Perez E. et al, 2005. Chemical composition, mineral... *Plant Foods Hum Nutr.*

Sabelli H.C. et al, 1995. Phenylethylamine modula-
tion of...*J Neuropsychiatry Clin Neurosci.*

Tiku A.B. et al, 2008. Protective effect of... *Environ
Mol Mutagen.*

Yokozawa T. et al, 2003. Protective effects of... *J
Nutr Sci Vitaminol.*

Subject Index

food alternatives, 128–129, 130–131
foods to avoid, 127, 130
and fruits, 122, 128, 131, 132
and GI health, 8, 65, 133
and heart health, 10, 18, 110
and hidden sugar, 44–47, 124, 127, 130
intuitive eating tools, 99–101
and liver health, 9–10, 18, 110, 123
and memory, 7, 36, 112
and metabolism, 8, 17–18, 48, 125
and mood improvement, 8–9, 17–18, 32–33, 102–105, 121, 124
natural ways to raise dopamine, 35–39
and overcoming cravings, 48, 102–105, 133–137
plan, 127–131
and recognizing hunger, 43, 100–101
stages of, 121–131
and taste buds, 9, 93, 99, 121–122
and therapy, 106–107

and vagus nerve, 107–112
and weight loss, 8, 97, 125–126
supplements, to balance blood sugar, 133–137
syrups, as sweeteners
    agave, 74, 127, 130, 132
    birch, 84
    brown rice, 63–64, 90
    maple, 62, 86, 124, 130
    sorghum, 64, 90
    tapioca, 74–75, 93

tapioca syrup, 74–75, 93
taste buds, and sugar-free lifestyle, 9, 93, 99, 121–122
therapy, and going sugar-free, 106–107
tiger nuts, 60–61, 83
tree saps, 62–63, 84, 86
tubers, natural sweeteners derived from, 59–61, 80–81, 83–84
turbinado sugar, 88, 127, 130, 132
turmeric, 135
tyrosine, 35

ubiquinol, 136–137

vagus nerve, 107–112
vegetables, and sugar-free lifestyle, 48, 128
vitamin D
    for dopamine, 36
    and insulin sensitivity, 41

weight gain, from artificial sweeteners, 68, 78–79, 88
weight loss
    and sugar-free lifestyle, 8, 97, 125–126
    supplements, 134–135, 137

xylitol, 71–72, 87

yacón, 61, 62, 84, 131
yoga, 42, 104, 110–111

zinc, 41, 133

Recipe Index